Computers in Biology and Medicine

Series Editor: George P. Moore
University of Southern California, Los Angeles

COMPUTER ANALYSIS OF NEURONAL STRUCTURES
Edited by Robert D. Lindsay

ANALYSIS OF PHYSIOLOGICAL SYSTEMS:
The White-Noise Approach
Panos Z. Marmarelis and Vasilis Z. Marmarelis

INFORMATION TECHNOLOGY IN HEALTH SCIENCE EDUCATION
Edited by Edward C. DeLand

In preparation:

COMPUTER-ASSISTED EYE EXAMINATION
Edited by Elwin Marg

A Continuation Order Plan is available for this series. A continuation order will bring delivery of each new volume immediately upon publication. Volumes are billed only upon actual shipment. For further information please contact the publisher.

Analysis of
Physiological Systems

The White-Noise Approach

Analysis of Physiological Systems

The White-Noise Approach

Panos Z. Marmarelis, M.D., Ph.D.
University of California, Los Angeles, School of Medicine
Los Angeles, California

and

Vasilis Z. Marmarelis, Ph.D.
School of Engineering and Applied Science
California Institute of Technology
Pasadena, California

PLENUM PRESS • NEW YORK AND LONDON

Library of Congress Cataloging in Publication Data

Marmarelis, Panos, Z.
  Analysis of physiological systems.

  (Computers in biology and medicine)
  Includes index.
  1. Physiology – Data processing. 2. Physiology – Mathematical models. 3. System analysis. I. Marmarelis, Vasilis Z., joint author. II. Title. III. Series: Computers in biology and medicine (New York, 1977-   ) [DNLM: 1. Physiology – Laboratory manuals. 2. Systems analysis – Laboratory manuals. QT25.3.M351a]
  QP44.5.M37   596'.01'028   78-497
  ISBN 0-306-31066-X

© 1978 Plenum Press, New York
A Division of Plenum Publishing Corporation
227 West 17th Street, New York, N.Y. 10011

Printed in the United States of America

To an ambitious new breed:

SYSTEMS PHYSIOLOGISTS

Preface

In studying physiological systems bioscientists are continually faced with the problem of providing descriptions of cause–effect relationships. This task is usually carried out through the performance of stimulus–response experiments. In the past, the design of such experiments has been ad hoc, incomplete, and certainly inefficient. Worse yet, bioscientists have failed to take advantage of advances in fields directly related to their problems (specifically, advances in the area of systems analysis). The raison d'être of this book is to rectify this deficiency by providing the physiologist with methodological tools that will be useful to him or her in everyday laboratory encounters with physiological systems.

The book was written so that it would be practical, useful, and up-to-date. With this in mind, parts of it give step-by-step descriptions of systematic procedures to be followed in the laboratory. It is hoped that this will increase the usefulness of the book to the average research physiologist and, perhaps, reduce the need for in-depth knowledge of some of the associated mathematics. Even though the material deals with state-of-the-art techniques in systems and signal analysis, the mathematical level has been kept low so as to be comprehensible to the average physiologist with no extensive training in mathematics. To this end, mathematical rigor is often sacrificed readily to intuitive simple arguments.

The main theme treated is the use of white-noise signals in identifying physiological systems. The reason for this emphasis is the plethora of advantages that these signals provide. However, other, more traditional methods are also covered—sine wave analysis, describing functions, etc. In general, the state of the art in system identification is adapted to the idiosyncrasies of physiological systems in a way that should be very useful to graduate students and researchers grappling with physiological systems. The book could also be used as a graduate-level textbook for courses in systems physiology, bioengineering, and biosignal analysis.

Chapter 1 discusses the problem of systems analysis in physiology, including the various philosophical as well as analytical approaches to it.

Chapter 2 discusses issues related to the analysis of physiological signals. Thus, it forms the background necessary for the developments in the following chapters. Both the time-domain and frequency-domain descriptions are covered, with emphasis on the statistical approach.

Chapter 3 covers the traditional approaches to system identification in physiology: gain and phase measurements, describing functions, spectral analysis, and feedback systems.

Chapter 4 introduces the Volterra–Wiener theory and related methodology. It also includes an exposition on the interpretation of Wiener kernels, the extension of the theory to multi-input systems, and a comparative discussion of other approaches.

Chapter 5 presents certain practical variants of the white-noise method (quasiwhite test signals) and their applicability. It also presents various methods of designing noise generators for use in experiments and the tests necessary to assess their suitability for system identification.

Chapter 6 discusses various computational approaches to the efficient estimation of the system kernels. Both time-domain and frequency-domain (fast Fourier transform) computer techniques are presented.

Chapter 7 discusses the various sources of error inherent in the identification process and how they may be minimized. These include effects of record length, system noise, bandwidth, system nonlinearity, etc.

Chapter 8 discusses the preliminary tests and considerations prior to the execution of the identification experiment, e.g., system stationarity, response drift removal, system memory, etc.

Chapter 9 concerns itself with the synthesis problem, i.e., how to identify interconnections between linear and nonlinear subsystems, e.g., cascade, feedback, etc.

Chapter 10 presents several applications of the white-noise method to physiological systems. These include the catfish retina, the fly visual system, the semicircular canal of the guitarfish, the abdominal ganglion of the seahare, and the lobster cardiac ganglion.

Chapter 11 covers various classes of physiological systems that require special treatment, e.g., neural systems with point process (action potentials) inputs and outputs, nonstationary systems, systems with spatiotemporal inputs, etc.

The final chapter is an exposition in dialogue form on specific aspects of the identification process. These points have often been a matter of lively discussion between us and our colleagues.

Acknowledgments

Even though the responsibility for some of the wilder views expressed in this book lies exclusively with us, we acknowledge with pleasure and appreciation helpful discussions with a number of colleagues: H. Bryant, T. K. Caughey, D. H. Fender, G. P. Moore, G. D. McCann, K.-I. Naka, D. O'Leary, T. A. Reichert, J. P. Segundo, and L. Stark.

We are especially indebted to Professor G. D. McCann for his generous support and encouragement at Caltech, to Professor K.-I. Naka for his great contribution and diligent efforts to enlighten biologists regarding the merits of systems analysis, and to Professor T. A. Reichert for providing one of us (P. Z. M.) with a warm and conducive atmosphere in a cold Pittsburgh winter (at Carnegie-Mellon University), where portions of this work were written.

Special thanks are due to Professor G. P. Moore, editor of this book, for sound advice on many aspects of this undertaking and his warm friendship.

Pasadena, California   Panos Z. Marmarelis, Ph.D., M.D.
                                          Vasilis Z. Marmarelis, Ph.D.

Contents

The Problem of System Identification in Physiology

Words ought to be a little wild
for they are the assault of
thoughts on the unthinking.

John Maynard Keynes

Introduction

Even though the epistemology of the life sciences has a distinctly hierarchical organization—extending from the subcellular level to the
behavioral—the main thrust of research up to now has focused on each
particular level of this organization, e.g., at the molecular, cellular, or
behavioral level. The relationships and interdependences between the
various levels have been relatively neglected. This latter endeavor belongs
to the realm of systems analysis. In addition, a great part of the
methodology employed within each particular level (and being equally
applicable to all of them) belongs to systems analysis. Thus, systems analysis, as a methodological tool, has both a "vertical" and a "horizontal"
component in the hierarchy of physiological systems.

The decade of the sixties saw massive application of engineering,
mathematical, and computer techniques to problems in the life sciences;
however, the significant results produced were far below expectations,
given the magnitude of this effort. Accordingly, the early seventies justifiably witnessed a developing skepticism as to the usefulness of this
large-scale invasion of the methodology of the physical sciences into
biology and medicine. In spite, however, of any sins of overenthusiasm
committed during the sixties, the inescapable conclusion was reached—and
emphasized—that living systems, including the human body, are such
complex collections of dynamically interacting components that their
efficient study could not be accomplished in piecemeal fashion, but
required their treatment as an organic whole; this necessitated the
employment of sophisticated systems analysis techniques.

1.1. The Problem of Systems Analysis in Physiology

In talking about physiological systems we will employ repeatedly the concepts of *system, element,* and *signal.*

A *system* is a set of connected and interacting "elements," conceived as a whole, and intended to achieve a certain objective. For example, the retina, at a certain level of approach, can be conceived as a set of connected and interacting neurons whose objective is to translate light patterns cast onto it into the matrix of ganglion responses that are sent to the brain.

An *element* is a conceptual entity that exhibits some measurable dimensions. The mathematical representation of such a measure is realized through a "variable." Continuing on the same example as before, a neuron is an element and its electrical activity is the variable.

A *signal* is the mathematical description of some quantity changing in time, e.g., in the example of the retina, the time history of a neuron potential is a signal. The change in the measurement of an element within a system may proclaim a change in the measure of another element of the system *if and only if* an interconnection exists between these two elements, e.g., the existence of a synaptic (or other) connection between two neurons. In this sense, *interconnection* between two elements of a system can be considered as the "path" that allows the flow of a "physiological change in time," i.e., a signal, from one element to another in the system.

It is evident that a system always has interconnections with elements (or systems) not belonging to itself. The possible signals "flowing" through such "boundary interconnections" are the so-called "inputs" and "outputs" of the system, according to the corresponding *direction of flow of the signal* at each "boundary interconnection": When the "flow" is directed inward to the system the "signal" is called *"input"* (stimulus); if the "flow" is directed outward it is called *"output"* (response).

According to this conceptualization of a system we can represent it as shown in Fig. 1.1. In general, the system will have many inputs (and therefore stimuli) and many outputs (i.e., possible recordable responses) in most cases. From the cause–effect point of view, however, and with regard to describing the transformations (by the system) of the stimuli $x_i(t)$ into the responses $y_i(t)$, we may consider each response separately. That is, we have

$$y_k(t) = F[x_1(t), x_2(t), \ldots, x_n(t)] \tag{1.1}$$

i.e., any of the responses could be a function of (may be due to) all the inputs. Following again the example of the retina mentioned above, the response of the ganglion cell can conceivably be described in terms of all the inputs impinging upon the "retina" (light, temperature, circulatory effects, other neuronal inputs from outside the retina, etc.), and so could all

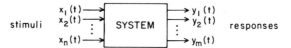

Fig. 1.1. Multi-input–multi-output system.

the other retinal neural responses. Alternatively, we could, of course, describe the ganglion responses in terms of the photoreceptor responses plus all these other inputs. However, the photoreceptor responses can in turn be described in terms of these retinal inputs (light, temperature, etc.); therefore, the ganglion responses are describable solely in terms of these inputs to the "retinal system." This should clarify our conceptualization of a system in terms of Eq. (1.1).

In the study of a system we seek to identify the functional transformation F depicted in Eq. (1.1). Experimentally this entails the measurement of all extrinsic variables (inputs) affecting the system (e.g., in the case of the retina, light, temperature, blood flow, etc.). Clearly, this is infeasible or extremely difficult in practice. Therefore, what is done is to simply ignore most of the inputs and concentrate on the few major ones with respect to their effect on each particular response. The relative effect of the ignored inputs can often be assessed approximately. These "minor" inputs are termed *noise* and are simply ignored in practice.

The first motivation in the study of a physiological system is our concern with the system's "expected" behavior, i.e., response to a known excitation. The justification of such a concern is something that the authors consider self-evident.

For example, in studying the retina the researcher will be concerned with the behavior of the retinal neurons and other retinal elements in such a way that he or she can *predict* their responses under normal or abnormal physiological operation.

The above comments apply quite generally to the analysis of systems. Our concern however is with *physiological* systems and the special problems associated with *their* analysis. Relative to physical and artificial systems, living systems are "great unknowns" to us. We are relatively ignorant of their function, structure, and modes of operations. Part of our problem is due to the fact that, experimentally, we are usually unable to break them up into their fundamental components and study them separately and/or while these are interacting. Thus, we are called upon, from the beginning of our efforts, to understand and describe phenomena that are quite complex. This forces us to take a *phenomenological approach* at the start of the study, which leads us directly and logically to the *functional identification* problem for the system—as posed in the next section. In short, this is the task of describing, as completely as possible, the system response to any given stimulus, i.e., identifying the function of the system in processing physiological signals from its inputs to its outputs. In conclusion, our relative ignorance about the workings of a physiological system is why this task—functional identification—is a first objective in approaching physiological systems through the systems analysis methodology.

The next question concerns the special conditions—experimental and other—that have to be dealt with in carrying out the functional identification task on physiological systems, i.e., the constraints and idiosyncracies of such systems as a set that will be encountered in practice (in experimental situations) during the identification process. This is discussed in the next sections.

1.2. Functional and Structural Identification of Physiological Systems

Bound by both inductive and deductive reasoning in our logic, we approach the study of physiological systems in terms of cause–effect relationships. These relationships are often manifested as stimulus–response relationships, where the stimulus is either applied externally by the experimenter or is simply observed as it occurs naturally during the operation of the physiological system.

Given this conceptualization in terms of stimulus–response relationships, two questions face the researcher immediately. The first is "What does the system do? That is, how does the system respond to various stimuli?" To answer this question in the absence of detailed information about the system's inner structure, we must perform stimulus–response experiments. From the results of these experiments we aim to deduce a complete description of the system, which will allow us to describe its response to each arbitrary stimulus. This task is the so-called *functional identification* of the system.

A natural question, following the functional identification question and a logical sequel to it, is "How does the system do this? That is, how are the various components of the system interconnected and how do they interact so as to produce the observed responses?" Obviously, this question concerns the structure of the system, and we, therefore, term it *structural identification* of the system. In practice, it is usually carried out by performing anatomy, that is, breaking open the "black box" and looking inside at the various components. Another way is to develop the ability to measure new system state variables, i.e., responses from points within the black box. However, this may prove to be a difficult task in practice for certain biological systems, for example, aggregates of neurons.

The system identification objectives, as outlined above, imply, up to a point, a "black box" approach, because they aim at the determination of the transfer characteristics at one approach level and largely ignore issues at underlying levels. For example, in studying a neuron network we would aim at the description of the transformation of incoming spike trains and/or continuous potentials into outgoing spike trains and/or continuous potentials while ignoring to a great extent the underlying physicochemical, molecular transformations. This is not a "limitation," as sometimes is mistakenly thought, but a necessary methodological feature. First, the analysis of a system into its "ultimate" components is a necessary but not a sufficient step for understanding thoroughly its operation and role; it may, in fact, be illusory to think that the smaller the pieces into which a system is dissected the better we will understand it. Second, in practice any investigator selects a certain approach level and deals with variables therein as with elementary quantities, as dictated by practical considerations (experimental observability) as well as conceptual ones. In any case, for any choice of an approach level, there would be an infinite number of more basic ones underlying it; description of the system's functioning at these lower levels may often becloud the issues involved at the higher levels of functioning by simply deflecting attention from these latter ones. Third, and most important, the system identification approach is compatible with our desire (this desire is clearly motivated again by the cause–effect nature of our logic) to explain higher-level functioning through descriptions at lower levels; in fact, it is a natural way to achieve it and the ones employed in practice *anyway*. Let us explain this statement: The system identification approach results in the determination of the system transfer characteristics without specifying its internal topological structure. However, as the experimental ability is developed to measure more "state variables," some heretofore "hidden" in the "black box," the system is broken up into smaller subsystems whose organization reflects more and more closely its topological structure. In spite of current common belief (more accurately, misconception), it should be stressed that no stimulus–response experiment can reveal the "internal structure" of a system without making assumptions about certain alternative configurations; that is, a stimulus–response experiment could conceivably, in certain cases, distinguish between two or more possible structural configurations but usually cannot determine precisely the system structure without *a priori* information about it. The task of *decomposing* a system into smaller component subsystems can be accomplished through the combination (and interplay) of functional identification (through stimulus–response experiments) and structural identification (through histology and anatomy).

To concretize the above general comments, let us consider a specific example, as it would be encountered in experimental research: the study and modeling of the vertebrate retina. The actual model to be described below is not necessarily accurate (even though it might be plausible), but it

is used as a vehicle to demonstrate the functional and structural identification procedures and how their employment might be carried out in
practice.

This study evolves by the interplay of stimulus–response experiments
(i.e., functional identification) and anatomical information (i.e., structural
identification). The process is described in Fig. 1.2.

The first experiment identifies the functional relationship between
light stimulus and ganglion response, i.e., between the input to the whole
retina and its signal to the brain (Fig. 1.2A).

In the next experiment the response of the horizontal cell, r_1, is
recorded, which, combined with anatomical information that the horizontal cell is intermediate in the signal processing chain from light to ganglion,
allows us to decompose the "black box" S as shown in Fig. 1.2B. From
these two stimulus–response experiments we can now describe quantitatively system transformation S_1 of light-to-horizontal-cell response, and
S_2, of horizontal-cell-response-to-ganglion-cell-response.

The following experiment depicts how the model of the retina evolves
when we develop the experimental ability to record the response r_2 of the

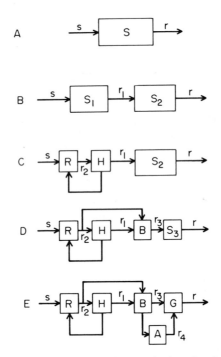

Fig. 1.2. Black box decomposition of the vertebrate retina based on functional and structural
identification.

photoreceptors (Fig. 1.2C). An experiment in which the horizontal cell is excited extrinsically (e.g., by injecting current intracellularly) and recording the response r_2 of the photoreceptors establishes a connecting feedback path from the horizontal cells to the photoreceptors as shown in Fig. 1.2C. This model is, of course, verified with the aid of anatomical evidence as to this structural configuration. From these identification experiments it is now possible to determine the characteristics of subsystems R and H.

Similar procedures, i.e., functional identification through stimulus–response experiments and structural identification through anatomy, are followed in arriving at the retinal models depicted in Figs 1.2D and 1.2E. This development is, of course, contingent upon the experimental ability to record the light-induced responses from bipolar cells, r_3, and amacrine cells, r_4—coupled with anatomical identification of these cells as such, as well as of the existence of the paths receptor-to-bipolar and bipolar-to-amacrine-to-ganglion, as shown in Fig. 1.2E.

In this whole process of modeling the retina, based upon functional and structural identification experiments, we note how the black box is gradually broken up into component subsystems whose organization reflects intimately the structure of this system, i.e., "what's going on inside the black box." This procedure would, therefore, seem to contradict the often heard comment that "functional identification through stimulus–response experiments cannot tell me what's going on inside the system!" In fact, with some extrapolation (and good will!) one can see that, indeed, little more than that can be done in practice *anyway*.

On the other hand, there is often a common implicit misconception among bioscientists (the optimistic ones!) that stimulus–response experiments will reveal the structure of the system; unfortunately, this is chasing a chimera. All that one can do is, based on the results of the stimulus–response experiments, to make certain hypotheses as to alternative structural configurations of the system, and then, on the basis of these hypotheses and additional stimulus–response experiments and/or information otherwise obtained, to choose one of them as most likely. This, therefore, brings us to a very important point: the need to design stimulus–response experiments in such a way that the information (knowledge) obtained about the functional characteristics of the system will allow us to make good hypotheses on its structure.

One may ask at this point: Why can we not simply keep on doing more and more experiments? And, indeed, often this is what is done in practice. However, it clearly behooves us to seek a strategy that will allow us to gather as much information as possible about the stimulus–response behavior of the system, under the experimental difficulties present and commonly encountered in studying physiological systems. This point is a central theme of the book. Such common difficulties, usually encountered in practice, include nonlinear behavior, short experimental lifetimes over which the identification experiment can take place, signals that are heavily corrupted by noise, and great variability in the data from preparation to preparation. Traditionally in biology, step and sine wave stimuli have been used in studying systems. We will argue in this book that these are not the most efficient stimuli that can be used for purposes of identification.

With regard to research methodology in physiology, much attention has been devoted in the past to developing techniques for measuring the system's state variables (e.g., various transducers such as microelectrodes for recording intracellular neuron responses and other), and, recently, much effort has been expended in acquiring and employing very sophisticated data analysis and processing equipment (digital computers). However, the link between these two facets of research is the types and richness (with regard to the above-stated objectives of identification) of these stimulus–response data flowing from the transducers to the powerful computer. This, in the opinion of the authors, has been a weak link in this chain of research. That is, the power and sophistication of modern laboratory computers has been vastly underused by the paucity of data types and analysis techniques employed in most laboratories of physiology.

1.3. *"Black Box" vs. Parameter Identification in Physiological Systems*

Since the study of physiological systems is usually encumbered by fragmentary knowledge of their underlying microstructure, the problem of analysis is tightly coupled to the so-called problem of "system identification" ("characterization" or "evaluation"). Identification of a system is the complete determination of the dynamic characteristics of its processes ("functioning") by performing suitable stimulus–response experiments. This task has general applicability and is closely related to our thinking in causal terms ("cause–effect," "input–output," "stimulus–response," "y is related to x," etc.)

Identification of a system comprises two main tasks: *specification* and *estimation*. The task of specification comprises the selection and determination of a mathematical form that would be convenient and successful in describing the system functioning. This form will generally contain a set of parameters that will have to be determined. This results in the *estimation* task.

Thus, "system identification" usually is formulated in two different but not mutually exclusive ways:

A. Parameter Estimation. The structural configuration of the system is assumed (or sometimes known), but the parameters of the describing differential (or other, such as integrodifferential, difference, algebraic, etc.) equations are unknown. The identification task becomes a search in "parameter space," where it attempts to minimize a certain error function, i.e., measuring "goodness" of fit.

B. *"Black Box" Estimation.* The structural configuration of the system is unknown and no assumptions about it are made. The identification task becomes a search in "function space," i.e., the space of system functionals.

As an example of A, suppose the specified model for the description of the system is

$$\frac{dy}{dt} + \alpha y = x$$

where $x(t)$ is the system stimulus and $y(t)$ is the system response, the identification task consists of estimating α, which constitutes the parameter space. Such an equation may arise from a patch of passive membrane that we describe as an RC circuit for which we do not know the value of RC (i.e., α). As an example of B, suppose the specified model for the membrane is

$$y(t) = \int_0^\infty h(\tau)x(t-\tau)\, d\tau$$

that is, we assume that the membrane is a linear system but not necessarily representable as a simple RC circuit. The identification task consists of estimating the function $h(\tau)$, which constitutes the function space.

In modeling physiological systems, approach A has often been used and consists of the following: A set of differential equations is chosen, which is assumed to describe the different processes taking place within the system; this set is picked on the basis of limited information about these processes and in order to provide for some of the system features; a set of experimental system responses is chosen, usually step and/or sinusoidal responses; the differential equation model responses to these same inputs (step and/or sines) are then compared with the experimental ones; based on this comparison, the parameters and/or the form of the equations or the equations themselves are changed, trying to obtain a better fit to the data; the process is terminated when the modeler decides that a satisfactory fit has been obtained. This approach has been very popular among modelers of biological systems. The whole procedure (and its outcome) depends solely on the skill and imagination of the modeler, and it is not systematic beyond what is described above. It usually involves many arbitrary assumptions about the system structure as it is reflected by the form of the postulated equations. In general, it tends to be time-consuming in designing the differential equations in order to fit the given set of data. The resulting model is usually good only for the chosen set of stimuli (steps/sines) and not satisfactory for other types of input. Often, as new information about the system is found by the experimenter it is necessary to change radically all the equations and start the modeling process from the beginning.

Approach B is that most often used by bioscientists, commonly by testing the system with step and sine wave stimuli. This leads to a representation over a limited and predetermined region of the function space (operational range). The main theme of this book (identification through "white-noise" testing) belongs also to the second category (approach B). However, the testing regions are picked randomly (or pseudo randomly) over the entire input space and the resulting characterization is obtained, in the average statistical sense, over all these tested regions. Therefore, it results in a representation of the system over its entire function space, i.e., for all possible stimuli.

In contrast to approach A, the white-noise method is a systematic procedure of characterizing a system; it provides global characterizations of the system over all possible inputs; it is uncomplicated to apply, once certain preliminary decisions are made; and it gives good results.

Finally, identification of physiological systems has to take into account the following inherent characteristics of these systems: (a) nonlinearities, which often are essential for optimal functioning; (b) limited durations of experiments because of nonstationarity conditions for the "dying" biological preparations; (c) low signal-to-noise ratios in the measurement of the system state variables; (d) great variability in the data.

Since the identification task is carried out through stimulus–response experiments, it is extremely *important to design* these stimulus–response experiments so as to *maximize the information* obtained from the system under study, within the constraints imposed by these idiosyncratic features.

Analysis of Physiological Signals

Introduction

In this chapter we discuss briefly the nature of signals encountered in physiological systems and some of the analytical tools used to study them. We avail ourselves of this opportunity to present the mathematical preliminaries necessary for the development of the methodology of functional identification of systems (primarily the white-noise approach) that will be discussed in the remainder of this book. In the course of this discussion we present examples of analysis of physiological signals through the use of these tools and concepts of signal analysis.

2.1. Physiological Systems Data: Deterministic and Stochastic Descriptions

The subject of whether nature is deterministic or probabilistic in character runs deep in almost all disciplines. This question is often resolved in favor of a probabilistic description, since physiological systems are very complex and relatively unknown to us in their structure and modes of interaction of their multiple components. Thus they necessitate a macroscopic, "average" description. This probabilistic point of view is further strengthened by the hierarchical organization in the epistemology of *living systems*, which embraces all levels of description from the cellular to behavioral, each level depending for its description on the action and interaction of a great number of components at the immediately lower level.

We call a signal *deterministic* when we know it will assume some specific value at a given (future) time instant t. When the signal does not necessarily assume a specific value at a given (future) time instant t, but the values of the signal follow a probabilistic pattern, then we call the signal *stochastic*.

In practice, a signal is considered deterministic if its values as a function of future time can be predicted with accuracy. For example, the coordinates of a stone thrown in the air on a windless day can be described *a priori* with good accuracy. However, the future values of an EEG recording from a human starting at 10:00 a.m. every day, even under controlled conditions, cannot be described with the same degree of accuracy; therefore, in this latter case we are forced to describe the signal in terms of probability statements and statistical measures (averages).

Of course, from the point of view of the purist—depending on his or her philosophical inclinations—it can be argued that all physical data are deterministic but we cannot describe them predictably because we are ignorant of their underlying microscopic mechanisms; or it can be argued that all physical data are stochastic because scientific law has evolved empirically and is itself a statistical procedure. As fundamental and fascinating as they are, we will not concern ourselves with these arguments in this book. We *are* concerned, though, with choosing a suitable description in a practical situation in the laboratory when we are faced with the task of analyzing a particular physiological system. Then the decision, in practice, of whether to employ a deterministic or statistical description of the data at hand would depend on our ability to reproduce the system data by controlled experiments to a satisfactory degree of accuracy.

2.2. Some Statistical Tools and Concepts

Physiological signals usually exhibit great variability among similar experimental preparations of the same system. In addition, they may be corrupted by high noise content. These features necessitate their stochastic representation.

Before entering the discussion of the stochastic properties of signals, we need to define the basic statistical concepts of random variable, random (or stochastic) process, and probability distribution. A *random variable* is a mathematical description of all the possible outcomes of a certain observable experiment. The *probability distribution* is the mathematical description of the relative likelihood of those possible outcomes. A *random process* is a time function (signal) the value of which at every time instant is a random variable.

Consider, as an example, the following experiment: Every hour, on the hour, the electroretinogram (ERG) signal of an experimental subject is recorded for several minutes. Typical results are shown in Fig. 2.1. There are several statistical quantities of interest which we may compute. These quantities should be evaluated on the basis of the collection of *sample* signals, such as those shown in Fig. 2.1. The set of sample signals is called an *ensemble*. For any time t_0 the values of these sample signals $\{x_1(t_0), x_2(t_0), \ldots, x_n(t_0)\}$ would constitute a random sample drawn from the population of the random variable $x(t_0)$. The sample $\{x_1(t_0), x_2(t_0), \ldots, x_n(t_0)\}$, then, would enable us to obtain all the desired

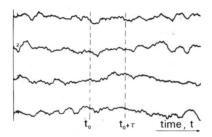

Fig. 2.1. Electroretinographic (ERG) signals obtained every hour.

estimates of the statistical quantities in which we are interested, according to standard procedures of statistics.

2.2.1. Stationarity and Ergodicity of Signals

If, in the example of Fig. 2.1, the "statistical behavior" of the signal is exactly the same for every t_0 arbitrarily chosen, then the stochastic signal will be called *stationary*. If it is not, the signal is called *nonstationary*. However, estimation of the desired statistical quantities would require a very large collection of data, which in practice may be neither feasible nor economical. For this reason, it is highly desirable that the signal exhibit the property of *ergodicity*, which allows us to substitute the statistical procedures of estimation over the several sample signals of the ensemble with an estimating procedure defined in time over only one member (one sample signal) of the ensemble. We now proceed to make these ideas more quantitative.

Several statistical quantities of interest may be computed from the data of Fig. 2.1. For example, the *mean* value of the ERG signal, t_0 sec after the hour, is given (estimated) by

$$\mu_{1,x}(t_0) = \frac{1}{N} \sum_{i=1}^{N} x_i(t_0) \tag{2.1}$$

Or, similarly, any of the *moments* of $x(t)$ would be estimated from

$$\mu_{n,x}(t_0) = \frac{1}{N} \sum_{i=1}^{N} x_i^n(t_0) \tag{2.2}$$

We can also compute the *correlation function*

$$\phi_{xx}(t_0, t_0 - \tau) = \frac{1}{N} \sum_{i=1}^{N} x_i(t_0) x_i(t_0 - \tau) \tag{2.3}$$

and higher-order correlation functions

$$\phi_{x\cdots x}(t_0, t_0-\tau_1, \ldots, t_0-\tau_n) = \frac{1}{N} \sum_{i=1}^{N} x_i(t_0)x_i(t_0-\tau_1)\cdots x_i(t_0-\tau_n) \qquad (2.4)$$

Note that all these averages are computed from the various signals of the "ensemble" of ERG signals; they are called "ensemble averages." Now, if $\mu_{1,x}(t_0)$ and $\phi_{xx}(t_0, t_0-\tau)$ vary with the choice of time t_0, then the signal ensemble is *nonstationary*. However, if they do not depend on the choice of t_0, then the ensemble is *weakly stationary*. If, in addition, to the two quantities $\mu_{1,x}$ and $\phi_{xx}(\ )$, the higher-order moments and correlation functions are also independent of the choice of t_0, then the signal ensemble is called *strongly stationary* or simply stationary. Usually, in practice, we test whether the signal ensemble is weakly stationary and then assume that it is also strongly stationary—a reasonable assumption in most practical situations. We then simply refer to it as *stationary*.

Instead of computing averages *across* the ensemble of signals we can also compute averages within a single member of the ensemble. For example, we can estimate the mean and autocorrelation for the kth ERG signal:

$$\mu_{1,x_k} = \frac{1}{T} \int_0^T x_k(t)\, dt \qquad (2.5)$$

$$\phi_{x_k x_k}(\tau) = \frac{1}{T} \int_0^T x_k(t)x_k(t-\tau)\, dt \qquad (2.6)$$

If it turns out that the two statistical quantities $\mu_{1,x}$ and $\phi_{xx}(\ )$ are the same for the different ensemble members $\{x_i(t)\}$, and if, in addition, the ensemble is stationary, then the stochastic process—i.e., the collection of $x_i(t)$'s— is called *ergodic*. In this case, these statistical quantities, i.e., the moments and correlations, are the same whether computed over the ensemble members or over a single member of the ensemble. For example,

$$\mu_{1,x_k} \cong \frac{1}{T} \int_0^T x_k(t)\, dt \cong \frac{1}{N} \sum_{i=1}^{N} x_i(t_0) \cong \mu_{1,x}(t_0) \qquad (2.7)$$

for any t_o since the ensemble is stationary.

It is exactly this feature that allows us, in practice, to compute from a single sample signal of the ensemble all the statistical quantities of interest for the ensemble. That is, each sample signal is representative of all signals of the ensemble as far as statistical averages are concerned.

Another statistical question of interest is how the amplitude values of the signal are distributed. Consider the ERG signal shown in Fig. 2.2. To

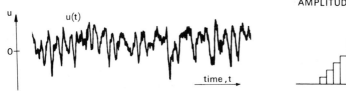
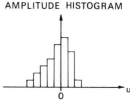

Fig. 2.2. Portion of ERG signal and its amplitude histogram.

find its amplitude distribution we do the following: (i) We sample the signal at fine enough intervals Δt to represent the highest frequencies present in the signal, obtaining a series of amplitudes for the signal

$$x_0, x_1, x_2, \ldots, x_n$$

where $x_k = x(k \, \Delta t)$ and the record length is $n \, \Delta t$; (ii) We divide the total range of the amplitudes into equal intervals (bins) and determine what fraction of the sample set $\{x_0, x_1, \ldots, x_n\}$ falls into each bin. This procedure results in an *amplitude histogram* for the signal $x(t)$ (Fig. 2.2). As the size of the amplitude bin is reduced and the record length of the signal $x(t)$ is increased, in the limit a continuous curve is obtained, which is the probability distribution of the signal amplitude. In a similar fashion we could estimate the amplitude probability distribution for the ensemble of signals, at a given instant of time t_0.

As will be discussed later, it should also be noted that the probability distribution of a random variable determines uniquely (and is determined by) all the moments of the random variable, e.g., mean, second moment, third moment, etc. This fact is used in the next example.

The amplitude distribution of a physiological signal often provides insight into the underlying mechanisms generating the signal. For example, for the ERG signal of Fig. 2.2, we note that at high amplitudes the histogram falls abruptly, indicating the possible presence of a saturating mechanism (we discuss this point further, later in this section). In Fig. 2.3 are shown the amplitude histograms of several physiological signals. Since physiological mechanisms usually are integrative, i.e., depend on the action of a large number of submechanisms, the law of large numbers often applies, resulting in signals with a Gaussian amplitude distribution, e.g., Fig. 2.3A. If the amplitude histogram is like the one in Fig. 2.3B then we may suspect that the system has a cutoff nonlinearity at low amplitudes. If the histogram is like the one in Fig. 2.3C then we can hypothesize that either the signal has two "preferable" states or we are recording a signal coming from two different populations—hence the bimodal (two-peak) nature of the histogram.

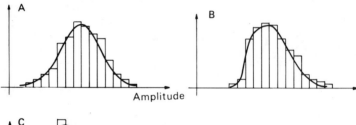

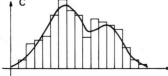

Fig. 2.3. Types of amplitude histograms of various signals encountered in practice.

Example. Consider an ensemble of stochastic signals such as that shown in Fig. 2.4. It consists of a collection of sine waves of constant amplitude A but random initial phase ϕ. Let us define two random variables* $\tilde{x}$ and $\tilde{\psi}$ by

$$\tilde{x}(t) = A \sin \tilde{\psi}$$
$$\tilde{\psi}(t) = \omega t + \tilde{\phi}$$

(2.8)

where ϕ is the initial random phase of the signal and ψ is the total argument (angle) of the sine wave.

The question that we pose is: What is the probability distribution of $\tilde{x}(t)$ (at a given time t) for given probability distribution of $\tilde{\phi}$? Obviously the range of values for ϕ is from 0 to 2π. We note that for a given value x of $\tilde{x}$ there are, in general, two corresponding values of $\tilde{\psi}$, viz., ψ_1 and ψ_2, in the interval $(\omega t, \omega t + 2\pi)$. Therefore, the problem we are faced with is a problem of transformation of a random variable.

Let $p_\phi(\phi)$, $p_x(x)$, and $p_\psi(\psi)$ be the probability distributions of $\tilde{\phi}$, $\tilde{x}$, and $\tilde{\psi}$, respectively. Then

$$\Pr\{x < \tilde{x} < x + dx\} = \Pr\{\psi_1 < \tilde{\psi} < \psi_1 + d\psi\} + \Pr\{\psi_2 < \tilde{\psi} < \psi_2 + d\psi\}$$

and consequently

$$p_x(x)\, dx = p_\psi(\psi_1)\, d\psi + p_\psi(\psi_2)\, d\psi$$

(2.9)

or, taking into account Eqs. 2.8 and 2.9,

$$p_x(x)\left(\frac{dx}{d\psi}\right) = p_\phi(\psi_1 - \omega t) + p_\phi(\psi_2 - \omega t)$$

(2.10)

Noting that

$$\frac{dx}{d\psi} = A \cos \psi = (A^2 - x^2)^{1/2}$$

(2.11)

we finally have

$$p_x(x) = \begin{cases} \dfrac{p_\phi(\psi_1 - \omega t) + p_\phi(\psi_2 - \omega t)}{(A^2 - x^2)^{1/2}} & \text{for } -A \leqslant x \leqslant A \\ 0 & \text{elsewhere} \end{cases}$$

(2.12)

Note that the above expression for $p_x(x)$ depends, in general, on t, and therefore the mean and other moments of the signal depend on the time t. Hence, $x(t)$ is a nonstationary process.

---

*We use the symbol $\tilde{x}$ to indicate a random variable that takes on specific values x.

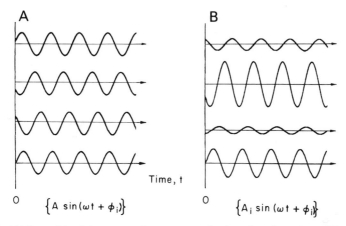

Fig. 2.4. (A) Ensemble of sine waves of constant amplitude and random phase; (B) ensemble of sine waves of random amplitude and random phase.

However, $x(t)$ could be stationary if $p_\phi(\phi)$ is chosen properly. For example, if $p_\phi(\phi)$ is chosen to be uniform over the interval $[0, 2\pi]$, then Eq. (2.12) becomes

$$p_x(x) = \begin{cases} \dfrac{1}{\pi(A^2 - x^2)^{1/2}} & \text{for } -A \leq x \leq A \\ 0 & \text{elsewhere} \end{cases} \tag{2.13}$$

and, therefore, $x(t)$ is stationary. This implies that all the moments of the ensemble, which are uniquely determined by the amplitude probability distribution are independent of time. Similarly, the autocorrelation function of the ensemble is

$$\phi_{xx}(t_0, t_0 - \tau) \cong \frac{1}{N} \sum_{i=1}^{N} A^2 \sin(\omega t_0 + \tilde{\phi}_i) \sin(\omega t_0 - \omega \tau + \tilde{\phi}_i) \tag{2.14}$$

which, for large N and recalling that $\tilde{\phi}$ is uniformly distributed in $[0, 2\pi]$, becomes

$$\phi_{xx}(t_0, t_0 - \tau) \cong \tfrac{1}{2} A^2 \cos \omega \tau \tag{2.15}$$

i.e., it is independent of the time t_0. Therefore, the signal $x(t)$ in this case (where the initial phase is uniformly distributed) is stationary. Moreover, it is easily seen that the amplitude probability distribution and autocorrelation of each sample signal is the same and equal to those of the ensemble, given by Eq. (2.15). Therefore, $x(t)$ is also ergodic.

Now, if the amplitude A of the sine wave is also a random variable, as shown in Fig. 2.4B, the stationarity of $x(t)$ is not affected. However, the process is not ergodic any more. This can be shown easily if we compute the autocorrelation function for the kth sample signal (by averaging in time):

$$\phi_{x_k x_k}(\tau) = \frac{\omega}{2\pi} \int_0^{2\pi/\omega} \tilde{A}_k^2 \sin(\omega t + \tilde{\phi}_k) \sin(\omega t + \omega \tau + \tilde{\phi}_k) \, dt$$

$$= \frac{\omega}{2\pi} \int_0^{2\pi/\omega} \tfrac{1}{2} \tilde{A}_k^2 [\cos \omega \tau - \cos(2\omega t + \omega \tau + 2\tilde{\phi}_k)] \, dt$$

$$= \tfrac{1}{2} \tilde{A}_k^2 \cos \omega \tau \tag{2.16}$$

Since this depends on k, it is not the same for all the sample signals and consequently the process is nonergodic. However, the signal (process) is stationary since the ensemble autocorrelation and amplitude probability distribution do not depend on time t.

2.2.2. Certain Statistical Quantities of Interest

We consider now certain statistical quantities often used in the description and evaluation of physiological signals. We assume that the signals are stationary and ergodic unless otherwise stated.

The *mean* of $x(t)$ at time t_0 is simply the ensemble *average* value of $x(t)$ at any time t_0'. We have

$$\mu_x(t_0) = E[x(t_0)] \tag{2.17}$$

where $E[\ ]$ denotes the "statistically expected value" of the quantity inside the brackets.

Since the signal $x(t)$ is stationary, the mean is independent of t_0, i.e., $\mu_x(t_0) = \mu_x$. Since $x(t)$ has, in addition, the ergodicity property, the ensemble average is equal to a sample signal time average:

$$\mu_x = \lim_{R \to \infty} \frac{1}{R} \int_0^R x_k(t)\, dt \tag{2.18}$$

where R is the record length of sample signal $x_k(t)$. This quantity can, of course, be computed from any of the sample signals $x_k(t)$. Of course, in practice we always compute an *estimate* of this average:

$$\hat{\mu}_x = \frac{1}{R} \int_0^R x(t)\, dt \tag{2.19}$$

Often, however, we will refer to this estimate as the mean of x for the sake of brevity, since we deal exclusively with physical signals, which are finite in length anyway.

If the signal is sampled, as is the case when the data are processed by a digital computer, then

$$\hat{\mu}_x = \frac{1}{N} \sum_{k=1}^N x_k \tag{2.20}$$

where $x_k = x(k\Delta t)$; Δt is the sampling interval and $R = N\Delta t$.

The *variance* is a measure of how much the signal value deviates from its mean value. It is given by

$$\sigma_x^2 = E[(x - \mu_x)^2] \cong \frac{1}{R} \int_0^R [x(t) - \mu_x]^2\, dt = \hat{\sigma}_x^2 \tag{2.21}$$

From this relation it is easily seen that

$$\sigma_x^2 = \mu_2 - \mu_x^2 \tag{2.22}$$

i.e., the variance is expressible in terms of the first and second moments. For an ergodic process $x(t)$, the *moments* are found either as a statistical ensemble average or as a time average. They are defined as

$$\mu_n = E[\![x^n]\!] = \lim_{R \to \infty} \frac{1}{R} \int_0^R x^n(t)\, dt \tag{2.23}$$

Of course in practice we can only obtain an estimate of the moments:

$$\hat{\mu}_n = \frac{1}{R} \int_0^R x^n(t)\, dt \tag{2.24}$$

for some finite record length R. Clearly the mean is the first moment of $x(t)$, and the variance is the second moment minus the square of the mean.

As an example, the moments of an ergodic Gaussian process with zero mean and amplitude probability distribution

$$p(x) = \frac{1}{(2\pi)^{1/2}\sigma} e^{-x^2/2\sigma^2} \tag{2.25}$$

are

$$\mu_n = \int_{-\infty}^{\infty} x^n p(x)\, dx$$

$$= \begin{cases} 0 & \text{for } n \text{ odd} \\[2mm] \dfrac{n!}{(\frac{1}{2}n)!\,2^{n/2}}\sigma^n & \text{for } n \text{ even} \end{cases} \tag{2.26}$$

Note that all the moments are expressible in terms of σ^2, the variance.

2.3. Autocorrelation and Crosscorrelation Functions

Throughout this work the concept of correlation function is predominant. For the signal $x(t)$ the *second-order autocorrelation function* (or simply, autocorrelation function) is defined as

$$\phi_{xx}(\tau) = E[\![x(t)x(t-\tau)]\!] = \lim_{R \to \infty} \frac{1}{2R} \int_{-R}^R x(t)x(t-\tau)\, dt \tag{2.27}$$

and practically estimated as

$$\hat{\phi}_{xx}(\tau) = \frac{1}{R-\tau} \int_0^R x(t)x(t-\tau)\, dt \tag{2.28}$$

The signal $x(t)$ is shifted by τ sec, multiplied by the unshifted $x(t)$, and then averaged. Thus, $\phi_{xx}(\tau)$ is a measure of how "correlated" $x(t)$ is with its value τ sec earlier *on the average*. For example, if $x(t)$ is formed by taking

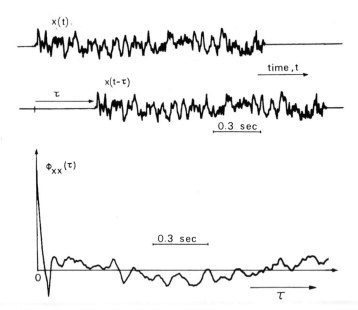

Fig. 2.5. ERG signal and its autocorrelation function.

independent samples from a certain probability distribution sampled every Δt sec, then we would expect, for $\tau > \Delta t$ sec,

$$\phi_{xx}(\tau) = E[\![x(t)x(t-\tau)]\!] = E[\![x(t)]\!]E[\![x(t-\tau)]\!] = \mu_x^2 \qquad (2.29)$$

a constant.

Figure 2.5 shows a portion of an ERG signal recorded at constant diffuse illumination and the autocorrelation function computed from it.

A related quantity that is often calculated instead is the *autocovariance* given by

$$E[\![[x(t)-\mu_x][x(t-\tau)-\mu_x]]\!] = \phi_{xx}(\tau) - \mu_x^2 \qquad (2.30)$$

Notice how the autocorrelation and autocovariance are analogous to the second moment and variance but with an additional parameter: time displacement τ. Also, the mean is analogous to the first-order correlation.

In a fashion similar to that of defining the higher moments of $x(t)$, we can define the higher-order autocorrelation function of $x(t)$. As will be seen later, it is exactly these higher-order autocorrelation functions that allow us to describe the nonlinearities of a system. The third-order autocorrelation function is

$$\phi_{xxx}(\tau_1, \tau_2) = E[\![x(t)x(t-\tau_1)x(t-\tau_2)]\!] \qquad (2.31)$$

and the $(n+1)$th-order autocorrelation function for stationary $x(t)$ is

$$\phi_{xx\cdots x}(\tau_1, \tau_2, \ldots, \tau_n) = E[\![x(t)x(t-\tau_1)\cdots x(t-\tau_n)]\!] \qquad (2.32)$$

In this exposition we assume that all these averages exist, i.e., there are no problems of convergence. This is actually the case since we restrict our attention to physical signals of finite duration and amplitude.

If $x(t)$ is ergodic, as is often assumed in practice, then these auto-correlations are estimated by a time average:

$$\hat{\phi}_{xx\cdots x}(\tau_1, \ldots, \tau_n) = \frac{1}{R - \max_{i=1,\ldots,n}\{\tau_i\}} \int_0^R x(t)x(t-\tau_1)\cdots x(t-\tau_n)\,dt$$

$$(2.33)$$

where R is the record length.

In a fashion similar to that used in defining and estimating functions of a signal $x(t)$, we can define and estimate the crosscorrelation function between two signals $x(t)$ and $y(t)$ as follows:

$$\phi_{yx}(\tau) = E[\![y(t)x(t-\tau)]\!] = \lim_{R\to\infty} \frac{1}{2R} \int_{-R}^{R} y(t)x(t-\tau)\,dt$$

$$(2.34)$$

$$\hat{\phi}_{yx}(\tau) = \frac{1}{R-\tau} \int_0^R y(t)x(t-\tau)\,dt$$

Obviously, this is a measure of how "correlated" are values of $x(t)$, τ sec before, with the present values of $y(t)$. Also, we can define and estimate similarly higher-order crosscorrelation functions such as

$$\phi_{yxx}(\tau_1, \tau_2) = E[\![y(t)x(t-\tau_1)x(t-\tau_2)]\!]$$

$$= \lim_{R\to\infty} \frac{1}{2R} \int_{-R}^{R} y(t)x(t-\tau_1)x(t-\tau_2)\,dt \qquad (2.35)$$

$$\hat{\phi}_{yxx}(\tau_1, \tau_2) = \frac{1}{R - \max\{\tau_1, \tau_2\}} \int_0^R y(t)x(t-\tau_1)x(t-\tau_2)\,dt$$

These higher-order correlation functions will be used extensively throughout this book. They form the basis for measuring the *nonlinear* characteristics of a system through the white-noise stimulation technique. If $\phi_{yx}(\tau) = \text{const}$, then the signals $x(t)$ and $y(t)$ are said to be "uncorrelated." In fact it is easily seen that if $x(t)$ and $y(t)$ are statistically independent then $\phi_{yx}(\tau) = 0$ for all τ, provided that μ_x or μ_y is zero; otherwise, $\phi_{yx}(\tau) = \mu_x\mu_y$. However, it should be noted that the converse is not true, i.e., if $\phi_{yx}(\tau) = 0$ then it does not necessarily follow that $x(t)$ and $y(t)$ are statistically independent.

2.3.1. Certain Properties of the Auto- and Crosscorrelation Functions

The autocorrelation function has the following properties:

$$\phi_{xx}(\tau) = \phi_{xx}(-\tau) \tag{2.36}$$

$$\phi_{xx}(0) > |\phi_{xx}(\tau)| \tag{2.37}$$

The crosscorrelation function exhibits the following properties:

$$\phi_{yx}(\tau) = \phi_{xy}(-\tau) \tag{2.38}$$

$$|\phi_{yx}(\tau)|^2 \leq \phi_{xx}(0)\phi_{yy}(0) \tag{2.39}$$

$$|\phi_{yx}(\tau)| \leq \tfrac{1}{2}[\phi_{xx}(0) + \phi_{yy}(0)] \tag{2.40}$$

To illustrate these basic properties of correlation functions, consider the two-terminal linear circuit shown in Fig. 2.6. The relation between the input (stimulus) and the output (response) of this system is given by the convolution integral [a linear transformation of the input $x(t)$]:

$$y(t) = \int_0^\infty h(\tau)x(t-\tau)\,d\tau \tag{2.41}$$

where

$$h(\tau) = \frac{1}{\alpha}e^{-\tau/\alpha} \qquad (\tau \geq 0)$$

$$\alpha = RC \tag{2.42}$$

The function $h(\tau)$ is called the "impulse response" of the system. Obviously, the impulse response constitutes a complete functional description of the input–output relation of the system. This is only true for a linear system.

Now, let us consider an input $x(t)$ that is ideal white noise. The ideal white noise is a stationary random process, which has the fundamental

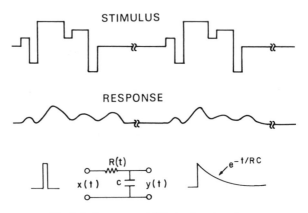

Fig. 2.6. Response of RC circuit to impulse.

property that any two samples of it are statistically independent. It also has a zero average value. Therefore, its second-order autocorrelation function is

$$\phi_{xx}(\tau) = E[x(t)x(t-\tau)]$$
$$= P\delta(\tau) \tag{2.43}$$

where the function $\delta(\tau)$ (delta function) is defined as being zero whenever $\tau \neq 0$ and as having an integral of 1 over any interval that includes the origin. The coefficient P is a scalar called the "power level" of the white-noise signal.

Consider the crosscorrelation between the white-noise input and the output of the system:

$$\phi_{yx}(\sigma) = E[x(t)y(t+\sigma)]$$
$$= E\left[\int_0^\infty h(\tau)x(t+\sigma-\tau)x(t)\,d\tau\right] \tag{2.44}$$

It can be shown that the operations of "expected value" and "linear transformation" are commutative (as long as the impulse response is absolutely integrable); thus

$$E\left[\int_0^\infty h(\tau)x(t)x(t+\sigma-\tau)\,d\tau\right] = \int_0^\infty h(\tau)E[x(t)x(t+\sigma-\tau)]\,d\tau \tag{2.45}$$

Then it follows that

$$\phi_{yx}(\sigma) = \int_0^\infty h(\tau)\phi_{xx}(\tau-\sigma)\,d\tau = \int_0^\infty h(\tau)P\delta(\tau-\sigma)\,d\tau$$
$$= Ph(\sigma) = (P/\alpha)\,e^{-\sigma/\alpha} \tag{2.46}$$

For the autocorrelation function of the system response we have ($\sigma > 0$)

$$\phi_{yy}(\sigma) = E[y(t)y(t+\sigma)]$$
$$= \int_0^\infty \int_0^\infty h(\mu)h(\nu)E[x(t-\mu)x(t+\sigma-\nu)]\,d\mu\,d\nu$$
$$= \int_0^\infty \int_0^\infty h(\mu)h(\nu)P\delta(\mu+\sigma-\nu)\,d\mu\,d\nu$$
$$= P\int_0^\infty h(\mu)h(\mu+\sigma)\,d\mu$$
$$= \frac{P}{\alpha^2}e^{-\sigma/\alpha}\int_0^\infty e^{-2\mu/\alpha}\,d\mu$$
$$= \frac{P}{2\alpha}e^{-\sigma/\alpha} \tag{2.47}$$

Now we can easily verify from Eqs. (2.46) and (2.47) all the properties for
the correlation functions mentioned before.

2.3.2. Correlation Measurement from Underlying Probability Distribution

Correlation functions can be measured alternatively from the joint
probability distribution of the signal amplitude.

The joint probability distribution is a mathematical description of the
relative likelihood of observing a specific set of values attainable by two or
more random variables. If these random variables are statistically independent, then the joint probability density function is simply the product of
the individual probability density functions of each and every variable.
However, if these random variables are statistically dependent, then the
joint probability density function is, in general, a nonseparable function of
those variables. In the case of a random process $x(t)$, the statistical interdependence of its values in time can be described by appropriate joint
probability density functions. Thus the second-order autocorrelation function can be evaluated as

$$\phi_{xx}(\tau) = \int\int_{-\infty}^{\infty} x_1 x_2 p(x_1, x_2; \tau) \, dx_1 \, dx_2 \tag{2.48}$$

where $x_1 = x(t)$, $x_2 = x(t+\tau)$, and $p(x_1, x_2, \tau)$ is the joint probability density
for (x_1, x_2) if they are separated by τ sec. Similarly,

$$\mu_x = E[\![x]\!] = \int_{-\infty}^{\infty} x p(x) \, dx \tag{2.49}$$

$$\sigma_x^2 = \int_{-\infty}^{\infty} (x - \mu_x)^2 p(x) \, dx \tag{2.50}$$

where $p(x)$ is the amplitude probability density function of $x(t)$. Also, in
this fashion, we can evaluate the crosscorrelation function as

$$\phi_{yx}(\tau) = \int\int_{-\infty}^{\infty} y_1 x_2 p(y_1, x_2; \tau) \, dy_1 \, dx_2 \tag{2.51}$$

An example will help clarify the use of the underlying amplitude probability distribution to compute the correlation functions.

Consider a "train" of impulse events that occur in time according to a
Poisson probability law. The Poisson probability law requires that the
probability of an event occurring in an infinitesimal time interval dt be
proportional to the duration dt. The impulse train looks like Fig. 2.7, where
the probability of an impulse between the time instants t_0 and $t_0 + dt$ is

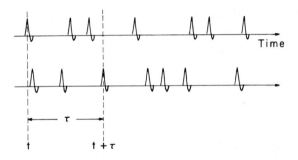

Fig. 2.7. Train of Poisson impulses (neuron spikes).

(λdt), where λ is the average number of impulses per time unit. It is obvious that the occurrence of an event in a Poisson process does not depend on previous occurrences (since it *only* depends on the time interval under consideration). Therefore the signal is *stationary*. Neural spike trains are often modeled as Poisson processes.

The autocorrelation function *for a given* τ must be found by computing the expected value of the product of the values that the signal attains at two time instants separated by a time interval equal to τ. Thus, according to Eq. (2.48) above we have

$$\phi_{xx}(\tau) = \sum_{i,j} x_i x_j \Pr \{x(t) = x_i \text{ and } x(t+\tau) = x_j\} \qquad (2.52)$$

where the summation is carried out over all possible values of x_i and x_j of $x(t)$. To facilitate the understanding of the computations that will follow, let us treat the impulses as the limiting case of a pulse of height P and duration Δt, where $\Delta t \to 0$, $P \to \infty$ so that $P\Delta t = 1$. Then, the possible values of $x(t)$ are 0 and P, and the probability of $x(t)$ attaining the value P per unit time is $\lambda \Delta t$. Now, if $\tau \neq 0$, then $x(t)$ and $x(t+\tau)$ are statistically independent and $\Pr \{x(t) = x_i \text{ and } x(t+\tau) = x_j\} = \Pr \{x(t) = x_i\} \Pr \{x(t+\tau) = x_j\}$. Thus,

$$\phi_{xx}(\tau) = \begin{cases} \lambda^2 & \text{for } \tau \neq 0 \\ \lambda P & \text{for } \tau = 0 \end{cases} \qquad (2.53)$$

which means that $\phi_{xx}(0)$ has an infinite value, since P tends to infinity. Therefore, we finally find

$$\phi_{xx}(\tau) = \lambda \delta(\tau) + \lambda^2 \qquad (2.54)$$

2.3.3. Summary of Definitions of Auto- and Crosscorrelation Functions

We summarize here the definition for auto- and crosscorrelation for the three classes of signals: periodic, transient, and random.

Periodic. The period of $x(t)$ is T sec. Therefore we have

$$\phi_{xx}(\tau) = \frac{1}{T} \int_0^T x(t)x(t-\tau)\,dt \tag{2.55}$$

For crosscorrelation, assuming $x(t)$ and $y(t)$ have the same period T,

$$\phi_{yx}(\tau) = \frac{1}{T} \int_0^T y(t)x(t-\tau)\,dt \tag{2.56}$$

If $x(t)$ and $y(t)$ have different periods $T_x \neq T_y$, then the integration is carried out over an interval T which is the smallest integral multiple of both T_x and T_y.

Transient. A signal is called transient if it is absolutely integrable from $-\infty$ to $+\infty$. Therefore we have

$$\phi_{xx}(\tau) = \int_{-\infty}^{\infty} x(t)x(t-\tau)\,dt \tag{2.57}$$

$$\phi_{yx}(\tau) = \int_{-\infty}^{\infty} y(t)x(t-\tau)\,dt \tag{2.58}$$

Random. A stationary random signal is not absolutely integrable from $-\infty$ to $+\infty$. Therefore we have

$$\phi_{xx}(\tau) = \lim_{T\to\infty} \frac{1}{2T} \int_{-T}^T x(t)x(t-\tau)\,dt \tag{2.59}$$

$$\phi_{yx}(\tau) = \lim_{T\to\infty} \frac{1}{2T} \int_{-T}^T y(t)x(t-\tau)\,dt \tag{2.60}$$

From the amplitude probability distribution we have

$$\phi_{xx}(\tau) = \int\int_{-\infty}^{\infty} x_1 x_2 p(x_1, x_2; \tau)\,dx_1\,dx_2 \tag{2.61}$$

$$\phi_{yx}(\tau) = \int\int_{-\infty}^{\infty} y_1 x_2 p(y_1, x_2; \tau)\,dy_1\,dx_2 \tag{2.62}$$

where $p(x_1, x_2; \tau)$ and $p(y_1, x_2; \tau)$ are the joint probability densities of $[x(t), x(t+\tau)]$ and $[y(t), x(t+\tau)]$, respectively.

2.3.4. Use of Correlation Functions

The autocorrelation function can be used, in general, to find the "interdependence" or "coupling" between signal values at any time with values at any other time. For example, if the signal consists of a deterministic periodic signal buried in noise, autocorrelation can sometimes recover the deterministic signal. This is easily seen. We measure a physiological signal $x(t)$, such that

$$x(t) = a(t) + n(t) \tag{2.63}$$

where $a(t)$ is a deterministic signal, e.g., a sine wave, and $n(t)$ is noise. Computing the autocorrelation, we have

$$\phi_{xx}(\tau) = E[[a(t) + n(t)][a(t-\tau) + n(t-\tau)]]$$
$$= \phi_{aa}(\tau) + \phi_{an}(\tau) + \phi_{na}(\tau) + \phi_{nn}(\tau) \tag{2.64}$$

Often the noise $n(t)$ is independent of the signal $a(t)$, in which case

$$\phi_{an}(\tau) = \phi_{na}(\tau) = \mu_a \mu_n \tag{2.65}$$

which is zero if either μ_a or μ_n is zero. Therefore we have

$$\phi_{xx}(\tau) = \phi_{aa}(\tau) + \phi_{nn}(\tau) \tag{2.66}$$

The two autocorrelation functions can often be separated by inspection since the contaminating noise $n(t)$ usually has a broad frequency bandwidth, i.e., $\phi_{nn}(t)$ is significant only for small values of t. For example, if $a(t)$ is a sine wave, then its autocorrelation is also a sine wave of the same frequency. Thus, if $a(t)$ is contaminated by broadband uncorrelated noise $n(t)$ then the sine wave form can be easily detected by looking at $\phi_{xx}(\tau)$ for large τ [cf. Eq. (2.66)].

In the study of physiological systems the use of crosscorrelation has found wide application (P. Z. Marmarelis and Naka, 1972, 1973a,b,c,d, 1974a,b; P. Z. Marmarelis and McCann, 1973; V. Z. Marmarelis and McCann, 1977b; G. D. McCann, 1974; Naka et al., 1975; Lipson, 1975a,b,c; O'Leary and Honrubia, 1975; Bryant and Segundo, 1976). A frequent use of crosscorrelation is in establishing an anatomical or functional coupling between subsystems. For example, recordings from two different neurons can be crosscorrelated to give an indication of whether there is a signal path between them.

The crosscorrelogram can also be used to measure the transit time as signals travel from one point to another. This is easily seen, assuming for simplicity that the system is linear. Figure 2.8 shows three possible cases of systems that are often encountered in practice. Since causality demands that the response of the system follow the stimulus, we expect that the crosscorrelation $\phi_{yx}(\tau)$ will be zero for $\tau < 0$ and will become significantly different from zero at the time τ that is equal to the travel (delay) time from the stimulus site to the response site. This is shown in Fig. 2.8A. If the system has two paths, as in Fig. 2.8B, then we expect to have two distinct

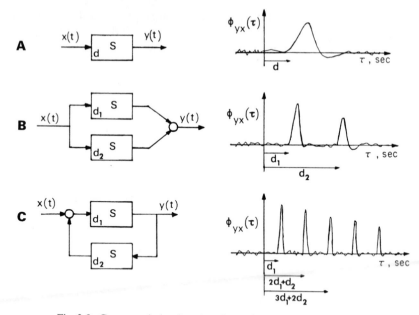

Fig. 2.8. Crosscorrelation functions for various system configurations.

peaks if the delays d_1 and d_2 associated with the two paths are significantly different. Measurement of the crosscorrelation $\phi_{yx}(\tau)$ allows us to measure these two delays of interest also in the case of a system with feedback (Fig. 2.8C) in which the forward and feedback paths have delays d_1 and d_2 respectively. Then the crosscorrelogram is expected to exhibit peaks at $d_1, 2d_1+d_2, 3d_1+2d_2$, etc. In fact, if the feedback is negative then we would expect the peak at $2d_1+d_2$ to be negative, the one at $3d_1+2d_2$ to be positive, the next peak to be negative, and so on. If, on the other hand, the feedback is positive, then all the peaks would be of the same polarity (all positive or all negative).

Another use of the crosscorrelogram is in detecting a signal that is buried in noise when the waveform of this signal is known. We have

$$x(t) = a(t) + n(t) \tag{2.67}$$

where $a(t)$ is the signal and $n(t)$ the noise. Crosscorrelation of $x(t)$ with $a(t)$ gives

$$\phi_{xa}(\tau) = \phi_{aa}(\tau) + \phi_{na}(\tau) \tag{2.68}$$

Often $n(t)$ is independent of $a(t)$. Then $\phi_{na}(\tau) = 0$ provided that the mean of $n(t)$, or the mean of $a(t)$, is zero; and the crosscorrelogram will produce a replica of $\phi_{aa}(\tau)$ at each occurrence of $a(t)$. Notice that since we know $a(t)$ we also know $\phi_{aa}(\tau)$. This is easily seen to be directly applicable to the detection of an ECG signal where $a(t)$ is the waveform in Fig. 2.13.

Another use of crosscorrelation, one directly related to a main theme of this book, is in finding the system dynamic characteristics. This was indicated previously [Eq. (2.46)], where we found that, for a linear system,

$$\phi_{yx}(\tau) = \int_0^\infty h(\nu)\phi_{xx}(\tau - \nu)\, d\nu \tag{2.69}$$

where $h(\nu)$ is the "impulse response" of the system. The Laplace transform $H(s)$ of $h(\nu)$ is the transfer function of the system; thus, knowledge of $h(\nu)$ for a system completely identifies its dynamic stimulus–response relationship. If the stimulus $x(t)$ is sufficiently broadband with respect to the system bandwidth, then $\phi_{xx}(u) \cong P\delta(u)$ and Eq. (2.69) becomes

$$\phi_{yx}(\tau) \cong Ph(\tau) \tag{2.70}$$

i.e., the crosscorrelation measures directly the system impulse response function. In fact, we argue later (Chapters 3 and 4) that the measurement of the system transfer function through this avenue has considerable practical advantages (e.g., it is relatively unaffected by the presence of noise, etc.).

In the case where the system has two parallel paths with widely different delays, as shown in Fig. 2.8B, the transfer characteristics (dynamics) of each can be found from the crosscorrelation. For example, consider the crosscorrelation $\phi_{yx}(\tau)$ obtained for such a system and shown in Fig. 2.9. The impulse response functions for each path are well separated and clearly exhibited. Using a guess-and-check procedure, we find that the system impulse response function is approximately of the form

$$h(\tau) = A_1(e^{-a\tau} - e^{-b\tau})u(\tau - d_1) + A_2 e^{-c\tau}(\sin \omega\tau)u(\tau - d_2)$$

where $u(t)$ is the unit step function:

$$u(t) = \begin{cases} 1 & \text{for } t \geq 0 \\ 0 & \text{for } t < 0 \end{cases}$$

The parameters $A_1, a, b, d_1, A_2, c, \omega, d_2$ can be found by curve-fitting procedures on the crosscorrelogram of Fig. 2.9.

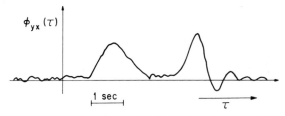

$\phi_{yx}(\tau)$

1 sec

τ

Fig. 2.9. Crosscorrelation function obtained with stimulus whose bandwidth is much larger than the system bandwidth (and therefore it approximates the system impulse response).

2.4. Frequency Domain Description of Signals

Often in the study of physiological systems we encounter signals that are nearly periodic, i.e., they repeat themselves about every T sec. The electrocardiogram (ECG) is such an example (Fig. 2.13). We examine briefly, here, the tools available for the study of periodic signals.

2.4.1. Fourier Series

Given a periodic signal of period T, i.e.,

$$x(t) = x(t \pm nT), \qquad n = 1, 2, 3, \ldots \tag{2.71}$$

we can represent this signal by an infinite sum of sine and cosine waves whose frequencies are integral multiples of the fundamental frequency $f_0 = 1/T$,

$$x(t) = \frac{a_0}{2} + \sum_{k=1}^{\infty} (a_k \cos k\omega_0 t + b_k \sin k\omega_0 t), \qquad \omega_0 = 2\pi f_0 \tag{2.72}$$

and the coefficients $\{a_k\}, \{b_k\}$ are given by

$$a_k = \frac{2}{T} \int_0^T x(t) \cos k\omega_0 t \, dt, \qquad k = 0, 1, 2, \ldots$$
$$b_k = \frac{2}{T} \int_0^T x(t) \sin k\omega_0 t \, dt, \qquad k = 1, 2, 3, \ldots \tag{2.73}$$

By combining the sine and cosine at each frequency we can rewrite Eq. (2.72) as

$$x(t) = C_0 + \sum_{k=1}^{\infty} C_k \cos (k\omega_0 t - \theta_k) \tag{2.74}$$

where

$$C_k = (a_k^2 + b_k^2)^{1/2}, \qquad \theta_k = \tan^{-1} (b_k/a_k)$$

To illustrate, let us consider the signal shown in Fig. 2.10. This waveform is periodic, repeating about every 1 sec. It was obtained as a recording indicating the mechanical movement of the human myocardium, using a noninvasive device. This device records the tissue movement by exploiting changes occurring in an induced electromagnetic field due to the movement of the tissue in the field. In any case, the waveform periodicity, of about 1 sec, reflects the cardiac cycle.

The coefficients of the Fourier series expansion are computed for this signal according to Eqs. (2.73) and the harmonic amplitudes obtained are

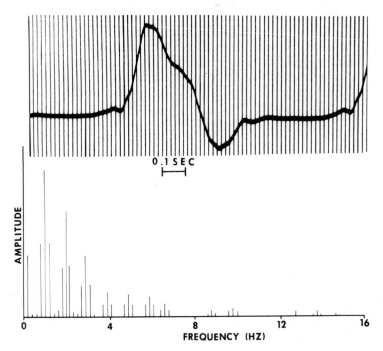

Fig. 2.10. Periodic electrocardiographic (ECG) signal and its Fourier amplitudes.

shown in the figure. A question may arise as to how the very low frequencies (lower than about 1 Hz) were obtained, since the waveform has a periodicity of about 1 Hz. This can easily be accomplished by choosing as the period T, in the above equations (2.73), a multiple of the obvious period of about 1 sec. This procedure then permits measurement of frequencies lower than 1 Hz, the lowest being $1/T$, for the chosen T. A procedure often used in the case of physiological signals is to (a) choose the period T about 1 sec or longer, (b) then average the signal cycles of period T to obtain a signal of duration T, and (c) perform Fourier analysis on this signal as described in the following paragraphs. This procedure may result—depending on how the fundamental interval of expansion is chosen—in frequency components lower than $1/T$.

The Fourier analysis results for the cardiac signal of Fig. 2.10 indicate the presence of strong frequencies around 1, 2, and 3 Hz and somewhat weaker, but significant ones, at 4, 5, and 6 Hz. The one at 1 Hz reflects the periodicity of the cardiac cycle. The peak at 2 Hz reflects the nearly sinusoidal time course of the off-baseline signal, which has a duration of about 0.5 sec. The smaller peak of the Fourier amplitude plot at 3 Hz reflects the ripple present in the off-baseline signal.

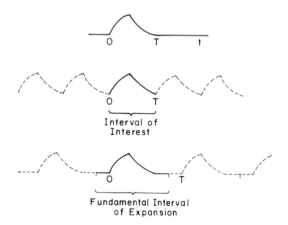

Fig. 2.11. Various fundamental intervals of expansion of a finite-duration signal.

If the signal is given only over a finite interval of time, as must always be the case in practice, then periodicity is not necessary in order to describe the function by a Fourier series over this limited interval. With reference to Fig. 2.11 the Fourier coefficients $\{a_k, b_k\}$ can be computed using the interval $[0, T]$ for integration. The resulting Fourier representation, then, represents the signal exactly over the interval $[0, T]$. However, the resultant expression, if extrapolated to predict values outside this interval, replicates the waveform in a periodic manner, with period T. If, though, we had chosen to use as the interval of expansion a larger one such as shown in Fig. 2.11, then, again, the resulting Fourier representation describes the signal within this interval and also as a periodic waveform outside this interval—with a period equal to the interval of expansion.

Thus, we can have an infinite number of representations of a signal within the interval of interest by choosing the outside interval properly.

If the basic interval of expansion is chosen symmetrically with respect to the origin and the signal is an even function, i.e., $x(t) = x(-t)$, then the Fourier series contains only cosine terms, as seen in Fig. 2.12A. Similarly, if the signal is an odd function, i.e., $x(t) = -x(-t)$, then it contains only sine terms (Fig. 2.12B). This follows from Eq. (2.72).

In a similar fashion, if a signal is given over the interval $[0, T]$, as shown in Fig. 2.12A, we can represent it by a series of cosines:

$$x(t) = \frac{a_0}{2} + \sum_{k=1}^{\infty} a_k \cos k\omega_0 t \tag{2.75}$$

where $\omega_0 = \pi/T$, and

$$a_k = \frac{2}{T} \int_0^T x(t) \cos k\omega_0 t \, dt \tag{2.76}$$

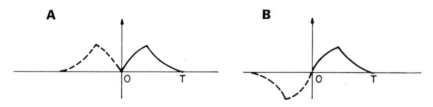

Fig. 2.12. Even and odd expansions of finite-duration signal.

This series represents the signal in $[0, T]$ and also produces copies of it outside this interval—as shown by Fig. 2.12A. In a similar way we can represent this same signal by a *sine* series,

$$x(t) = \sum_{k=1}^{\infty} b_k \sin k\omega_0 t \, dt \qquad (2.77)$$

where

$$b_k = \frac{2}{T} \int_0^T x(t) \sin k\omega_0 t \, dt \qquad (2.78)$$

The difference is that in the sine representation the copies of the signal are such as to make the periodic signal an *odd* function. The resulting signal is shown in Fig. 2.12B. Whether a cosine or a sine representation is chosen is usually dictated by such practical considerations as whether an average value of zero or nonzero is desirable (notice that in the example of Fig. 2.12 the sine representation will have a zero average value while the cosine expansion will not).

   In practice, of course, we can only evaluate a finite number of coefficients in the Fourier series with which to represent the signal. The question arises: How good is the representation of the signal if only the first n terms are used? This question is very crucial in a practical sense and it is directly related to the work described later in this book. For this purpose, we will make the argument a little more general.

   Starting from the expansion idea in vector spaces, where any vector of an n-dimensional space can be expressed in terms of a coordinate set of n linearly independent basis vectors, we can generalize to arrive at the idea of function expansion. A function within any continuous range of its independent variable is considered to be a vector of infinite dimensionality. Thus the concept of linear expansion can be extended to cover function expansions (Lanczos, 1956). This requires the definition of inner product between functions. The inner product of two functions $f(t)$ and $g(t)$ is defined in a way similar to the vector case:

$$\langle f(t), g(t) \rangle = \int_a^b w(t) f(t) g(t) \, dt \qquad (2.79)$$

where $w(t)$ is a weighting function and $[a, b]$ is the domain of the independent variable. The concepts of linear independence, orthogonality, basis functions, and projections on subspaces are defined in a way directly analogous to the vector case. Two functions are linearly dependent whenever the one is a scalar multiple of the other. Two functions are orthogonal whenever their inner product is zero (for a certain weighting function and domain of independent variable). Basis functions are linearly independent functions of the space. If any function of a given space is exactly representable by a set of basis functions, then this basis is called complete. An incomplete basis spans only part of the space. An expansion of a function on an incomplete basis constitutes a projection of the function on the respective subspace. With these basic notions in mind we proceed to examine the case of orthogonal expansion of a signal.

Assume that the signal $x(t)$ is represented by a series of *orthogonal* signals, such as the sines and cosines of the Fourier series. We have

$$x(t) = \sum_{k=1}^{\infty} a_k f_k(t) \tag{2.80}$$

where $\{f_k(t)\}$ is a family of orthonormal (i.e., normalized orthogonal) functions, over the interval $[0, T]$, i.e.,

$$\int_0^T f_i(t) f_j(t)\, dt = \begin{cases} 1 & \text{if } i = j \\ 0 & \text{if } i \neq j \end{cases} \tag{2.81}$$

Incidentally, properly normalized sines and cosines have exactly this property. Because of the orthogonality of $f_k(t)$ the coefficients a_k of the representation are given by

$$a_k = \int_0^T x(t) f_k(t)\, dt \tag{2.82}$$

This is easily seen by substituting $x(t)$ from Eq. (2.80) into Eq. (2.82) and using the orthogonality of $\{f_k(t)\}$ as manifested by Eq. (2.81). Of course, in practice, we can only compute a finite number of coefficients. Thus, we usually approximate the signal $x(t)$ using the n first expansion coefficients:

$$x(t) \cong \sum_{k=1}^{n} a_k f_k(t) \tag{2.83}$$

To measure the "goodness" of this representation we consider the mean square error, ε,

$$\varepsilon = \int_0^T \left[x(t) - \sum_{k=1}^{n} a_k f_k(t) \right]^2 dt \tag{2.84}$$

and ask the question: For which coefficients a_k, $k = 1, \ldots, n$ is this error minimized for the expansion in terms of $\{f_k(t)\}$? By taking the derivative of ε with respect to each of a_m and setting it equal to zero we answer this latter question:

$$
\frac{1}{2} \frac{\partial \varepsilon}{\partial a_m} = \int_0^T \left[x(t) - \sum_{k=1}^n a_k f_k(t) \right] [-f_m(t)] \, dt
$$

$$
= - \int_0^T x(t) f_m(t) \, dt + \int_0^T dt \sum_{k=1}^n a_k f_k(t) f_m(t) = 0
$$

(2.85)

and because of orthogonality of the $\{f_k(t)\}$,

$$
\int_0^T x(t) f_m(t) \, dt - a_m = 0
$$

(2.86)

Therefore,

$$
a_m = \int_0^T x(t) f_m(t) \, dt
$$

(2.87)

That is, the *best* coefficients one could choose in minimizing the mean-square error in the truncated series representation of the signal are those obtained *in the first place* by the exact (infinite series) representation of the signal. This is a very important result, which, when generalized to the orthogonal representation of systems, is directly applicable to the main theme of this book—the white-noise approach to system characterization. In conclusion, for a given set of basis functions, the most accurate (in terms of mean-square error) representation of a signal using a finite series expansion is that obtained by an orthogonal series.

2.4.2. The Fourier Transform

In the example of Fig. 2.11, let us consider what happens as we increase the basic interval of expansion $[0, T]$. In the limit, as this interval is increased to infinity, the frequency representation of the signal becomes continuous and the Fourier series becomes a Fourier transform of $x(t)$. The Fourier transform (FT) of an integrable function $x(t)$ is defined by

$$
X(\omega) = \int_{-\infty}^{\infty} x(t) e^{-i\omega t} \, dt
$$

(2.88)

which in general is a complex quantity, i.e.,

$$
X(\omega) = |X(\omega)| e^{-i\theta(\omega)}
$$

(2.89)

having a magnitude and a phase. A signal $x(t)$ and its FT are uniquely

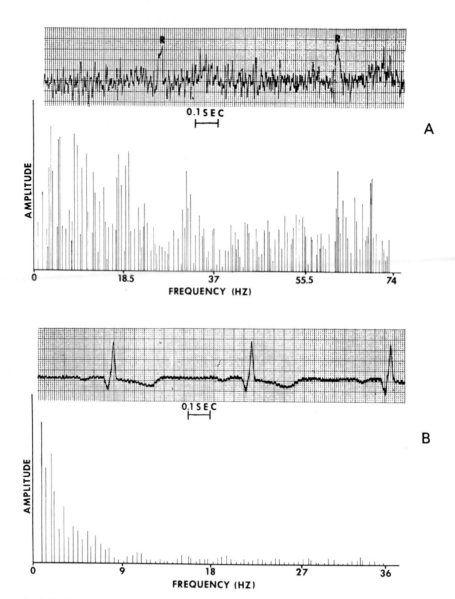

Fig. 2.13. Fourier amplitude spectra of (A) ECG signal with high-frequency noise and (B) low-pass filtered ECG.

related by Eq. (2.88) and by its inverse

$$x(t) = \frac{1}{2\pi} \int_{-\infty}^{\infty} X(\omega) e^{i\omega t} d\omega \qquad (2.90)$$

The Fourier series or transform analysis of physiological signals is often useful in detecting the frequency ranges of certain possible contaminating noise sources, e.g., main power supply 60-Hz noise, contributions of other neighboring physiological sources such as blood vessels or muscle electrical activity, etc. If the frequency ranges of these contaminating noise sources are identified, then it is sometimes possible to design a filter (as discussed later, in Sec. 2.8) that reduces unwanted frequency components. For example, Fig. 2.13A shows an ECG (electrocardiogram) signal that is heavily contaminated by noise. The frequency spectrum of this signal is shown in the same figure. Notice the substantial content around 60 Hz (main supply noise) and higher frequencies (probably "muscle artifact noise") that obstructs the detection of the R-wave complex. Figure 2.13B shows a portion of the same signal, along with its frequency spectrum, after it has been low-pass filtered.

2.4.3. Power Spectrum

As discussed previously, we describe and analyze random signals by measuring certain statistical quantities, either on the ensemble or a particular sample. Such statistical quantities include the moments of the signal (underlying amplitude probability distribution) and correlation functions. It is desirable, however, to have a description of a stochastic signal in the frequency domain, in much the same way that the Fourier series and Fourier transform serve for periodic and transient signals. It can be shown that a similar measure of the stochastic signal is obtained by taking the FT of the autocorrelation function, resulting in the so-called *power spectrum* of the signal:

$$\Phi_{xx}(\omega) = \int_{-\infty}^{\infty} \phi_{xx}(\tau) e^{-i\omega\tau} d\tau \qquad (2.91)$$

and, since the autocorrelation is an even function,

$$\Phi_{xx}(\omega) = \int_{-\infty}^{\infty} \phi_{xx}(\tau) \cos \omega\tau \, d\tau \qquad (2.92)$$

Conversely, we have

$$\phi_{xx}(\tau) = \frac{1}{2\pi} \int_{-\infty}^{\infty} \Phi_{xx}(\omega) e^{i\omega\tau} d\omega \qquad (2.93)$$

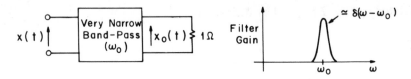

Fig. 2.14. Very narrow bandpass filter.

Assume that $x(t)$ is the voltage across a 1-Ω resistor. Then, from Eqs. (2.27) and (2.93), we have

$$\phi_{xx}(0) = \int_{-\infty}^{\infty} \Phi_{xx}(\omega)\, d\omega$$

$$= \lim_{R \to \infty} \frac{1}{2R} \int_{-R}^{R} x^2(t)\, dt \tag{2.94}$$

that is, the integral of the power spectrum over all frequencies gives the total power delivered to the resistor. Wiener has shown rigorously that, indeed, $\Phi_{xx}(\omega)$ is the "power density" at frequency ω. To show this (Fig. 2.14), consider that $x(t)$ is filtered through a very narrow bandpass filter whose output then is delivered to a 1-Ω resistor. The filtered output is

$$x_0(t) \simeq A_0 \sin(\omega_0 t + \theta_0) \tag{2.95}$$

whose autocorrelation function is

$$\phi_{x_0 x_0}(\tau) = \tfrac{1}{2} A_0^2 \cos \omega_0 \tau \tag{2.96}$$

and power spectrum is

$$\Phi_{x_0 x_0}(\omega) = \tfrac{1}{4} A_0^2 [\delta(\omega - \omega_0) + \delta(\omega + \omega_0)] \tag{2.97}$$

On the other hand, the power delivered by $x_0(t)$ is

$$\lim_{R \to \infty} \frac{1}{2R} \int_{-R}^{R} A_0^2 \sin^2(\omega_0 t + \theta_0)\, dt = \frac{A_0^2}{2} \tag{2.98}$$

as presaged by Eq. (2.94). Thus, $\Phi_{xx}(\omega)$ is indeed the power density at frequency ω. If we think of $x(t)$ as the sum of sine waves of all frequencies, such as ω_0, we see that $\Phi_{xx}(\omega)$ computed as the FT of the autocorrelation $\phi_{xx}(\tau)$ is a measure of the power content of the signal at each frequency. It should be noted that the reason we cannot use the FT of a random signal directly—and therefore we have to resort to the intermediate calculation of the autocorrelation—is that in general the FT of an infinitely long (stationary) stochastic signal does not exist (the Fourier integral does not converge). However, this is not the case *in practice*, where we deal only with finite-length signals; there, we can compute meaningfully the FT of the signal and get a consistent estimate of it. Also, it is easily shown that for such a signal

$$\Phi_{xx}(\omega) = X(\omega)X^*(\omega) = |X(\omega)|^2 \qquad (2.99)$$

where $X(\omega)$ is the FT of $x(t)$ and $X^*(\omega)$ is the complex conjugate of $X(\omega)$.

It should be noted that the power spectrum, like the autocorrelation, does not carry any phase information about the harmonic components of the signal. Instead, it only measures amplitudes at different frequencies. This is desirable in describing properties of an ensemble of signals, where the phases may vary among its various members (or be of no interest) while the amplitude properties are the same (or are of interest).

2.5. Certain Properties of Gaussian Signals

Signal ensembles with a Gaussian amplitude probability distribution are abundant in physiological systems. Often, the reason for this is that physiological processes are usually *integrative* (summative) of a great number of subprocesses. An important theorem of probability theory, the central limit theorem, states that if

$$x_1, x_2, \ldots, x_N$$

are independent random variables with almost any probability distribution (any distribution fairly concentrated around the mean value), having corresponding means and variances

$$(\mu_1, \sigma_1), (\mu_2, \sigma_2), \ldots, (\mu_N, \sigma_N)$$

then a random variable, formed by the summation of subprocesses corresponding to $x_1, x_2, \ldots, x_N$

$$X = \sum_{i=1}^{N} a_i x_i \qquad (2.100)$$

where the a_i are arbitrary constants, will have a Gaussian distribution with mean

$$\mu = \sum_{i=1}^{N} a_i \mu_i \qquad (2.101)$$

and variance

$$\sigma^2 = \sum_{i=1}^{N} a_i^2 \sigma_i^2 \qquad (2.102)$$

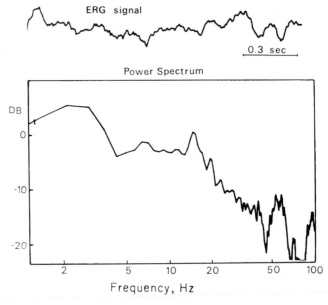

Fig. 2.15. ERG signal and its spectral density function.

The probability density function for a Gaussian random variable is

$$p(x) = \frac{1}{\sigma (2\pi)^{1/2}} \exp\left[-\frac{(x-\mu)}{2\sigma^2} \right] \qquad (2.103)$$

Figure 2.15 shows a portion of a physiological signal along with its power spectrum. The signal is an ERG (electroretinogram), a gross potential recorded from the retina and reflecting its average electrical activity. The power spectrum, shown in the figure, reveals (a) a strong contribution to the signal from 60-Hz noise, (b) another strong contribution at frequencies higher than 70 Hz (possibly due to high-frequency electrode noise), (c) a roll-off in the power starting at about 15 Hz, reflecting the fact that the neural elements in the retina act as low-pass filters with corner frequencies in the range of 10–15 Hz, and (d) a substantial power contribution at very low frequencies, 1–3 Hz, probably reflecting the slow adaptation mechanisms of the retinal neurons and the possible contributions from circulatory effects due to nearby blood vessels.

Thus, we see that the frequency spectrum of a signal could reveal many mechanisms that may be affecting the physiological system producing it. Such information is often not easily available from observation of the signal in the time domain alone. It should be noted that a Gaussian distribution is completely specified by its first two moments $\mu_1 = \mu$, $\mu_2 =$

$\mu^2+\sigma^2$. By the same argument, for a Gaussian, stationary, ergodic ensemble of signals, if the means and second-order autocorrelations (or cross correlations for a pair of ensembles) are independent of time—i.e., if the ensemble is weakly stationary—then it is also strongly stationary since all the higher-order correlations (moments) are completely specified by the first two, which are time invariant.

In general, to specify completely an arbitrary distribution, we need to know all of its moments. This is easily shown. Given a probability distribution $p(x)$, its *characteristic function* is

$$P(\omega) = \int_{-\infty}^{\infty} p(x)\, e^{i\omega x}\, dx$$

$$= \int_{-\infty}^{\infty} p(x)\left[1 + i\omega x + \frac{(i\omega x)^2}{2!} + \cdots + \frac{(i\omega x)^n}{n!} + \cdots\right] dx$$

$$= 1 + i\omega\mu_1 + \frac{(i\omega)^2}{2!}\mu_2 + \cdots + \frac{(i\omega)^n}{n!}\mu_n + \cdots \qquad (2.104)$$

The term-by-term integration holds if the moments are finite and the series converges absolutely near $\omega = 0$. Therefore, we need to know all the moments in order to be able to specify $p(x)$ uniquely in the general case. As seen above, however, for a Gaussian distribution the first two moments suffice.

Consider an ergodic Gaussian process with zero mean. Then, for any sample signal of the process, we have

$$p(x) = \frac{1}{\sigma(2\pi)^{1/2}}\, e^{-x^2/2\sigma^2} \qquad \text{(at a time } t\text{)} \qquad (2.105)$$

and

$$\sigma^2 = E[\![x^2(t)]\!] = \phi_{xx}(0) = \frac{1}{2\pi}\int_{-\infty}^{\infty} \Phi_{xx}(\omega)\, d\omega \qquad (2.106)$$

Therefore, we can find the variance σ^2 and hence the probability distribution $p(x)$ from knowledge of the power spectrum $\Phi_{xx}(\omega)$. If the mean is nonzero it will be manifested in the power spectrum as a δ function at the origin ($\omega = 0$) whose strength is a measure of this mean. Also, from Eq. (2.106) it is seen that the variance of $x(t)$ is equal to the total power of the signal.

For a random process we may consider also a quantity related to the autocorrelation function in the same manner that the *variance* is related to the second moment. This is the *covariance* function

$$C_{xx}(\tau) = E[\![[x(t) - \mu_x][x(t-\tau) - \mu_x]]\!] \qquad (2.107)$$

and for two random signals the crosscovariance function

$$C_{yx}(\tau) = E[[y(t) - \mu_y][x(t-\tau) - \mu_x]] \tag{2.108}$$

Obviously, these quantities are the same as the corresponding correlation functions except that the mean has been subtracted from the signals. Similarly we may define the *correlation coefficient function*

$$\rho_{yx}(\tau) = \frac{C_{yx}(\tau)}{[C_{xx}(0)C_{yy}(0)]^{1/2}} \tag{2.109}$$

For two Gaussian processes with zero mean we then have

$$\phi_{yx}(\tau) = E[[y(t)x(t-\tau)] = \rho_{yx}(\tau)\sigma_x\sigma_y$$

$$= \int\limits_{-\infty}^{\infty}\!\!\int x_1 x_2 p(x_1, x_2; \tau)\, dx_1\, dx_2 \tag{2.110}$$

where $x_1 = y(t)$ and $x_2 = x(t-\tau)$. Letting $\rho_{yx}(\tau) = \rho(\tau)$, $\sigma_x = \sigma_y = \sigma$, we have

$$p(x_1, x_2; \tau) = \frac{1}{2\pi\sigma^2[1-\rho^2(\tau)]^{1/2}} \exp\left\{-\frac{1}{2\sigma^2[1-\rho^2(\tau)]}[x_1^2 - 2\rho(\tau)x_1 x_2 + x_2^2]\right\} \tag{2.111}$$

It should be noted that if $\rho(\tau) = 0$ then

$$p(x_1, x_2; \tau) = p(x_1)p(x_2) \tag{2.112}$$

that is, if $x(t)$ and $y(t)$ are uncorrelated, then they are independent, provided they are Gaussian signals.

2.5.1. High-Order Moments of Gaussian Signals

Of crucial importance in the "white-noise" method of nonlinear system analysis are certain properties of the higher-order correlation functions of Gaussian signals. It can be shown that (cf. Laning and Battin, 1956) for Gaussian random variables $x_1, x_2, \ldots, x_N, \ldots$ that have zero mean,

$$E[x_1 x_2 \cdots x_N] = 0 \tag{2.113}$$

if N is odd. If N is even,

$$E[x_1 x_2 \cdots x_N] = \sum\prod E[x_i x_j] \tag{2.114}$$

where $\sum\prod$ means the sum of the products of $E[x_i x_j]$, the pairs $x_i x_j$ being taken from $\{x_1, x_2, \ldots, x_N\}$ in all the possible distinct ways. The number of ways is $(2N)!/N!2^N$. Thus we have

$$E[x_1] = 0$$

$$E[x_1 x_2] = C_{x_1 x_2}$$

$$E[x_1 x_2 x_3] = 0 \qquad (2.115)$$

$$E[x_1 x_2 x_3 x_4] = E[x_1 x_2]E[x_3 x_4] + E[x_1 x_3]E[x_2 x_4] + E[x_1 x_4]E[x_2 x_3]$$

$$E[x_1 x_2 x_3 x_4 x_5] = 0, \quad \text{etc.}$$

It should be noted that the higher-order moments, and hence correlations, of Gaussian signals are either zero (for odd ones) or expressible (for even ones) in terms of the second-order correlations. Thus, for example, if $x(t)$ is a Gaussian signal with autocorrelation $\phi_{xx}(\tau)$, then

$$\begin{aligned}
\phi_{xxxx}(\tau_1, \tau_2, \tau_3) &= E[x(t)x(t-\tau_1)x(t-\tau_2)x(t-\tau_3)] \\
&= E[x(t)x(t-\tau_1)]E[x(t-\tau_2)x(t-\tau_3)] \\
&\quad + E[x(t)x(t-\tau_2)]E[x(t-\tau_1)x(t-\tau_3)] \\
&\quad + E[x(t)x(t-\tau_3)]E[x(t-\tau_1)x(t-\tau_2)] \\
&= \phi_{xx}(\tau_1)\phi_{xx}(\tau_2-\tau_3) + \phi_{xx}(\tau_2) \\
&\quad \times \phi_{xx}(\tau_1-\tau_3) + \phi_{xx}(\tau_3)\phi_{xx}(\tau_1-\tau_2) \qquad (2.116)
\end{aligned}$$

2.5.2. Stationarity and Ergodicity of Gaussian Signals

As we saw above, if a signal has a Gaussian amplitude distribution then all higher moments and autocorrelation functions are determined by the mean and covariance functions. Therefore, it follows that if a Gaussian signal is *weakly stationary* it is also *strongly stationary*.

In addition, if a Gaussian signal is *weakly stationary* then its ergodic character can be easily checked by showing first that the mean and autocorrelation functions of sample signals from a Gaussian ensemble are the same and then invoking the property of Gaussian signals stated in the previous paragraph.

2.5.3. Gaussian Signals through Linear Systems

An important property—to be used later in our exposition of the white-noise method—is the fact that if the random input to a linear system is Gaussian then the output is also Gaussian (cf. Davenport and Root, 1958, for proof of this result). Further, if the linear system is time invariant (i.e., having time-independent parameters), then the stationarity and ergodicity of the input signal is also preserved in the output.

2.5.4. Gaussian White Noise

White noise is a stationary random process that possesses the special property that *any* two samples of it are statistically independent. If, in addition, the amplitude probability distribution of the process is Gaussian (with zero mean), then the process is called Gaussian white noise.

Clearly, the autocorrelation function of Gaussian white noise is a delta function. This implies that its power spectrum is constant over all frequencies. Consequently, Gaussian white noise is a physically unrealizable signal, since it involves infinite power. In practice, Gaussian white noise is approximated by Gaussian random processes that have sufficiently broad frequency bandwidth for the application at hand.

2.6. Sampling Considerations

The considerations of choosing a sampling rate for the signal records are related to the so-called *aliasing* problem. This is a problem inherently present in records that have been digitized, and it results from the fact that, if samples are used to represent signals, there may be more than one frequency present described by these samples. This is illustrated in Fig. 2.16. Accordingly, in order to describe *any* sinusoidal wave accurately at least two samples are required per cycle of the sine wave. Therefore, if the sampling interval is Δt, the highest frequency that can be described by sampling at this interval is $1/(2\Delta t)$ cycle/sec. Therefore, any frequencies present in the data that are above $1/(2\Delta t)$ cycle/sec will not be described accurately but will be "folded back" into the frequency range of 0 to $1/(2\Delta t)$ cycle/sec and will be confused with the data in this low range. Thus, the estimates of the low frequencies [within 0 to $1/(2\Delta t)$] will be aliased by the presence of these frequencies. This is illustrated in Fig. 2.17. The frequency $f_c = 1/(2\Delta t)$ is called the Nyquist frequency or folding frequency.

Simply stated, the problem of aliasing can be understood as follows. If a sinusoidal frequency higher than $1/(2\Delta t)$ Hz is sampled at the rate of

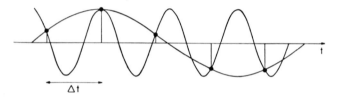

Fig. 2.16. Aliasing: More than one frequency may correspond to the samples (indicated by the solid circles) taken at intervals Δt.

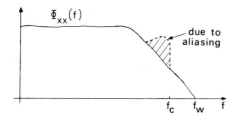

Fig. 2.17. Illustration of aliasing in the power spectrum.

$1/\Delta t$ samples per second, then this sinusoidal wave will appear as one of a lower frequency. This is illustrated in Fig. 2.16. Therefore, any measurement of this lower frequency will be misestimated or aliased by the contribution of the higher frequency, which is mistaken for the lower frequency because of sampling. Computations affected by this phenomenon would include estimation of the power spectrum, correlation, etc.

Now the question arises: *Which* of the frequencies in the range $(0, f_c)$ are thus aliased by which of the higher frequencies $f > f_c$? Or, put in another way, given the samples such as in Fig. 2.16, which ones are the frequencies that can be obtained from the sampled record and thus be indistinguishable from the frequencies actually present in the original record? Obviously there is an infinite number of them. It can easily be shown that for any frequency f in the range $(0, f_c)$ the frequencies that will be indistinguishable from the sampled record are

$$\tilde{f} = (2f_c n \pm f), \qquad n = 1, 2, \ldots \tag{2.117}$$

Thus, for example, if $f = 20$ Hz and $\Delta t = 0.01$, then $f_c = 50$ Hz and the frequencies aliased with $f = 20$ Hz are 80, 120, 180, 220, 280, 320 Hz, etc.

A familiar example of aliasing is the stroboscope and how movements appear in its light. That is, if a periodic movement is faster than the sampling rate of the stroboscope then this movement appears as a much slower movement. This is *aliasing* of the high frequency into a low frequency.

2.7. Statistical Estimation from Physiological Signals

Statistical averages, such as the moments and correlation functions, that are parameters of a signal are theoretically calculated from sums or integrals involving "infinities." In practice, however, we are forced to estimate these parameters from sample signals of finite length. Because of this and other imperfections necessarily encountered in the practical estimation of parameters—or identification of systems—we wish to examine the errors resulting from a finite length of record and a finite bandwidth.

Consider a class of physiological signals $\{x(t)\}$, which under controlled conditions can be assumed stationary and ergodic. We wish to find the average value of $\{x(t)\}$. The record length of the signal is T sec. We can estimate, therefore, the true mean μ by the statistic $\hat{\mu}$, found as

$$\hat{\mu} = \frac{1}{T} \int_0^T x(t)\, dt \tag{2.118}$$

The question arises: How good is this estimate? How close is $\hat{\mu}$ to μ? Since $\hat{\mu}$ is computed from a single member of the ensemble, $\hat{\mu}$ itself can be thought of as a random variable whose value depends on the particular member chosen and the particular time period T used in computing it. Therefore, if $\hat{\mu}$ is seen as a random variable, then a measure of the error we are committing, on the average, in taking it as an estimate of μ is given by the variance of this random variable,

$$\text{Var}\,[\![\hat{\mu}]\!] = E[\![(\hat{\mu} - \mu)^2]\!] = E[\![\hat{\mu}^2]\!] - \mu^2 \tag{2.119}$$

since the estimate is unbiased, i.e., $E[\![\hat{\mu}]\!] = \mu$. We can calculate

$$E[\![\hat{\mu}^2]\!] = E\!\left[\!\left[\left[\frac{1}{T}\int_0^T x(t)\,dt\right]^2\right]\!\right]$$

$$= \frac{1}{T^2} \int\!\!\int_0^T E[\![x(u)x(v)]\!]\, du\, dv$$

$$= \frac{1}{T^2} \int\!\!\int_0^T \phi_{xx}(u - v)\, du\, dv \tag{2.120}$$

Hence, from Eq. (2.119)

$$\text{Var}\,[\![\hat{\mu}]\!] = \frac{1}{T} \int_{-T}^T \left(1 - \frac{|u|}{T}\right)\phi_{xx}(u)\, du - \mu^2 \tag{2.121}$$

From the signal record we can estimate

$$\mu \approx \hat{\mu}$$

and for $u > 0$

$$\phi_{xx}(u) \approx \hat{\phi}_{xx}(u) = \frac{1}{T - u} \int_u^T x(t)x(t - u)\, dt \tag{2.122}$$

and, therefore, find approximately the variance of $\hat{\mu}$.

Often in this book we will be interested in these kinds of estimation errors. They occur naturally because the white-noise approach of system identification depends on the estimation of cross correlations from finite stimulus–response records. To find a measure of the error incurred in computing crosscorrelations we follow a similar procedure and compute the variance assuming that the estimate itself is a random variable. Therefore, we have (for an unbiased estimate)

$$\text{Var}\,[\hat{\phi}_{yx}(\tau)] = E[[\hat{\phi}_{yx}(\tau) - \phi_{yx}(\tau)]^2]$$

$$= E[\hat{\phi}_{yx}^2(\tau)] - \phi_{yx}^2(\tau) \tag{2.123}$$

Then, substituting $\hat{\phi}_{yx}$ in terms of $y(t)$ and $x(t)$ we obtain

$$\text{Var}\,[\hat{\phi}_{yx}(\tau)] \cong E\left[\frac{1}{T^2}\int_0^T\!\!\int y(\mu)x(\mu - \tau)y(\nu)x(\nu - \tau)\,d\mu\,d\nu\right] - \phi_{yx}^2(\tau)$$

$$\tag{2.124}$$

Now, let us assume that the signals $x(t)$ and $y(t)$ are Gaussian; if they are not, the following argument holds approximately in most cases. According to Eq. (2.115) we have

$$E[y(\mu)x(\mu - \tau)y(\nu)x(\nu - \tau)]$$

$$= E[y(\mu)x(\mu - \tau)]E[y(\nu)x(\nu - \tau)] + E[y(\mu)y(\nu)]E[x(\mu - \tau)x(\nu - \tau)]$$

$$+ E[y(\mu)x(\nu - \tau)]E[y(\nu)x(\mu - \tau)]$$

$$= \phi_{yx}^2(\tau) + \phi_{yy}(\mu - \nu)\phi_{xx}(\mu - \nu) + \phi_{yx}(\mu - \nu + \tau)\phi_{yx}(\nu - \mu + \tau) \tag{2.125}$$

Then the expression for the variance of the crosscorrelation estimate, after an appropriate change of variable, similar to that used for estimating the variance of the mean, becomes

$$\text{Var}\,[\hat{\phi}_{yx}(\tau)] \cong \frac{1}{T}\int_{-T}^{T}\left(1 - \frac{|u|}{T}\right)[\phi_{xx}(u)\phi_{yy}(u) + \phi_{yx}(\tau + u)\phi_{yx}(\tau - u)]\,du$$

$$\tag{2.126}$$

2.7.1. Variance of the Mean for Sampled Signals

In practice, signal records are sampled in order to be processed by a digital computer. Let us consider therefore, a signal $x(t)$ sampled every Δt, resulting in N sample values: $x_i(i = 1, \ldots, N)$. Then the sample mean will be (note that the sample mean is a random variable dependent upon the sample)

$$\hat{\mu} = \frac{1}{N}(x_1 + x_2 + \cdots + x_N) \tag{2.127}$$

Note that $E[\![\hat{\mu}]\!] = \mu$ (unbiased estimate), and

$$E[\![\hat{\mu}^2]\!] = \frac{1}{N^2} \sum_{i=1}^{N} \sum_{j=1}^{N} E[\![x_i x_j]\!] \qquad (2.128)$$

The values $E[\![x_i x_j]\!]$ depend on the autocorrelation function $\phi_{xx}(\ )$, i.e.,

$$E[\![x_i x_j]\!] = \phi_{xx}[(i-j)\Delta t] \qquad (2.129)$$

Notice that the total number of cross terms $E[\![x_i x_j]\!]$ in Eq. (2.128) is $N(N-1)$ and the number of cross terms where $i-j=k$ is $2(N-k)$. Thus,

$$\sum_{i=1}^{N} \sum_{j=1}^{N} E[\![x_i x_j]\!] = \sum_{k=1}^{N-1} 2(N-k)\phi_{xx}(k\Delta t) + N\phi_{xx}(0) \qquad (2.130)$$

If σ^2 is the variance of $x(t)$ and μ the mean, then

$$\phi_{xx}(0) = \sigma^2 + \mu^2 \qquad (2.131)$$

Therefore, Eq. (2.128) becomes

$$E[\![\hat{\mu}^2]\!] = \frac{1}{N}(\sigma^2 + \mu^2) + \frac{1}{N^2} \sum_{k=1}^{N-1} 2(N-k)\phi_{xx}(k\Delta t) \qquad (2.132)$$

and the variance of the sample mean becomes

$$\begin{aligned}
\text{Var}[\![\hat{\mu}]\!] &= E[\![\hat{\mu}^2]\!] - \mu^2 \\
&= \frac{\sigma^2}{N} - \frac{(N-1)}{N}\mu^2 + \frac{2}{N^2} \sum_{k=1}^{N-1} (N-k)\phi_{xx}(k\Delta t)
\end{aligned}$$
$$(2.133)$$

Given that

$$\sum_{k=1}^{N-1} 2(N-k) = N(N-1) \qquad (2.134)$$

It follows that

$$\text{Var}[\![\hat{\mu}]\!] = \frac{\sigma^2}{N} + \frac{2}{N^2} \sum_{k=1}^{N-1} (N-k)[\phi_{xx}(k\Delta t) - \mu^2] \qquad (2.135)$$

Note that if the samples are considered independent, then

$$\begin{aligned}
\phi_{xx}(k\Delta t) &= E[\![x(t)x(t-k\Delta t)]\!] \\
&= E[\![x(t)]\!]E[\![x(t-k\Delta t)]\!] \\
&= \mu^2
\end{aligned}$$
$$(2.136)$$

and Eq. (2.135) becomes

$$\text{Var}[\![\hat{\mu}]\!] = \sigma^2/N \qquad (2.137)$$

a relation familiar from elementary statistics.

2.7.2. Confidence Interval of Estimates

As we discussed, the estimate of a parameter of correlation function can itself be though of as a random variable. Its variance gives us a measure of how good the estimate is. Therefore, it seems more reasonable, instead of giving a single value as the estimate, to give a range (interval) within which the true parameter value will lie with a given degree of confidence. That is, a probability statement will be made about the degree of certainty with which the true parameter value lies within a specified range.

Assume that we are trying to estimate the mean value, μ, of a signal $x(t)$. The signal is sampled every Δt seconds, producing a sequence of samples

$$x_1, x_2, \ldots, x_N$$

where $x_k = x(k\,\Delta t)$. However, because of limitations of the system bandwidth not all of these samples are statistically independent. Let us say that M of them, where $M < N$, are independent. Let us further assume that $x(t)$ has a Gaussian distribution with mean μ. This mean is estimated by taking

$$\hat{\mu} = \frac{1}{M} \sum_{i=1}^{M} x_i \qquad (2.138)$$

over all the independent samples of $x(t)$. In practice, of course, both dependent and independent samples are used in estimating μ. However, only the independent ones contribute significantly in improving the estimation. It can be shown that the random variable, t_m,

$$\frac{\hat{\mu} - \mu}{s} M^{1/2} = t_m, \qquad m = M - 1 \qquad (2.139)$$

where

$$s^2 = \frac{1}{M-1} \sum_{i=1}^{M} (x_i - \hat{\mu})^2 \qquad (2.140)$$

has a Student t-distribution with $(M-1)$ degrees of freedom (cf. Bendat and Piersol, 1971). Therefore, we can make the following probability statement about the value of the estimate:

$$\Pr\left\{ |\hat{\mu} - \mu| > \frac{s}{M^{1/2}} t_{m;\alpha/2} \right\} = \alpha \qquad (2.141)$$

where α is a measure of the risk we assume by determining a confidence interval and possibly having the true value μ lying outside of it. Thus,

$$\Pr\{ |t_m| > t_{m;\alpha/2} \} = \alpha \qquad (2.142)$$

Or, slightly differently,

$$\Pr\left\{t_{m;1-\alpha/2}<\frac{(\hat{\mu}-\mu)M^{1/2}}{s}<t_{m;\alpha/2}\right\}=1-\alpha \tag{2.143}$$

that is, a probability statement can be made about the certainty with which we can expect the estimate of mean within a certain interval. Rearranging Eq. (2.143) we have

$$\Pr\left\{\hat{\mu}-\frac{s}{M^{1/2}}t_{m;\alpha/2}<\mu<\hat{\mu}+\frac{s}{M^{1/2}}t_{m;\alpha/2}\right\}=1-\alpha \tag{2.144}$$

which says that the true mean falls within the interval noted in the equation with probability $(1-\alpha)$ (usually in practice $1-\alpha=0.95$). Note that the quantities denoting the limits of this interval can be readily found from the sample record; these are $\hat{\mu}, s, M^{1/2}$. The quantity $t_{m;\alpha/2}$ is chosen to conform with our choice of degree of confidence—usually 90%, 95%, or 99%.

We summarize here the successive computational steps required for the determination of the confidence interval of any kind of estimate resulting from a set of sample values.

Consider a sample record $\{x_i\}$ of N samples. We illustrate the case of an estimate of the mean.

(1) We compute the estimate of the mean:

$$\hat{\mu}=\frac{1}{N}\sum_{i=1}^{N}x_i \tag{2.145}$$

(2) We compute the estimate of the autocorrelation function:

$$\hat{\phi}_{xx}(k\,\Delta t)=\frac{1}{N-k}\sum_{i=1}^{N-k}x_i x_{i+k}, \qquad k=0, 1, 2, \ldots, N-1 \tag{2.146}$$

(3) We determine the M independent samples in the record. This can be done approximately here by inspecting the estimate of the autocorrelation function and thus determining the samples that are weakly or not at all correlated.

(4) We compute an estimate of the variance of x_i;

$$s^2=\frac{1}{M-1}\sum_{i=1}^{M}(x_i-\hat{\mu})^2 \tag{2.147}$$

using the M independent samples found at step (3).

(5) A significance level α is chosen (usually 0.10 or 0.05) and the critical value $t_{m;\alpha/2}$ is determined using a Student t-distribution with m degrees of freedom such that

$$\Pr\{t>t_{m;\alpha/2}\}=\alpha/2, \qquad m=M-1 \tag{2.148}$$

(6) The confidence interval bounds are now determined as

$$\text{upper bound} = \hat{\mu} + \frac{s}{M^{1/2}} t_{m;\alpha/2}$$

$$\text{lower bound} = \hat{\mu} - \frac{s}{M^{1/2}} t_{m;\alpha/2}$$

(2.149)

It is evident that the "sensitive" point of this procedure is step (3), where the M independent samples are determined. This step is amenable to arbitrary subjective judgement, which may become sometimes crucially unfortunate. Therefore we propose an alternative, more rigorous procedure:

(3') We compute an estimate of the variance of $\hat{\mu}$ [see Eq. (2.135)]:

$$s_\mu^2 = \frac{\hat{\phi}_{xx}(0)}{N} + \frac{2}{N^2} \sum_{k=1}^{N-1} (N-k)[\hat{\phi}_{xx}(k\Delta t) - \hat{\mu}^2]$$

(2.150)

(4') Since the number of independent samples is usually in practice greater than 30, the $t_{m;\alpha/2}$ statistic becomes approximately a standard Gaussian variable, and therefore the cirtical value $z_{\alpha/2}$ is determined from a standard Gaussian distribution, such that

$$\text{Pr}\{z > z_{\alpha/2}\} = \alpha/2$$

(2.151)

(5') The confidence interval bounds are now determined as

$$\text{upper bound} = \hat{\mu} + s_\mu z_{\alpha/2}$$

$$\text{lower bound} = \hat{\mu} - s_\mu z_{\alpha/2}$$

(2.152)

Similar steps can be followed for the determination of the confidence interval of any other estimate (resulting from averaging of samples) with special attention at step (3'), where the variance of the estimate is computed.

For more extensive discussion on estimators and statistical analysis of random signals, the reader may consult the literature (Bendat and Piersol, 1971; Jenkins and Watts, 1968; Bogdanoff and Kozin, 1963; Brownlee, 1965).

2.8. Filtering of Physiological Signals

We briefly describe here a few of the signal-filtering schemes most often employed in analyzing physiological signals. Some of these will be used in preprocessing the stimulus–response data of a white-noise experiment.

2.8.1. Averaging Responses to Identical Stimuli

Since the response signals obtained from physiological systems commonly exhibit large variability and high noise content, they are often averaged; i.e., the same stimulus is applied repeatedly and corresponding evoked responses are averaged in an attempt to minimize the "unwanted" noise components. The assumption usually underlying this operation is, of course, that the noise component is simply additive and has zero mean. With reference to Fig. 2.18 we assume that the noise signal $\varepsilon(t)$ is a stationary ergodic signal. The averaging of N experiments, in which the same stimulus $x(t)$ is applied, produces

$$\text{Aver } \{y^*(t)\} = y(t) + \frac{1}{N} \sum_{i=1}^{N} \varepsilon_i(t) \qquad (2.153)$$

where $y^*(t)$ is the observed response and $y(t)$ is the "true" response to the input $x(t)$. Therefore, if N becomes large, this error term becomes small provided that the $\varepsilon_i(t)$ noise signals are independent (in fact, it is easily shown that the signal-to-noise ratio improves with $N^{1/2}$).

Figure 2.19A shows the stimulus, a pulse, and the evoked response of a physiological system to three repetitions of this stimulus. Figure 2.19B shows the resulting average response after ten repetitions and after twenty repetitions. Note the high-frequency smoothing occurring as the number of averaged responses increases (indicating the presence of high-frequency noise).

2.8.2. Low-Frequency Trend Removal

Because of the limited length of signal records, very-low-frequency components are difficult to remove by high-pass filtering without distorting the signal significantly with the filter action. Moreover, physiological signals often exhibit a slow-varying nonstationarity, due, for example, to deterioration of the preparation, which is best removed by fitting least-squares-error polynomials to the data and subtracting them from the record. The polynomials most commonly used in practice are the linear and quadratic ones. We consider here, for illustration, the quadratic one. Given a signal $x(t)$ that is sampled

$$x_1, x_2, x_3, \ldots, x_N$$

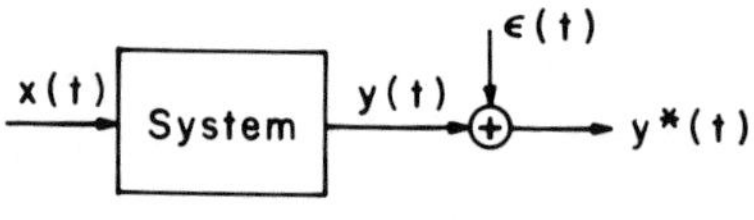

Fig. 2.18. System whose response is contaminated by additive noise.

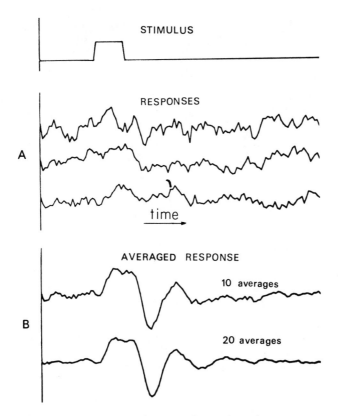

Fig. 2.19. Illustration of the effect of averaging noisy responses.

we fit the polynomial

$$p(t) = a_0 + a_1 t + a_2 t^2 \qquad (2.154)$$

by taking the error

$$\mathscr{E} = \sum_{i=1}^{N} [p(t_i) - x(t_i)]^2, \qquad t_i = i\Delta t \qquad (2.155)$$

and choosing the coefficients a_0, a_1, and a_2 in order to minimize this error. To do this we set

$$\frac{\partial \mathscr{E}}{\partial a_0} = 0, \qquad \frac{\partial \mathscr{E}}{\partial a_1} = 0, \qquad \frac{\partial \mathscr{E}}{\partial a_2} = 0 \qquad (2.156)$$

Then it is easily found that the coefficients that minimize this error are given as solutions of the following set of linear equations:

$$a_0 + a_1 \sum_i t_i + a_2 \sum_i t_i^2 = \sum_i x(t_i)$$

$$a_0 \sum_i t_i + a_1 \sum_i t_i^2 + a_2 \sum_i t_i^3 = \sum_i t_i x(t_i) \qquad (2.157)$$

$$a_0 \sum_i t_i^2 + \alpha_1 \sum_i t_i^3 + a_2 \sum_i t_i^4 = \sum_i t_i^2 x(t_i)$$

where the summation runs from $i = 1$ to $i = N$.

Once these a_i have been found, the new filtered signal $x^*(t)$ is computed by taking

$$x^*(t) = x(t) - p(t) \qquad (2.158)$$

where $p(t)$ is given by Eq. (2.154). Often it is advisable to carry out the computations of Eq. (2.157) in double precision to avoid overflow or underflow problems.

Figure 2.20 shows two examples of physiological signals corrupted by two commonly encountered types of low-frequency noise. The first, case A, arises, for example, in recording intracellularly from neurons and may reflect an adaptation process or deterioration of the experimental preparation. The second, case B, can arise when a strong low-frequency, nearly periodic, physiological source happens to contribute components to response recording (e.g., respiratory signal noise in recording cardiac electrical signals, circulatory blood-flow noise in recording neuroelectrical signals from sites near blood vessels, etc.). The first type of noise (case A) can be removed by the trend-removal procedure outlined above. To remove the second type of noise (case B) we must resort to high-pass filtering in spite of the phase distortion that results if a physical (analog) filter is used. (This last procedure is discussed in the next section.)

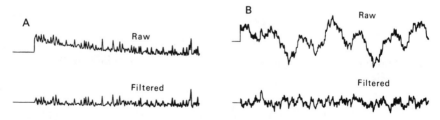

Fig. 2.20. Raw and filtered signals. (A) Parabolic trend; (B) low-frequency noise.

2.8.3. Digital Filters

The action of a linear filter can be represented by the convolution integral, whose output $y(t)$ is related to the filter input $x(t)$ by

$$y(t) = \int_{-\infty}^{\infty} h(\tau)x(t-\tau)\, d\tau \tag{2.159}$$

For physically realizable filters, causality requires $h(\tau) = 0$, for $\tau < 0$, i.e., the filter cannot operate on *future* values of the signal $x(t)$. Given the desired frequency response of the filter, $H(\omega)$, the impulse response $h(\tau)$ is found from

$$h(\tau) = \frac{1}{2\pi} \int_{-\infty}^{\infty} H(\omega) e^{i\omega\tau}\, d\omega \tag{2.160}$$

Unlike analog electronic filters, in designing a digital filter it is not necessary that the filter be physically realizable, since it is not required that $h(\tau) = 0$ for $\tau < 0$. Data may be stored in computer memory and both past and future values of the signal are available. For example, consider a symmetric moving-average filter. For it, we have

$$h(\tau) = h(-\tau) \tag{2.161}$$

and in digitized form

$$h(k) = h(-k) \qquad \text{for } k = 0, 1, 2, \dots, M \tag{2.162}$$

Then, the output $y(t)$ is found from

$$y(n) = \sum_{i=1}^{M} h(i)[x(n+i) + x(n-i)]\Delta t \qquad \text{for } i = 1, 2, \dots, N \tag{2.163}$$

Note that future values of the input are involved. For a symmetric digital filter of this type there is a zero phase characteristic since

$$H(\omega) = 2 \sum_{k=1}^{M} h(k) \cos \omega k \Delta t \tag{2.164}$$

Having the phase information unaltered is very desirable in practice because it reduces greatly the distortion problem associated with high-pass filtering of physiological signals such as shown in Fig. 2.20B. Consider the case of the ideal low-pass filter

$$H(\omega) = \begin{cases} 1, & -\omega_0 < \omega < \omega_0 \\ 0, & \text{otherwise} \end{cases} \tag{2.165}$$

Then, it is found that

$$h(\tau) = \frac{\sin \omega_0 \tau}{\pi \tau} \tag{2.166}$$

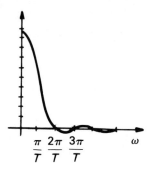

Fig. 2.21. Frequency characteristic of Hanning filter.

which, of course, is not physically realizable since $h(\tau) \neq 0$ for $\tau < 0$. However, this is not a restriction if the data exist in a computer memory, thus making both the past and future values of the signal available for filter action.

In digitized form, this filter is approximated by taking $M + 1$ terms

$$h(k) = \frac{\sin \omega_0 k \Delta t}{\pi k \Delta t} \tag{2.167}$$

i.e., there is a truncation error in approximating $h(\tau)$. Note that this filter, $h(k)$, does not attenuate very quickly—only as $1/k$. Therefore, in practice, many terms of it are required for use in Eq. (2.163). Also, since $H(\omega)$ has an abrupt transition at $\omega = \omega_0$, the truncation error between the desired $H(\omega)$ and that found by the approximation of Eq. (2.164) will cause a "ringing" effect near the ω_0 frequency (Gibbs phenomenon). To avoid this latter effect in practice we usually employ low-pass filters, which have a smoother transition at the ω_0 frequency (cutoff frequency).

A widely used filter is the so-called Hanning filter:

$$h(\tau) = \frac{1}{2}\left(1 + \cos\frac{\pi\tau}{T}\right), \qquad -T \leqslant \tau \leqslant T \tag{2.168}$$

with frequency response

$$H(\omega) = \frac{\sin \omega T}{\omega(1 - \omega^2 T^2 / \pi^2)} \tag{2.169}$$

as shown in Fig. 2.21. Its bandpass version has an impulse response function

$$h(\tau) = \frac{1}{2}\left(1 + \cos\frac{\pi\tau}{T}\right) \cos \omega_0 \tau \tag{2.170}$$

Better performance can be obtained by *recursive* digital filters. These are filters that operate on previous *outputs*, as well as inputs, i.e., through feedback. For example,

$$y(n)= \sum_{i=1}^{L} g(i)x(n-i)+ \sum_{k=1}^{M} h(k)y(n-k) \qquad (2.171)$$

uses M previous outputs and L previous inputs. Then

$$Y(\omega)= G(\omega)X(\omega)+ Y(\omega) \sum_{k=1}^{M} h(k)e^{-i\omega k \Delta t} \qquad (2.172)$$

and

$$H(\omega)=\frac{Y(\omega)}{X(\omega)}=\frac{G(\omega)}{1-\sum_{k=1}^{M} h(k)e^{-i\omega k \Delta t}} \qquad (2.173)$$

As in the study of feedback control systems, we need to study the poles of $H(\omega)$ in order to study its behavior. This is beyond the scope of this book. We present, however, some simple examples of recursive digital filters in order to compare them with nonrecursive ones.

A low-pass filter can be obtained by operating on only one value of the input and the output. We have, for example.

$$y(n)= (1-\alpha)x(n)+\alpha y(n-1) \qquad (2.174)$$

whose transfer function is

$$H(\omega)=\frac{1-\alpha}{1-\alpha e^{-i\omega \Delta t}} \qquad (2.175)$$

For low frequencies ω we can always choose Δt small enough so that

$$\omega \Delta t \ll 1$$

and then

$$e^{-i\omega \Delta t} \cong 1- i\omega \Delta t$$

resulting in

$$H(\omega) \cong \left(1+i\frac{\alpha \Delta t}{1-\alpha}\omega\right)^{-1} \qquad (2.176)$$

which, for $0<\alpha<1$ is the common RC-type low-pass filter. However, it should be noted that this recursive filter is constructed by operating on only two values—one input and one output value—while the equivalent non-recursive low-pass filter would have required more values for $h(k)$— typically about 100, in practice. This implies significant advantages of recursive filters in processing physiological signals by the usual small laboratory computer.

To construct a simple high-pass recursive filter we take

$$y(n) = (1+\alpha)x(n) + \alpha y(n-1), \qquad -1 < \alpha < 0 \qquad (2.177)$$

Then

$$H(\omega) = \frac{1+\alpha}{1-\alpha e^{-i\omega \Delta t}} \qquad (2.178)$$

At $\omega = 0$

$$H(0) = \frac{1+\alpha}{1-\alpha} \qquad (2.179)$$

which is a small number if α is negative and close to -1. At the high-frequency end, when $f = 1/(2\Delta t)$ $(\omega = \pi/\Delta t)$ we have

$$H(\pi/\Delta t) = 1 \qquad (2.180)$$

as it should be for a high-pass filter.

The above are simple, first-order, recursive digital filters. Of course, recursive filters with better performance can be constructed as higher-order schemes are considered, i.e., more values of the input and output are employed in the recursive relation. Discussion of these filters can be found in the literature (Rabiner and Rader, 1972) and the reader should consult these sources if he or she intends to employ these filtering techniques.

2.8.4. Analog Filtering

The necessity for analog filtering usually arises in cases where online analysis of physiological signals is needed in the laboratory. As an illustrative example consider the filtering of electrocardiograms for the detection of the R wave.

The basic structure of the filter used in this example is of the bandpass type. As will be demonstrated, noise in biological measurements is usually a combination of various sources, with frequencies lower, higher, and within the range of the desired signal. With analog filtering it is only possible to eliminate noise outside the range of the signal. The upper curve of Fig. 2.22A shows an ECG (chest lead) with superimposed 60-Hz noise. The lower curve shows the same ECG filtered with a passband from 5 to 20 Hz. It is clear that the 60-Hz noise has completely disappeared. However, the contour of the filtered ECG waveform is of little clinical value since it is distorted by the frequency-dependent amplitude gain and phase shift introduced by the filter.

Figure 2.22B shows an artificial spike introduced onto the ECG (lead III) (marked S on the figure) and the filtered ECG, again with a bandwidth of 5–20 Hz. The frequency content of the spike is such that even after

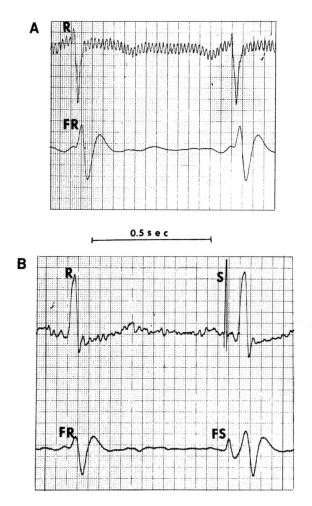

Fig. 2.22. ECG corrupted by technical noise (upper curves) and with the noise filtered (lower curves). (A) 60 Hz; (B) spikes. (Courtesy of R. Vas.)

vigorous filtering it is very much present (*FS* in the figure). The amplitude ratio of *R* to *S* has increased, thereby reducing the chance of falsely detecting the spike as an *R* wave.

Figure 2.23A shows high-frequency muscle tremor potentials superimposed on a lead III ECG and the same ECG filtered by an analog filter (5–20 Hz bandwidth). Almost complete elimination of the muscle potential is achieved. The ECG, however, loses its diagnostic value and a time shift of 50 msec appears. The detection of the *R* wave is still very easy.

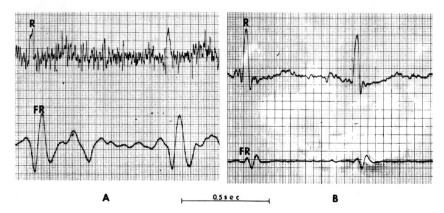

Fig. 2.23. ECG corrupted by physiological noise. (A) high-frequency muscle tremor artifact; (B) muscle artifact during vigorous handgrip exercise. (Courtesy of R. Vas.)

Figure 2.23B shows an ECG (lead II) taken from a subject during a vigorous hand-grip exercise. The detection of the *R* waves here is clearly possible. After filtering, the *R* waves are still detectable but a significant phase-shift has occurred.

Figure 2.24A shows an ECG (lead AVR) with baseline shifts due to respiration artifacts. It is very important to note that peak detection

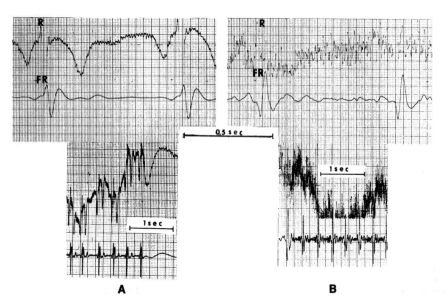

Fig. 2.24. ECG corrupted by physiological noise. (A) Respiration artifact; (B) respiration plus muscle artifact. (Courtesy of R. Vas.)

devices for the identification of R waves would not be sufficient in such cases, as is obvious from this figure. Eliminating the baseline drift alone would be easy using a simple high-pass filter. However, this would preserve any other high-frequency noise. The clinical situation almost always combines multiple sources of noise, as can be seen in Fig. 2.24B. Therefore, a simple high-pass filter would not be sufficient for the detection of the R waves here. Thus, the use of a bandpass filter is essential. It can be seen from Fig. 2.24B that very good extraction of the R waves can be achieved with the use of a simple band-pass filter; the lower cutoff eliminates the baseline shifts due to respiration, and the higher cutoff reduces the high-frequency muscle artifacts.

2.9. Considerations in Computing Power Spectra

There are several subtle problems in the calculation of power spectra that, if not considered, may lead to gross inaccuracies. We discuss them since they are directly applicable to our main theme, the white-noise approach of testing physiological systems and their characterization in terms of crosscorrelation functions.

Before the rediscovery of the fast Fourier transform (FFT) by Cooley and Tukey (1965), the computation of power spectra was always done by first computing the autocorrelation (or crosscorrelation in the case of cross spectra) function, which in itself is usually a data-reducing operation, and then performing a Fourier transformation on it. The reason was that the computation of the Fourier transform (FT) on a digital machine was a time-consuming operation. Thus, given a signal $x(t)$ over a time period from 0 to T sec, its autocorrelation $\phi_{xx}(\tau)$ was first computed by (for $\tau > 0$)

$$\phi_{xx}(\tau) = \frac{1}{T-\tau} \int_{\tau}^{T} x(t)x(t-\tau)\, dt \tag{2.181}$$

and then its power spectrum by

$$\Phi_{xx}(\omega) = \int_{-\infty}^{\infty} \phi_{xx}(\tau)\, e^{-i\omega\tau}\, d\tau$$

$$= \int_{-\infty}^{\infty} \phi_{xx}(\tau) \cos \omega\tau\, d\tau \tag{2.182}$$

since $\phi_{xx}(\tau)$ is an even function. However, the introduction in the mid-sixties of the FFT algorithm drastically reduced the computer time required for the computation of the FT. Therefore, it became more economical and practical to compute the power spectrum of a signal $x(t)$

directly by utilizing the property that

$$\Phi_{xx}(\omega) \cong FT\left[\frac{1}{T}\int_0^T x(t)x(t-\tau)\,dt\right] \cong X(\omega)X^*(\omega) = |X(\omega)|^2 \qquad (2.183)$$

where $X(\omega)$ is the FT of $x(t)$ and $X^*(\omega)$ is its complex conjugate. It should be noted that random signals do not present a problem in practice, if this route of computation is chosen, because they are finite in duration and, therefore, their FT can always be computed.

The signal $x(t)$ is sampled every Δt, giving

$$x(0), x(\Delta t), x(2\Delta t), \ldots, x(N\Delta t)$$

or

$$x(0), x(1), x(2), \ldots, x(N)$$

where $T = N\Delta t$ and the record has $N+1$ samples. Then we can represent the signal as a train of δ functions with strengths equal to the respective sample values of it (Fig. 2.25). That is,

$$x(t) = \sum_{k=0}^N x(k\Delta t)\delta(t-k\Delta t), \qquad 0 \le t \le T$$

Since this signal has a finite duration $(0, T)$, it can be represented by a Fourier series. Thus, the power spectrum of $x(t)$ is found to be

$$\Phi_{xx}(\omega) \cong |X(\omega)|^2 = \left|\sum_{k=0}^N x(k)\,e^{i\omega k\Delta t}\right|^2 \Big/ (N+1) \qquad (2.184)$$

We examine now some of the practical considerations entering into an accurate computation of the power spectrum.

2.9.1. Aliasing

We note that $\Phi_{xx}(\omega)$, as given by Eq. (2.184), does not go to zero for very high frequencies, even if none are existent in the original analog version of the signal. In fact the quantity described by Eq. (2.184) is

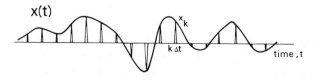

Fig. 2.25. Continuous signal discretized by sampling.

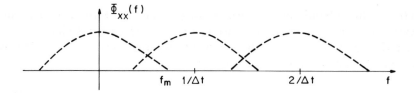

Fig. 2.26. Power spectrum of discretized signal.

periodic. Let

$$\omega_1 = \omega + 2\pi/\Delta t \qquad (2.185)$$

Then

$$i\omega_1 k \Delta t = i\omega k \Delta t + i2\pi k \qquad (2.186)$$

Therefore it repeats itself with period $2\pi/\Delta t$ rad/sec in frequency ($1/\Delta t$ in Hz). This is a direct consequence of representing the signal by its samples rather than continuously. Thus, Eq. (2.184) produces a spectrum description that consists of the actual spectrum $\Phi_{xx}(f)$ but "aliased" by copies of it that are centered at higher frequencies ($1/\Delta t, 2/\Delta t, \ldots$), as shown in Fig. 2.26.

Clearly, no harm will be done if the sampling frequency, $1/\Delta t$, is sufficiently high compared with the highest frequency f_m in $x(t)$ and if, in addition, we simply restrict our attention to the range of frequencies from 0 to f_m. Thus, for *no* overlap between the various copies of $\Phi_{xx}(f)$, $1/\Delta t$ (sampling frequency) must exceed twice the highest frequency present in $x(t)$, i.e.,

$$\text{Nyquist frequency} \doteq \frac{1}{2\Delta t} \geq \text{highest frequency in } x(t) \qquad (2.187)$$

This problem is inherent in sampling. To reduce the computationally taxing requirement of a high sampling rate, we can filter high frequencies out of $x(t)$ before we compute the spectrum, provided that these high frequencies are of no interest or of marginal value.

2.9.2. Statistical Errors

In practice, the signals are corrupted by noise. Therefore, the averages (sums) indicated by Eq. (2.184) have some statistical variation. Since the Fourier transformation of a signal is a numerically *ill-posed problem*, in the sense that small errors in the time domain produce large errors in the transform (frequency) domain, the variance of the estimates in the frequency domain can be very large. Let us consider a simple example:

$x(t)$ is a broadband Gaussian white-noise signal with zero mean and unit variance. Therefore, with reference to Eq. (2.184), each $x(k)$ has a Gaussian distribution and, since the bandwidth is large, they are also independent of each other. For $\omega = 0$, we have

$$\Phi_{xx}(0) = \frac{1}{N+1}\left[\sum_{k=0}^{N} x(k)\right]^2 = v^2 \tag{2.188}$$

The quantity

$$v = \left[\sum_{k=0}^{N} x(k)\right]/(N+1)^{1/2}$$

is itself a Gaussian variable. Note that even if the $x(k)$'s are not Gaussian, this quantity is still Gaussian because of the central limit theorem. We compute the variance of $\Phi_{xx}(0)$. For computational convenience let us assume that the $x(k)$'s are independent with mean zero and variance σ^2. Then v has also zero mean and variance σ^2. Thus the normalized quantity

$$z^2 = v^2/\sigma^2 \tag{2.189}$$

will be a χ^2 (chi-square) random variable with one degree of freedom. Therefore,

$$E[\![z^2]\!] = 1$$
$$\text{Var}\,[\![z^2]\!] = 2 \tag{2.190}$$

and consequently,

$$E[\![\Phi_{xx}(0)]\!] = \sigma^2$$
$$\text{Var}\,[\![\Phi_{xx}(0)]\!] = 2\sigma^4 \tag{2.191}$$

Thus, the normalized variance of the estimate of the spectrum density at $\omega = 0$ is

$$\varepsilon^2(0) = \frac{\text{Var}\,[\![\Phi_{xx}(0)]\!]}{\{E[\![\Phi_{xx}(0)]\!]\}^2} = 2 \tag{2.192}$$

which is considerably large. In fact, the $\omega = 0$ case is the worst, and for the other frequencies the statistical error gets smaller. More specifically, according to Eq. (2.184), for any frequency $\omega \neq 0$

$$\Phi_{xx}(\omega) = \frac{1}{N+1}\left[\sum_{k=0}^{N} x(k)\cos k\omega \Delta t\right]^2 + \frac{1}{N+1}\left[\sum_{k=0}^{N} x(k)\sin k\omega \Delta t\right]^2$$
$$= v_1^2 + v_2^2 \tag{2.193}$$

Each one of the random variables v_1^2 and v_2^2, properly normalized by its own variance, will be a chi-square variable with one degree of freedom.

However, v_1^2 and v_2^2 are clearly not independent. Let the variance of v_1 and v_2 be $\lambda_1\sigma^2$ and $\lambda_2\sigma^2$, respectively, where clearly both λ_1 and λ_2 are less than unity and positive. Then, we have

$$\text{Var } [\![\Phi_{xx}(\omega)]\!] < 2(\lambda_1\sigma^2)^2 + 2(\lambda_2\sigma^2)^2 \tag{2.194}$$

where the quantity on the right-hand side is the variance in the case where v_1^2 and v_2^2 are independent, which is clearly bigger than when they are positively correlated (that being the real situation). Also, we have

$$E[\![\Phi_{xx}(\omega)]\!] = \lambda_1\sigma^2 + \lambda_2\sigma^2 \tag{2.195}$$

Therefore, the normalized variance is

$$\varepsilon^2(\omega) = \frac{\text{Var } [\![\Phi_{xx}(\omega)]\!]}{\{E[\![\Phi_{xx}(\omega)]\!]\}^2} < \frac{2(\lambda_1^2 + \lambda_2^2)}{(\lambda_1 + \lambda_2)^2} < 2 \tag{2.196}$$

We also notice that

$$\frac{2(\lambda_1^2 + \lambda_2^2)}{(\lambda_1 + \lambda_2)^2} \geq 1 \tag{2.197}$$

which takes care of any premature enthusiasm that the above relation could provide a proper combination of λ_1 and λ_2 that would eliminate the error in the estimate. After this discussion, it becomes evident that the rms error in the estimate is at most $2^{1/2}$ at $\omega = 0$ and takes on values between 1 and $2^{1/2}$ for other frequencies. In practice, we usually take

$$\varepsilon^2 \cong 1 \tag{2.198}$$

which is still unpleasantly large (for more details cf. Blackman and Tukey, 1958). One obvious remedy would be to split the record into m segments, compute the spectra for each segment, and then average the results. Then we would expect

$$\varepsilon^2 \cong 1/m \tag{2.199}$$

thus significantly reducing the error.

2.9.3. Smoothing

From the above considerations of the statistical error it seems desirable to segment the record into m pieces. The question arises: What exactly is the effect of this segmentation in the frequency domain, i.e., on $\Phi_{xx}(f)$? It is easily shown that the effect of segmentation on the autocorrelation function of the signal is

$$\phi_m(\tau) = w(\tau)\phi(\tau) \tag{2.200}$$

where $\phi(\tau)$ is the autocorrelation of the original (unsegmented) signal of

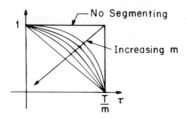

Fig. 2.27. "Window" function of segmenting-and-averaging procedure.

duration T; $\phi_m(\tau)$ is the autocorrelation resulting from averaging the autocorrelations of m segments (or of the original, finite-length signal, $m = 1$) and $w(\tau)$ is a "window" function accounting for the segmenting and averaging procedure on $\phi(\tau)$ and given by (Fig. 2.27)

$$w(\tau) = \begin{cases} \dfrac{T - m|\tau|}{T - |\tau|} & \text{when } |\tau| \leq T/m \\ 0 & \text{elsewhere} \end{cases} \tag{2.201}$$

Note that for large m, $w(\tau)$ is nearly a triangular window. In any case, from Eq. (2.200), we have that

$$\Phi_m(\omega) = \int_{-\infty}^{\infty} \Phi(\omega') W(\omega - \omega')\, d\omega' \tag{2.202}$$

where, in particular, for the *triangular window* we have

$$W(f) = \frac{m}{\pi^2 f^2 T} \sin^2\left(\frac{\pi f T}{m}\right), \qquad \omega = 2\pi f \tag{2.203}$$

That is, for any frequency ω the "segmented" signal spectrum results from weighting the unsegmented spectrum $\Phi(\omega')$ by the waveform shown in Fig. 2.28 (convolution operation). From this figure we see that segmented averaging introduces some sort of *spectral* smoothing (smearing or local averaging). Thus, reducing statistical variability introduces a reduction in

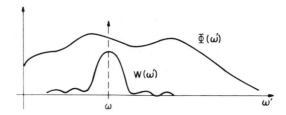

Fig. 2.28. Signal spectrum and smoothing window.

spectral resolution, as might be expected. This reduction in spectral resolution is approximately described by the relation

$$\Delta f \simeq m/T \tag{2.204}$$

where Δf is the "smearing" range or frequency resolution in the estimate. Thus, we cannot distinguish values of the spectrum for frequencies that are closer than Δf. This is a direct consequence of the finiteness of the record length (or record segment length, in case of segmenting).

We showed previously that the normalized mean-square statistical error for the spectral density estimate is bounded as [cf. Eqs. (2.196) and (2.197)]

$$1 \leq \varepsilon^2(\omega) \leq 2 \tag{2.205}$$

or, if we use m segments of the original record to compute the estimate,

$$1/m \leq \varepsilon^2(\omega) \leq 2/m \tag{2.206}$$

Recalling also Eq. (2.204) we get

$$1 \leq T\Delta f \varepsilon^2(\omega) \leq 2 \tag{2.207}$$

which states that accuracy and resolution of the spectral density estimate are two complementary characteristics (i.e., there is a trade-off between them). As we said before, in practice we usually take

$$\varepsilon^2 \cong 1/m$$

which in turn gives

$$\varepsilon^2 T\Delta f \cong 1 \tag{2.208}$$

From this relation we can specify the record length T needed to achieve a desired pair of values ε^2 and Δf.

These results have been derived for a Gaussian signal $x(t)$. Similar conclusions hold approximately for any other random signal that has an amplitude probability distribution that allows the employment of the central limit theorem in connection with the crucial relation (2.193), which determines the statistics of the power spectrum estimate. We know that most of the probability distributions that are used in practice allow the employment of the central limit theorem (which basically requires that the distribution be fairly concentrated around its mean value). In case of a statistically pathological signal, a particular and complete analysis of the statistics of the power spectrum estimate, as given by Eq. (2.193), must be made.

Segmental averaging is only one way, the naturally motivated way, to reduce the statistical error by a sacrifice in spectral resolution (uncertainty principle). Another way, rather indirect but achieving the same goal, would be to compute the original $\Phi(\omega)$ and then smooth it with some appropriate $W(\omega)$. Then we have

$$\Phi_w(f) = \int_{-\infty}^{\infty} \Phi(f') W(f-f') \, df' \tag{2.209}$$

From this relationship and with reference to Fig. 2.28 we see that the "smoothing" window $W(f)$ must have a *strong and narrow central lobe and small sidelobes* if we want to avoid significant distortion in our spectrum estimate. The sidelobes cannot be entirely eliminated because $g(\tau)$ vanishes for $|\tau| > T$, if not before, and a fundamental theorem of Fourier analysis implies that $W(f)$ must have nonzero values at arbitrarily high frequencies. Note that the smoothing operation can be done either in the time domain by $w(\tau)$ [cf. Eq. (2.200)] or in the frequency domain by $W(f)$ [cf. Eq. (2.209)].

The triangular window resulting from segmenting—for a large number of segments—has small positive sidelobes (about 5% of the main lobe). A window often used for smoothing is the Hamming window,

$$w_{\text{HM}}(\tau) = \begin{cases} 0.54 + 0.46 \cos(\pi\tau/T), & |\tau| < T \\ 0 & \text{elsewhere} \end{cases} \tag{2.210}$$

which has sidelobes with alternating signs, the largest of which accounts for about 1% of the main lobe. Also, the Hanning window is often used

$$w_{\text{HN}}(\tau) = \begin{cases} 0.5 + 0.5 \cos(\pi\tau/T), & |\tau| < T \\ 0 & \text{elsewhere} \end{cases} \tag{2.211}$$

For very small sidelobes and high attenuation in succeeding sidelobes the following Parzen window is often used:

$$W_P(f) = \frac{3T}{4} \left[\frac{\sin(\frac{1}{2}\pi fT)}{\frac{1}{2}\pi fT} \right]^4 \tag{2.212}$$

There are several other such spectral "smoothing" windows used in practice (Blackman and Tukey, 1958).

2.9.4. Practical Considerations

As we discussed at the beginning of this section, the maximum frequency f_m present in the signal determines the proper sampling interval Δt, i.e.,

$$\Delta t = 1/2f_m \tag{2.213}$$

On the other hand, a sufficiently small statistical error ε and a tolerable resolution in frequency Δf determine the record length T by

$$T \cong \frac{1}{\Delta f \varepsilon^2} \qquad (2.214)$$

Then the number of samples in the record are constrained to be

$$N = \frac{T}{\Delta t} \cong \frac{2 f_m}{\Delta f \varepsilon^2} \qquad (2.215)$$

If f_m is high and Δf should be small, for a given error ε, we may end up with very long computations. However, in practice, fine resolution is usually needed only at low frequencies. Therefore we can filter out the high frequencies, sample at lower rates, and then use a shorter portion of the original signal (higher resolution) sampled at a high rate to get the high-frequency spectrum.

... to determine the record length ...

$$\tag{1}$$

$$\tag{2}$$

3

Traditional Approaches to Physiological System Identification

Introduction

Having discussed the analysis of physiological signals, we must now discuss the specific ways in which they propagate through systems and the resulting transformation of a stimulus signal into a response signal.

In this chapter we discuss the methodology that has been prevalent among physiologists in describing transformations of the stimulus into response signals. This methodology has concentrated primarily on measuring the linear system transfer characteristics either by ignoring the nonlinearities and trying to obtain a "best" linear approximation to the transfer function or by searching for a stimulus domain (such as small signal amplitudes in certain cases) within which the system acts approximately linearly.

In most work on physiological systems these linear system descriptions have been made either in the frequency domain (gain and phase plots), or in the time domain (obtaining the system impulse, step, or ramp response). In this chapter we discuss briefly the relative merits of these two approaches, given the experimental realities of physiological systems, e.g., short stable records of stimulus–response data, high noise contamination of the recorded signals, etc. In addition, we describe a nonlinear system identification procedure that has been used, though rather rarely: the describing-function technique.

In the next chapter we embark upon the description and discussion of the main theme of this book: testing physiological systems with white-noise stimuli and describing their nonlinear dynamic characteristics in a systematic and experimentally efficient way.

3.1. Stimulus–Response Relations in Linear Systems

The concept of the *transfer characteristic* for a system is central in the theme of this book. It is the relationship that describes *how* the stimulus signals are transformed by the system into response signals (i.e., transferred to the system output).

These stimulus–response relationships can be expressed either in the time domain or the frequency domain. Descriptions in this latter domain, while achieved at the expense of being somewhat removed from our direct experience of these signals, are advantageous in many respects, both in terms of analytical convenience and often in terms of enhancing our information about signals in the presence of noise. In physiological systems the characteristics of signals are best described in stochastic terms and therefore are most easily described by their spectral composition, i.e., their content of various frequencies. In addition, examples abound in physiology, where the "information" of the signals is dependent on their frequency composition: acoustic signals, voice signals, perhaps even visual signals. A further justification for a signal description in the frequency domain arises from the high noise content usually encountered in physiological signals. If the frequency spectrum of the noise does not overlap with the spectrum of the signal then the noise can be conveniently filtered out by working in the frequency domain.

3.1.1. Time Domain

The response $y(t)$ of a *linear* system to a stimulus $x(t)$ is given by the convolution (superposition) integral

$$y(t) = \int_0^\infty h(\tau)x(t-\tau)\, d\tau \tag{3.1}$$

where $h(\tau) = 0$ for $\tau < 0$ since physical systems have to follow the principle of causality, i.e., the response cannot precede the stimulus that causes it. It should be stressed that relationship (3.1) holds whether the stimulus is periodic, transient, or random. From this general relation for the stimulus and response signals of a system, we can derive several relations involving the system "impulse response" $h(\tau)$ and the various auto- and cross-correlation of $x(t)$ and $y(t)$. For example, multiplying both sides of Eq. (3.1) by $x(t-\tau)$ and averaging (i.e., taking "expected values"), we find

$$\phi_{yx}(\tau) = \int_0^\infty h(\lambda)\phi_{xx}(\tau-\lambda)\, d\lambda \tag{3.2}$$

The assumptions underlying this result are that the system is a time-invariant (constant parameter) linear system with finite memory (cf. Sec. 4.2) and that the stimuli $x(t)$ are stationary signals. Then, of course, the response signals $y(t)$ are stationary. In a similar fashion and with the same assumptions we obtain

$$\phi_{yy}(\tau) = \int_0^\infty h(\mu)\left[\int_0^\infty h(\lambda)\phi_{xx}(\tau-\mu-\lambda)\, d\lambda\right] d\mu \tag{3.3}$$

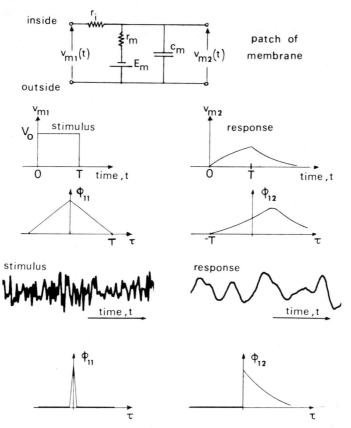

Fig. 3.1. Auto- and crosscorrelation functions for a patch of membrane subjected to deterministic and random stimuli.

relating the stimulus and response autocorrelations with the system impulse response $h(\tau)$.

To illustrate these system relationships we consider a patch of passive membrane shown in Fig. 3.1 and its response to both a deterministic stimulus (a pulse) and a random stimulus (a broadband white-noise signal).

The differential equation describing the stimulus–response relation of the membrane patch is

$$\frac{V_{m1} - V_{m2}}{r_i} = \frac{V_{m2} - E_m}{r_m} + C_m \frac{dV_{m2}}{dt} \tag{3.4}$$

which becomes

$$\frac{r_i r_m}{r_i + r_m} C_m \frac{dV_{m2}}{dt} + V_{m2} = \frac{r_i}{r_i + r_m} E_m + \frac{r_m}{r_i + r_m} V_{m1} \tag{3.5}$$

The time-varying response of this linear system can be computed without taking into consideration the dc source E_m, since it only contributes a dc component to the response. Thus, if we let

$$A = \frac{1}{r_i C_m}, \qquad \alpha = \frac{1}{C_m} \frac{r_i + r_m}{r_i r_m} \tag{3.6}$$

the differential equation that characterizes the time-varying response component becomes

$$\frac{d V_{m2}}{dt} + \alpha V_{m2} = A V_{m1} \tag{3.7}$$

The solution of this first-order linear differential equation is found (by standard methods) to be

$$V_{m2}(t) = \int_0^\infty A e^{-\alpha \tau} V_{m1}(t - \tau) \, d\tau + V_{m2}(0) \tag{3.8}$$

Therefore, the impulse response of this membrane patch is

$$h(\tau) = A e^{-\alpha \tau} \qquad (\tau \geqslant 0) \tag{3.9}$$

Consider now a stimulus voltage $V_{m1}(t)$, which is a pulse, of width T as shown in Fig. 3.1. Then the response of the system will be

$$V_{m2}(t) = \int_0^\infty h(\tau) V_{m1}(t - \tau) \, d\tau$$

$$= \begin{cases} (A V_0 / \alpha)(1 - e^{-\alpha t}), & 0 \leqslant t \leqslant T \\ (A V_0 / \alpha)(e^{-\alpha(t-T)} - e^{-\alpha t}), & t > T \end{cases} \tag{3.10}$$

for $V_{m2}(0) = 0$.

The autocorrelation function of $V_{m1}(t)$ is easily found to be

$$\phi_{11}(\tau) = \begin{cases} V_0^2 (T - |\tau|), & |\tau| \leqslant T \\ 0, & |\tau| > T \end{cases} \tag{3.11}$$

as shown in Fig. 3.1. The crosscorrelation function of $V_{m1}(t)$ and $V_{m2}(t)$ is found to be

$$\phi_{12}(\tau) = \begin{cases} \dfrac{A V_0^2}{\alpha}(T - \tau) + \dfrac{A V_0^2}{\alpha^2}[(1 - e^{-\alpha T})(e^{\alpha \tau} - 1) \\ \qquad - (1 - e^{-\alpha(T-\tau)})], & 0 \leqslant \tau \leqslant T \\[2mm] \dfrac{A V_0^2}{\alpha}(T + \tau) + \dfrac{A V_0^2}{\alpha^2}(e^{-\alpha(T+\tau)} - 1), & -T \leqslant \tau < 0 \end{cases} \tag{3.12}$$

as shown in Fig. 3.1.

One may arrive at the same expressions for these correlations by using Eq. (3.2).

We now consider a stimulus at $V_{m1}(t)$ that is stochastic, e.g., a broadband Gaussian white-noise signal. Then we have

$$\phi_{11}(\tau) \cong P\delta(\tau)$$

and

$$\phi_{12}(\tau) = \int_0^\infty h(\lambda)\phi_{11}(\tau-\lambda)\,d\lambda$$

$$= Ph(\tau)$$

$$= PA\,e^{-\alpha\tau} \qquad (\tau \geq 0) \tag{3.13}$$

Note that $V_{m2}(t)$ is also Gaussian noise but not white (because of the system's limited bandwidth). It is evident that we cannot give a closed-form expression for $V_{m2}(t)$ since it is a stochastic signal. Of course, $V_{m2}(t)$ may still be found using the equation

$$V_{m2}(t) = \int_0^\infty h(\tau)V_{m1}(t-\tau)\,d\tau \tag{3.14}$$

Then the autocorrelation function of $V_{m2}(t)$ can be found to be

$$\phi_{22}(\tau) = \int\!\!\int_0^\infty h(\mu)h(\lambda)\phi_{11}(\tau+\mu-\lambda)\,d\mu\,d\lambda$$

$$= \frac{PA^2}{2\alpha}e^{-\alpha|\tau|} \tag{3.15}$$

3.1.2. Frequency Domain

There are several advantages in describing system stimulus–response relationships in the frequency domain (through Fourier or Laplace transformations). The main advantage, from the analysis point of view, is the fact that the integral equations relating the stimulus and response in the time domain, described in the previous section, become algebraic equations in the frequency domain. This, in turn, greatly facilitates the description of composite systems, providing an easy way to combine (synthesize) subsystems by describing them in the frequency domain. This holds true for both linear systems (as shown in this chapter) and nonlinear ones (as shown in Chap. 9).

Taking the Fourier transform of relationships (3.2) and (3.3) of the previous section, we have

$$\Phi_{yx}(\omega) = H(\omega)\Phi_{xx}(\omega) \qquad (3.16)$$

$$\Phi_{yy}(\omega) = |H(\omega)|^2\Phi_{xx}(\omega) \qquad (3.17)$$

which relate the power spectra (and cross-power spectra) of the stimulus and response. From the point of view of "identifying" the system we note the following:

(1) Equation (3.16) will give $H(\omega)$, the system transfer function, directly, simply by measuring the stimulus–response cross-power spectrum $\Phi_{yx}(\omega)$ and stimulus power spectrum $\Phi_{xx}(\omega)$.

(2) Equation (3.17) will give $|H(\omega)|$, the magnitude (gain) of the system (but not the phase), by measuring the stimulus and response (auto-) power spectra. However, if the system has the special property of being a "minimum-phase system" then the magnitude $|H(\omega)|$ is sufficient for determining the transfer function $H(\omega)$, and the phase characteristic is uniquely determined by the gain characteristic (cf. Sec. 3.2).

As an example, consider again the patch of membrane shown in Fig. 3.1. We compute first the power spectrum of the pulse stimulus. The autocorrelation function of the pulse is shown in Fig. 3.1. The power spectrum is (see Fig. 3.2A)

$$\Phi_{11}(\omega) = \int_0^\infty \phi_{11}(\tau)e^{-i\omega\tau}\,d\tau = V_0^2 T^2\left[\frac{\sin(\omega T/2)}{\omega T/2}\right]^2 \qquad (3.18)$$

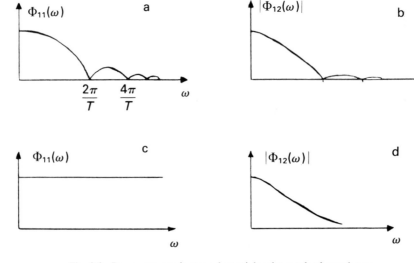

Fig. 3.2. Power spectra (auto and cross) for the patch of membrane.

The transfer function of the system is

$$H(\omega) = \frac{A}{\alpha + i\omega} \tag{3.19}$$

Thus, the cross-power spectrum, from Eq. (3.16) is (see Fig. 3.2B)

$$\Phi_{12}(\omega) = \frac{AV_0^2 T^2}{\alpha + i\omega} \left[\frac{\sin(\omega T/2)}{\omega T/2} \right]^2 \tag{3.20}$$

Also the power spectrum of the response is found, from Eq. (3.17), to be

$$\Phi_{22}(\omega) = \frac{A^2 V_0^2 T^2}{\alpha^2 + \omega^2} \left[\frac{\sin(\omega T/2)}{\omega T/2} \right]^2 \tag{3.21}$$

We can verify these expressions for $\Phi_{12}(\omega)$ and $\Phi_{22}(\omega)$ by taking the Fourier transform of $\phi_{12}(\tau)$ and $\phi_{22}(\tau)$, as found above [cf. Eqs. (3.11), (3.12) and (3.17)]. Let us compute the power spectra of the system in question for the case of a Gaussian white-noise input (see Figs. 3.2C and 3.2D):

$$\Phi_{11}(\omega) = P$$

$$\Phi_{12}(\omega) = \frac{AP}{\alpha + j\omega} \tag{3.22}$$

$$\Phi_{22}(\omega) = \frac{A^2 P}{\alpha^2 + \omega^2}$$

These expressions can also be derived by taking the Fourier transform of $\phi_{12}(t)$ and $\phi_{22}(t)$, given by Eqs. (3.13) and (3.15).

3.2. Transfer Functions and Bode Plots

We consider first the case of a linear system with one input and one output, as shown in Fig. 3.3. As we have seen, we have

$$y(t) = \int_0^\infty h(\tau) x(t - \tau) \, d\tau \tag{3.23}$$

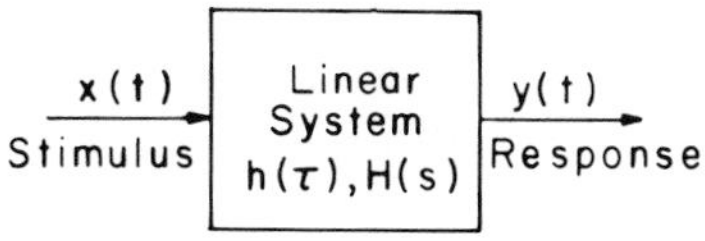

Fig. 3.3. Single-input, single-output linear system.

Taking the Laplace transform of both sides and assuming zero initial conditions—not a restrictive assumption in practice—we have

$$Y(s) = H(s)X(s), \qquad H(s) = Y(s)/X(s) \tag{3.24}$$

which describes how the input is transformed into the output. $H(s)$ is called the *transfer function* of the system.

3.2.1. Analysis

For a linear, stationary, constant parameter system without delays, the transfer function $H(s)$ can be written as a ratio of two polynomials:

$$H(s) = \frac{a_m s^m + \cdots + a_1 s + a_0}{b_n s^n + \cdots + b_1 s + b_0} \tag{3.25}$$

This derives directly from the fact that such systems are described by linear differential equations with constant coefficients. For physically realizable systems we must have $n > m$. Otherwise, i.e., if $n \leq m$, it would be implied that energy can be transferred instantaneously through the system.

By factoring the polynomials in Eq. (3.25) we have

$$H(s) = \frac{K'(s - z_1) \cdots (s - z_m)}{(s - p_1) \cdots (s - p_n)} \tag{3.26}$$

where the polynomial roots z_i, p_i can be zero, real or complex (if complex, they come as conjugate pairs). The "poles" p_i of the system must be negative (or, if complex, have negative real parts) for the system to be stable.

Since any waveform can be represented to an arbitrary degree of accuracy by a sum of sine waves, and since linear systems obey the principle of superposition, the response of a linear system to an arbitrary signal waveform can be deduced if we know the system response to sine wave signals of all frequencies. Thus, let us consider that we apply as a stimulus to the system a sine wave

$$x(t) = A \sin \omega t \tag{3.27}$$

Then, the response $y(t)$ in the frequency domain is

$$Y(s) = H(s) \frac{As}{s^2 + \omega^2} \tag{3.28}$$

since $s/(s^2 + \omega^2)$ is the Laplace transform of $\sin \omega t$. Using partial fraction expansion of the right-hand side of Eq. (3.28) we get

$$Y(s) = \frac{c_1}{s + i\omega} + \frac{c_2}{s - i\omega} + \frac{c_3}{s - p_1} + \frac{c_4}{s - p_2} + \cdots \tag{3.29}$$

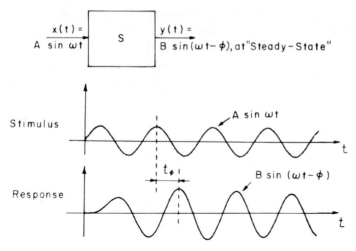

Fig. 3.4. Measurement of gain and phase.

and therefore

$$y(t) = c_1 e^{-i\omega t} + c_2 e^{i\omega t} + c_3 e^{p_1 t} + c_4 e^{p_2 t} + \cdots \qquad (3.30)$$

Providing that the system is stable (i.e., $p_i < 0$) the steady-state response is

$$y_{ss}(t) = c_1 e^{-i\omega t} + c_2 e^{i\omega t} \qquad (3.31)$$

Using standard partial fraction expansion techniques we find that

$$c_1 = \tfrac{1}{2} A H(-i\omega)$$
$$c_2 = \tfrac{1}{2} A H(i\omega) \qquad (3.32)$$

and therefore we easily see that

$$y_{ss}(t) = A |H(i\omega)| \cos \{\omega t + \theta[H(i\omega)]\} \qquad (3.33)$$

where $|H(i\omega)|$ denotes the magnitude of $H(i\omega)$ and $\theta[H(i\omega)]$ its angle. Therefore, we note that, for a linear system, the response to a sine-wave stimulus of fixed frequency is a sine wave of the same frequency, but with possibly different amplitude and phase (see Fig. 3.4).

The magnitude $|H(i\omega)|$ signifies the ratio of the response amplitude to the stimulus amplitude and the phase $\theta[H(i\omega)]$ denotes the phase difference between the stimulus and the response sine-wave signals.

If we combine (multiply) the complex-conjugate pairs of roots and normalize the constant term in each factor in Eq. (3.26) we find that

$$H(s) = \frac{K s^n (1 + T_1 s) \cdots (s^2 / \omega_{n1}^2 + 2\zeta_1 s / \omega_{n1} + 1) \cdots}{s^m (1 + T_\alpha s) \cdots (s^2 / \omega_{n\alpha}^2 + 2\zeta_\alpha s / \omega_{n\alpha} + 1) \cdots} \qquad (3.34)$$

We note that the numerator and denominator consist of three types of factors: powers of s, first-degree terms, and second-degree terms, the second-degree terms resulting from complex-conjugate pair roots. The parameters ζ and ω_n in the second-order terms are the familiar *damping* and *natural frequency* of a second-order linear system.

The Bode plots consist of plotting the quantities $20 \log |H(i\omega)|$ (these units of gain are called decibels) and $\theta[H(i\omega)]$, in degrees, as functions of frequency ω, where the frequency abscissa is in log ω scale. The reasons for this are that graphing of the transfer function then becomes easy and the mathematical realtionships become very simple, as we shall see shortly. The advantages resulting are as follows:

(1) The numerator (denominator) factor terms become simply additive (subtractive) terms, since the logarithm of the quantity is considered.

(2) For high and low frequencies the magnitude and phase plots can be accurately represented by straight-line asymptotes while for intermediate frequencies simple rules can facilitate greatly the task of plotting.

It should be noted that in the case of physiological sensory systems the logarithmic transformation of the Bode plots is, indeed, very convenient since most of these systems, e.g., vision, audition, perform logarithmic transformations on the stimulus intensity themselves.

Taking the logarithm in Eq. (3.34) we have

$$20 \log |H(i\omega)| = 20 \log K + 20 \log |(i\omega)^n| + 20 \log |1 + i\omega T_1| + \cdots$$

$$+ 20 \log |-\omega^2/\omega_{n1}^2 + 2i\omega\zeta_1/\omega_{n1} + 1|$$

$$+ \cdots - \text{(similar terms coming from the denominator)}$$

$$(3.35)$$

For the phase we have

$$\theta[H(i\omega)] = \theta(K) + \theta[(i\omega)^n] + \theta(1 + i\omega T_1) + \cdots$$

$$+ \theta(-\omega^2/\omega_{n1}^2 + 2i\omega\zeta_1/\omega_{n1} + 1)$$

$$+ \cdots - \text{(similar terms coming from the denominator)} \quad (3.36)$$

Therefore we see that the magnitude and phase of $H(i\omega)$ are composed of four types of factors: a constant, K, poles or zeros such as $(i\omega)^{\pm n}$, poles or zeros such as $(1 + i\omega T)$, and quadratic poles or zeros such as $(-\omega^2/\omega_n^2 + 2i\omega\zeta/\omega_n + 1)$.

We can see now the advantage of the Bode plot: Each of the four kinds of factors may be considered as a separate plot, with the final plot resulting from these plots being added or subtracted.

A constant K. We simply plot $20 \log_{10} K$, a constant, and

$$\theta(K) = 0°$$

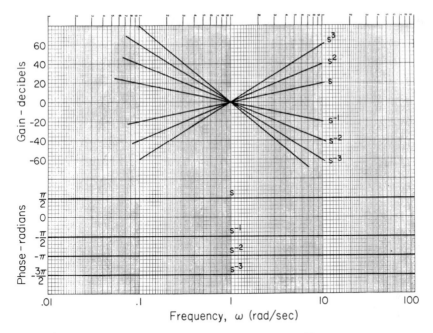

Fig. 3.5. Gain and phase plots of $(i\omega)^{\pm n}$.

Poles or zeros such as $(i\omega)^{\pm n}$. For the magnitude we have

$$20 \log_{10} |(i\omega)^{\pm n}| = \pm 20n \log_{10} \omega \quad \text{db} \tag{3.37}$$

This is the equation of a straight line as shown in Fig. 3.5. The slopes of these lines can be found by taking

$$\frac{d\{20 \log_{10} [(i\omega)^{\pm n}]\}}{d(\log_{10} \omega)} = \pm 20n \quad \text{db} \tag{3.38}$$

Therefore, if the frequency changes by ten times (a decade) we get a change of $\pm 20n$ db.

Often an octave of frequency is used. Frequencies ω_1 and ω_2 are separated by an octave if $\omega_2/\omega_1 = 2$. Therefore, it is easily seen that the slope of $20n$ db/decade corresponds to $6n$ db/octave.

For the phase we have

$$\theta[(i\omega)^n] = 90n \quad \text{degrees} \tag{3.39}$$

Both the magnitude and phase plots for this factor are shown in Fig. 3.5.

Factor $(1 + i\omega T)$. For the magnitude, we have

$$20 \log_{10} |H(i\omega)| = 20 \log_{10} (1 + \omega^2 T^2)^{1/2} \tag{3.40}$$

For the phase,

$$\theta[H(i\omega)] = \tan^{-1} \omega T$$

We note that for very low frequencies, $\omega T \ll 1$, thus

$$20 \log_{10} (1 + \omega^2 T^2)^{1/2} \approx 20 \log_{10} 1 = 0 \qquad (3.41)$$

Also, for very high frequencies, $\omega T \gg 1$, thus

$$20 \log_{10} (1 + \omega^2 T^2)^{1/2} \approx 20 \log_{10} \omega T \qquad (3.42)$$

Equation (3.42) is a straight line with a slope of 20 dbs/decade (or 6 db/octave). The intersection of the low-frequency and the high-frequency asymptotes is found easily since at that point

$$20 \log_{10} \omega T = 0 \quad db$$

Therefore, the frequency $\omega_c = 1/T$ at the "corner," or intersection, of the low-frequency and high-frequency asymptotes, is called the *corner frequency*. Of course, the approximation in terms of these straight-line asymptotes is not so good at intermediate frequencies. In that range, the actual magnitude curve is smoothly varying. However, the deviation from the straight-line asymptote approximation is not severe for most practical purposes.

Thus, the procedure in plotting the linear factor $(1 + i\omega T)$ is, first, to locate the corner frequency $\omega_c = 1/T$ and, second, to draw the 6-db/octave straight-line asymptotes through the corner frequency, with positive or negative slope depending on whether the term is in the numerator or denominator. If greater accuracy is required, then the corrections denoted in Table 3.1 should be used.

The Bode phase curve for this factor can similarly be plotted in terms of the straight-line asymptotes, as shown in Fig. 3.6. A straight line is

Table 3.1. Exact and Approximate Values of Gain and Phase of the Linear Factor in Bode Plots

ωT	$\begin{array}{c}\|1+i\omega T\| \\ \text{(db)}\end{array}$	$\|1+i\omega T\|$	Straight-line approximation $\|1+i\omega T\|$	$\theta(1+i\omega T)$ (deg)	Straight-line approximation $\theta(1+i\omega T)$ (deg)
0.1 one decade below	1.04	0.04	0	6	0
0.5 one octave below	1.12	1.00	0	27	22
1.0	1.41	3.00	0	45	45
2.0 one octave above	2.24	7.00	6	63	58
10 one decade above	10.50	20.40	20	84	90

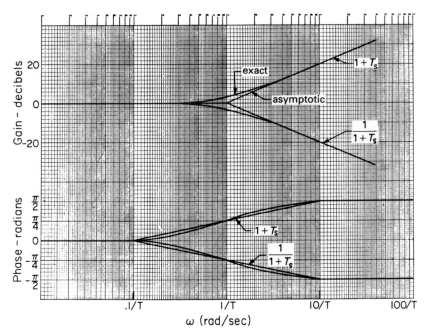

Fig. 3.6. Gain and phase plots of $(1 + i\omega T)^{\pm 1}$.

drawn from $0°$ at one decade below the corner frequency $\omega_c = 1/T$, i.e., at $\omega = 1/10T$, to $90°$ at $\omega = 10/T$, i.e., a decade higher than ω_c.

Quadratic factors: $-\omega^2/\omega_n^2 + i2\omega\zeta/\omega_n + 1$. For the magnitude of $H(i\omega)$ we have

$$20 \log_{10} |H(i\omega)| = 20 \log_{10} \left\{ \left[1 - \left(\frac{\omega}{\omega_n} \right)^2 \right]^2 + \left(\frac{2\zeta\omega}{\omega_n} \right)^2 \right\}^{1/2} \qquad (3.43)$$

For the phase plot we have

$$\theta[H(i\omega)] = 20 \tan^{-1} \left[\frac{2\zeta\omega/\omega_n}{1 - (\omega/\omega_n)^2} \right] \qquad (3.44)$$

We note that at very low frequencies, $\omega/\omega_n \ll 1$, thus

$$20 \log_{10} |H(i\omega)| \cong -20 \log_{10} 1 = 0 \quad \text{db} \qquad (3.45)$$

i.e., the low-frequency asymptote is, again, a straight line with zero slope. Also, at very high frequencies, $\omega/\omega_n \gg 1$, thus,

$$20 \log_{10} |H(i\omega)| = 20 \log_{10} \{ [1 - (\omega/\omega_n)^2]^2 + (2\zeta\omega/\omega_n)^2 \}^{1/2}$$

$$\cong 40 \log_{10} (\omega/\omega_n) \qquad (3.46)$$

The high-frequency asymptote is, therefore, a straight line with slope of 40 db/decade.

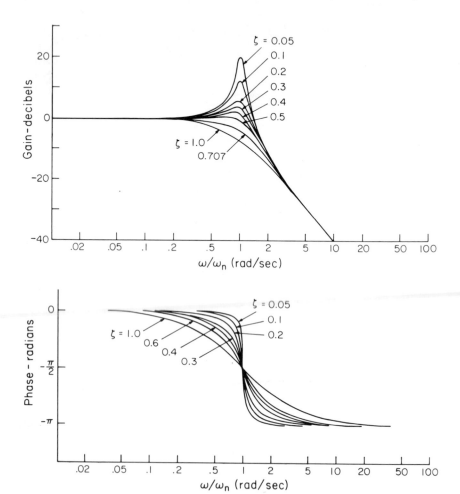

Fig. 3.7. Gain and phase plots of $-(\omega/\omega_n)^2 + i2\zeta\omega/\omega_n + 1$ for various values of damping ratio ζ.

The intersection of the two asymptotes is found from

$$40 \log_{10}(\omega/\omega_n) = 0 \quad db$$

which implies that $\omega = \omega_n$ at the intersection point. However, the actual magnitude plot in this case differs considerably from the asymptotic lines. The reason for this is that the amplitude and phase curves depend not only on the frequency ω_n, but also on the damping ratio ζ. The exact Bode magnitude and phase plots are shown in Fig. 3.7. In practice, if a transfer function of the quadratic form is encountered, first the values of ζ and ω_n are determined and then, by using the template curves shown in Fig. 3.7, the magnitude and phase curves are plotted. If the factor

$$(i\omega/\omega_n)^2 + 2\zeta(i\omega/\omega_n) + 1$$

appears in the numerator, the magnitudes of the Bode amplitude and phase angle are the same as those in Fig. 3.7 except that they have opposite signs.

The magnitude of a quadratic factor with $\zeta < 1$ has a peak value. The magnitude of this peak value and the frequency at which it occurs can easily be found to be

$$\text{magnitude of peak} = \frac{1}{2\zeta(1-\zeta^2)^{1/2}} \qquad (3.47)$$

$$\text{peak frequency} = \omega_n(1-2\zeta^2)^{1/2} \qquad (3.48)$$

We note that the peak value depends only on the damping ratio ζ, which is bounded as $0 < \zeta < 2^{1/2}/2$, since Eq. (3.48) is meaningful only for real values. This implies that the peak value is greater than unity. We also note that the frequency at which this peak value occurs depends on both the damping ratio and the undamped natural frequency. Therefore, the degree of damping in a system influences the frequency at which its response gain is maximum.

3.2.2. (Non-) Minimum-Phase Systems

The discussion thus far deals with minimum-phase factors (no delays and all poles and zeros are in the left-half of the complex plane). As can easily be seen, the magnitude curves for non-minimum-phase factors (poles and zeros in the right half of the complex plane) are the same as those for the corresponding minimum-phase factors; however, the angle curves are different. The angle for factor $(1 - i\omega T)$ varies from $0°$ to $90°$ as ω varies from zero to infinity. For the quadratic factor, if ζ is negative, we have a non-minimum-phase term; in this case the angle varies from $-360°$ to $-180°$ as ω varies from zero to infinity. These facts can easily be seen from the formulas above, following a similar discussion.

3.2.3. Synthesis

With these relations in mind for a single-input, single-output system we can now attack the identification problem for linear stationary systems. In fact, the gain and phase plot (Bode plot) approach has been extensively and almost exclusively used in identifying physiological systems in the past. The disadvantages of this approach in studying physiological systems lie in the assumptions of linearity and stationarity for the systems, conditions usually tenuously satisfied in biological systems. In addition, certain other experimental constraints usually encountered in the study of physiological systems, such as high noise content and short durations of the experiments, are not optimally managed by this approach.

The usual procedure followed in doing sinusoidal analysis in order to obtain the system Bode plots is as follows:

(1) A sinusoidal stimulus of frequency f is applied to the system, i.e.,

$$x(t) = A \sin (2\pi ft)$$

and the corresponding system response, when steady state is reached, is recorded (see Fig. 3.4):

$$y(t) = B \sin (2\pi ft - \phi)$$

(2) The ratio of amplitudes B/A of response over stimulus is computed and plotted on the Bode diagram for gain at frequency f. Similarly, the phase

$$\phi = (t_\phi/T)2\pi \quad \text{rad}$$

$$= (t_\phi/T)360° \tag{3.49}$$

is computed, where T is the period of the sine wave, i.e., $T = 1/f$.

(3) Steps 1 and 2 are repeated for different frequencies f, from very low to very high, so that the entire frequency range to which the system responds is covered. At the end, a sufficient number of points of the Bode curves have been obtained so that smooth curves can be drawn connecting them.

(4) The gain curve is fitted by straight-line asymptotes at high- and low-frequency ranges. The high-frequency asymptote should be an integer multiple of 6 db/octave. In case of noise, the choice between adjacent multiples of 6 db/octave, such as, for example, 18 db/octave and 24 db/octave, may be difficult in practice. Then, perhaps, the dispute can be settled by reference to the phase curve (since for 18 db/octave high-frequency slope the maximum phase would be 270° while for 24 db/octave the maximum phase would be 360°). This does not mean, of course, that noise cannot also distort the phase estimates. Finally, the segments of the Bode plots for intermediate frequencies are drawn with the help of Table 3.1 and the plots of Figs. 3.5, 3.6, and 3.7.

(5) The system transfer function can now be written by visual inspection of the Bode plots.

A few illustrative examples are presented below, which should clarify this procedure. In practical situations only one of the two Bode plots, either the gain or the phase, need be measured since the other is uniquely determinable from it—of course, under the assumption that the system is minimum-phase and has no delays. Usually, only the gain is measured.

However, a good case can be made also for measuring only the phase characteristic, since there are advantages resulting from the fact that the phase is a *normalized* measure of the transfer function and is convenient in neurophysiological applications where microelectrodes of high impedance are involved (cf. Valdiosera *et al.*, 1974).

Example. Figure 3.8 shows the gain plot obtained after stimulating a system with sine waves of various frequencies. Let us assume that the data obtained justify the approximation of this gain curve by the straight-line asymptotes shown in the figure. Following the procedure outlined above we find the transfer function for this system to be of the approximate form

$$H(s) = \frac{(1 + T_1 s)}{(1 + T_2 s)[(1 + T_3 s)(1 + T_4 s)]^2} \tag{3.50}$$

where $T_1 = 1/0.4\pi$, $T_2 = 1/0.8\pi$, $T_3 = 1/2\pi$, $T_4 = 1/10\pi$. It should be noted that T_1, T_2, T_3, T_4 are the various time constants of the system response.

In deriving the transfer function for this system we have not considered the phase measurements. As noted before, the phase curve is uniquely determined from the gain curve (and, vice versa, the gain curve is determinable from the phase curve), assuming that the system is a "minimum-phase" system. If the phase predicted from the gain is different from the one measured then the system is "non-minimum-phase" and additional analysis is required. This happens sometimes in the study of physiological systems; for example, the eye-movement control system is such (cf. Fender, 1964b; Young *et al.*, 1964; Stark, 1968).

Example. *Sinusoidal Analysis of a Retinal System.* Experiments were performed on the catfish retina (cf. P. Z. Marmarelis and Naka, 1973a,b,c). The stimulus was a light of variable intensity covering about 2/3 of the entire retinal surface, and the response was the resulting

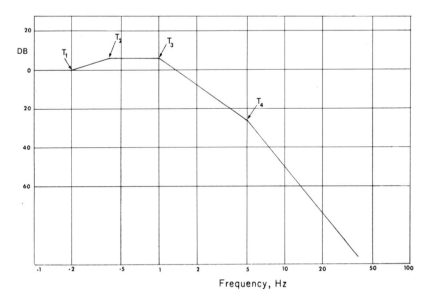

Fig. 3.8. Gain plot of a system.

potential change of a horizontal cell recorded intracellularly. The sine wave stimulus had a modulation depth of about 0.8 (modulation depth is the ratio I_m/I_{av}, where I_m is the amplitude of the sine wave modulation and I_{av} is the average intensity). Figure 3.9 shows the stimulus and horizontal cell responses for a wide range of frequencies.

The gain and phase data curves for this system are shown in Fig. 3.10.

Turning our attention to the gain curve, we see after some consideration that it is of the form

$$H(s) = \frac{K}{[s^2/\omega_n^2 + (2\zeta/\omega_n)s + 1]^2} \tag{3.51}$$

We came to this conclusion after noting that the upward (positive) slope of the gain curve is *not* close to a multiple of 6 db/octave while, on the other hand, the templates of Fig. 3.7 look very similar to it. Since the high-frequency asymptote is close to 24 db/octave we conclude that the denominator term should be squared, as shown in Eq. (3.51). The values of

$$\zeta = 0.5, \qquad \omega_n = 2\pi(10)$$

give a good fit to the gain curve of this system.

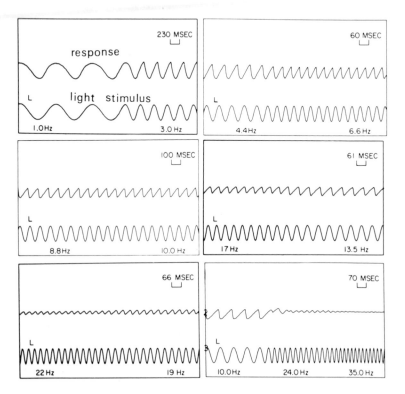

Fig. 3.9. Sinusoidal light stimulation data obtained from horizontal cell in the catfish retina.

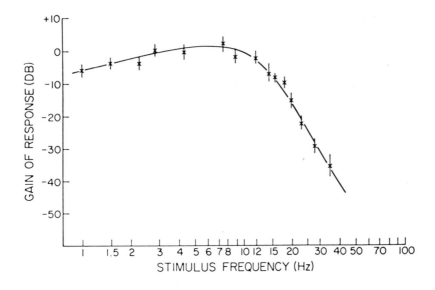

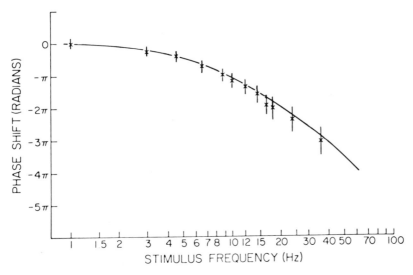

Fig. 3.10. Gain and phase plots of data from system light → horizontal cell.

We turn our attention, now, to the phase-shift data. We would expect the phase curve to approach -2π radius for high frequencies; instead, the phase keeps increasing as the frequency increases. This is due to the system latency (delay), i.e., the transit time of the stimulus signal as it propagates to the response site.

3.2.4. Delays in Transfer Functions

A linear system with a delay d can be represented by the configuration shown in Fig. 3.11. The output of the delay component is

$$z(t) = x(t-d) \tag{3.52}$$

and therefore the transfer function of the delay is

$$H_d(s) = e^{-sd} \tag{3.53}$$

Therefore, the overall transfer function of the system is

$$H(i\omega) = H_d(i\omega)G(i\omega)$$
$$= |G(i\omega)| \exp\left(i\{-\omega d + \theta[G(i\omega)]\}\right) \tag{3.54}$$

We note that (a) the delay has no effect on the gain of the system, which remains $|G(i\omega)|$, and (b) it does modify the phase of the system by adding an additional phase of $-\omega d$. Therefore, it is possible to measure the system delay d from the measured phase curve. Let θ_1 be the phase of the overall system and θ_2 be the phase of $G(i\omega)$. Then we have

$$\theta_1 = -\omega d + \theta_2(\omega) \tag{3.55}$$

We know, however, that $\theta_2(\omega)$ becomes constant (and a multiple of $\frac{1}{2}\pi$) for very high frequencies. Therefore, from Eq. (3.55) we get

$$\frac{\partial \theta_1}{\partial \omega} = -d + \frac{\partial \theta_2}{\partial \omega}$$
$$= -d \tag{3.56}$$

That is, the slope of the phase curve at high frequencies, where θ_2 does not vary, gives directly the delay d. Of course, any point of the phase θ_1 in this high-frequency region could give us an estimate of the delay d; however, in the presence of noise, the slope will generally provide a better estimate.

Naturally, the question now arises: What if the delay d is a function of frequency? How do we measure it? If $d = -d(\omega)$, then again the phase function is

$$\phi(\omega) = +\omega\, d(\omega) + \theta(\omega) \tag{3.57}$$

We said that $\theta(\omega)$ is known if the gain function of the system is known; however, its exact determination is not trivial and involves a considerable computational effort. Thus, the obvious solution

$$d(\omega) = (1/\omega)[\phi(\omega) - \theta(\omega)] \tag{3.58}$$

where $\phi(\omega)$ is known (measured) and $\theta(\omega)$ is computed (as the minimum-phase lag from the gain function) is not always practically achievable. In such cases, approximate relations can be obtained for very low frequencies

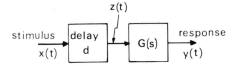

Fig. 3.11. System with delay.

and very high frequencies. Differentiating Eq. (3.57), we obtain

$$\frac{\partial \phi(\omega)}{\partial \omega} = \omega \frac{\partial d(\omega)}{\partial \omega} + d(\omega) + \frac{\partial \theta(\omega)}{\partial \omega} \qquad (3.59)$$

Now, for very low frequencies

$$\omega \frac{\partial d(\omega)}{\partial \omega} \cong 0$$

and

$$\frac{\partial \theta(\omega)}{\partial \omega} \cong \text{const}$$

(where the constant is usually determinable by inspecting the gain); thus

$$d(\omega) \cong \frac{\partial \phi(\omega)}{\partial \omega} - \text{const} \qquad (3.60)$$

for very low frequencies. Similarly, for very high frequencies,

$$\frac{\partial \theta(\omega)}{\partial \omega} \cong 0$$

and a linear differential equation results with respect to $d(\omega)$:

$$\omega \frac{\partial d(\omega)}{\partial \omega} + d(\omega) = \frac{\partial \phi(\omega)}{\partial \omega} \qquad (3.61)$$

This can be solved since $\partial \phi(\omega)/\partial \omega = \Psi(\omega)$ is known (measured). The solution for the delay is

$$d(\omega) = \frac{1}{\omega} [\phi(\omega) - \phi(0)] \qquad (3.62)$$

Returning to the analysis of the (light)→(horizontal cell response) system, we can utilize the measured phase curve in order to estimate the system delay (transit time of the signal from input to output). From Fig. 3.10 we obtain $\Delta \theta = \pi$ for $\Delta f = 30$ Hz and, therefore, using Eq. (3.56), we find that

$$\text{delay } d \cong \frac{\pi}{2\pi(30)} = 0.016 \text{ sec}$$

i.e., it takes approximately 16 msec for the light signal to first be "sensed" by the horizontal cell.

3.3. Transfer Functions from Stimulus–Response Spectra

Often, in practice, it is not possible to excite the biological system under study with sine wave stimuli. For example, this may be due to the fact that the system is a component subsystem of a larger system and we cannot disconnect it without seriously impairing it. Then, we are reduced to merely watching its input and output signals. In other situations, the same difficulty—inability to test with sine waves—may arise for other reasons, such as impracticalities in constructing a sinusoidal excitation source. However, even in such cases, we wish to be able to derive a transfer function description of the system. Again, we assume the system is linear; the nonlinear case is the main theme of this book and is examined in the following chapters.

The transfer function of the system can be found by utilizing the following two relations:

$$\Phi_{yy}(\omega) = |H(\omega)|^2 \Phi_{xx}(\omega) \qquad (3.63)$$

$$\Phi_{yx}(\omega) = H(\omega)\Phi_{xx}(\omega) \qquad (3.64)$$

The spectra $\Phi_{yy}(\omega)$ and $\Phi_{xx}(\omega)$ of the response and stimulus signals can be computed by recording $x(t)$ and $y(t)$, and then the magnitude of the system transfer function is given by

$$|H(\omega)| = [\Phi_{yy}(\omega)/\Phi_{xx}(\omega)]^{1/2} \qquad (3.65)$$

It should be noted that (auto-) spectra such as $\Phi_{yy}(\omega)$ and $\Phi_{xx}(\omega)$ are real quantities. Assuming a minimum-phase system the phase of $H(\omega)$ can be found directly from $|H(\omega)|$. Then, $H(\omega)$ is completely determined. Alternatively, if we do not wish to make the minimum-phase-system assumption, the second relation [Eq. (3.64)] can be used to obtain $H(\omega)$ both in magnitude and phase, i.e., as a complex quantity. This is found as

$$H(\omega) = \frac{\Phi_{yx}(\omega)}{\Phi_{xx}(\omega)} \qquad (3.66)$$

It should be noted that $\Phi_{yx}(\omega)$ is a complex quantity whose phase is the same as that of $H(\omega)$.

Figure 3.12 shows results obtained from an experiment on a system where the input stimulus was broadband. The stimulus spectrum $\Phi_{xx}(\omega)$ was computed as well as the magnitude of the stimulus–response cross spectrum, $|\Phi_{yx}(\omega)|$, as shown in Fig. 3.12. From these data the magnitude

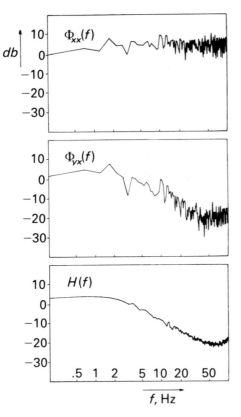

Fig. 3.12. Determination of transfer function from input spectrum and cross spectrum.

of the transfer function, $|H(\omega)|$ was found, under the assumption of linearity. Making the additional assumption that the system is also mini-mum-phase (a very reasonable assumption in most practical cases), we can find the transfer function of this system as

$$H(s) \simeq \frac{K}{(1 + Ts)^2}$$

where $K \simeq 1.5$ and $T \simeq 1/25$ sec. The values beyond 50 Hz are due to noise.

3.3.1. The Effect of Noise

In practice, the measurement of physiological signals by transducers is corrupted by noise. We assume, for the present discussion, that this noise is additive for both the stimulus and response signals, as shown in Fig. 3.13.

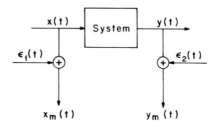

Fig. 3.13. System with input and output measurement noise.

Then the *measured* stimulus and response signals $x_m(t)$ and $y_m(t)$ are, respectively,

$$x_m(t) = x(t) + \varepsilon_1(t) \tag{3.67}$$

$$y_m(t) = y(t) + \varepsilon_2(t) \tag{3.68}$$

The two basic equations (3.63) and (3.64) are slightly altered in this case. Assuming statistical independence for the contaminating noise signals, each with zero mean, we have

$$\phi_{x_m x_m}(\tau) = E[[x(t) + \varepsilon_1(t)][x(t+\tau) + \varepsilon_1(t+\tau)]]$$

$$= \phi_{xx}(\tau) + \phi_{\varepsilon_1 \varepsilon_1}(\tau) \tag{3.69}$$

Similarly,

$$\phi_{y_m y_m}(\tau) = \phi_{yy}(\tau) + \phi_{\varepsilon_2 \varepsilon_2}(\tau) \tag{3.70}$$

and

$$\phi_{y_m x_m}(\tau) = \phi_{yx}(\tau) \tag{3.71}$$

Notice that in these relationships we assumed that the records were of sufficient length so that terms such as $\phi_{x\varepsilon_1}(\tau)$ became negligibly small.

Then, the two system equations become, in terms of the measured signals $y_m(t)$ and $x_m(t)$,

$$\phi_{y_m y_m}(\tau) - \phi_{\varepsilon_2 \varepsilon_2}(\tau) = \int_0^\infty h(\nu) \int_0^\infty h(\mu)$$
$$\times [\phi_{x_m x_m}(\tau + \mu - \nu) - \phi_{\varepsilon_1 \varepsilon_1}(\tau + \mu - \nu)] \, d\mu \, d\nu \tag{3.72}$$

$$\phi_{y_m x_m}(\tau) = \int_0^\infty h(\nu)[\phi_{x_m x_m}(\tau - \nu) - \phi_{\varepsilon_1 \varepsilon_1}(\tau - \nu)] \, d\nu \tag{3.73}$$

and, taking the FT, we get the power spectra relationships

$$\Phi_{y_m y_m}(\omega) = \Phi_{\varepsilon_2 \varepsilon_2}(\omega) + |H(\omega)|^2 [\Phi_{x_m x_m}(\omega) - \Phi_{\varepsilon_1 \varepsilon_1}(\omega)] \tag{3.74}$$

$$\Phi_{y_m x_m}(\omega) = H(\omega)[\Phi_{x_m x_m}(\omega) - \Phi_{\varepsilon_1 \varepsilon_1}(\omega)] \tag{3.75}$$

Knowledge, from experimental evidence, of the noise spectra $\Phi_{\varepsilon_1\varepsilon_1}(\omega)$ and $\Phi_{\varepsilon_2\varepsilon_2}(\omega)$ can be used in estimating accurately the system transfer function from Eqs. (3.74) and (3.75) above. It should be noted that in computing these spectra, in a practical situation, the considerations described in Sec. 2.9 should be taken into account. Thus, for example, to provide a small statistical error in the spectral estimates, the record should be segmented and the estimates obtained from the segments should be averaged—or, alternatively, a proper smoothing window should be used in the frequency domain.

Let us assume now that the noise $\Phi_{\varepsilon_1\varepsilon_1}(\omega)$ is either small or can be estimated and accounted for in Eq. (3.75). Then we would have

$$H(\omega) \cong \frac{\Phi_{y_m x_m}(\omega)}{\Phi_{x_m x_m}(\omega)} \cong \frac{\Phi_{yx}(\omega)}{\Phi_{xx}(\omega)} \tag{3.76}$$

It should be noted that the system measurement task becomes very simple if the stimulus signal $x(t)$ is white noise. For, in this case, we have

$$\phi_{xx}(\tau) = P\delta(\tau) \tag{3.77}$$

$$\Phi_{xx}(\omega) = P \tag{3.78}$$

Therefore, from Eqs. (3.71), (3.73), and (3.75) we obtain

$$h(\tau) = \phi_{yx}(\tau)/P \tag{3.79}$$

$$H(\omega) = \Phi_{yx}(\omega)/P \tag{3.80}$$

i.e., the system transfer characteristic is readily obtained in the time domain or the frequency domain. However, in practice $\Phi_{xx}(\omega)$ is not a constant for two reasons: (a) Most laboratory white-noise sources are not perfectly flat, and (b) because of the finite record and random nature of the signals, there is a deviation from constancy that is of statistical nature. If use is made of Eq. (3.66) instead of Eq. (3.80) then these problems are greatly alleviated since any deviations of the stimulus from whiteness are accounted in the final result, $H(\omega)$.

Finally, the determination of the system transfer function through Eq. (3.65) suffers from problems of "noise sensitivity" in its numerical analysis at high frequencies. We have

$$|H(\omega)|^2 = \Phi_{yy}(\omega)/\Phi_{xx}(\omega) \tag{3.81}$$

Let us assume that the stimulus spectrum is, for example,

$$\Phi_{xx}(\omega) = \frac{a^2}{a^2 + \omega^2} \tag{3.82}$$

Then, a small perturbation $\delta y(t)$ in the response, having the spectrum

$$\delta \Phi_{yy}(\omega) = \begin{cases} 1/\omega_0, & \omega_0 < \omega < \omega_0 + \Delta\omega \\ 0, & \text{elsewhere} \end{cases} \tag{3.83}$$

produces a perturbation $\delta |H(\omega)|^2$ in the determination of the transfer function which (for $\Delta\omega$ very small) is

$$\delta |H(\omega)|^2 = \begin{cases} (a^2 + \omega_0^2)/a^2\omega_0, & \omega_0 < \omega < \omega_0 + \Delta\omega \\ 0, & \text{elsewhere} \end{cases} \tag{3.84}$$

The difficulty now becomes obvious since even though

$$\delta \Phi_{yy}(\omega) \to 0 \quad \text{as } \omega_0 \to \infty$$

the perturbation in $H(\omega)$ behaves as

$$\delta |H(\omega)|^2 \to \infty \quad \text{as } \omega_0 \to \infty$$

Thus, at high frequencies the error in the estimate of $H(\omega)$ is large. This is the nature of this "ill-posed" numerical problem. To alleviate it, in practice we often filter the high frequencies out of the stimulus–response signals before applying Eq. (3.81). Of course, this filtering itself affects the high-frequency estimation of the transfer function.

3.3.2. Application to a Physiological System: Light → ERG

To illustrate the above procedure of determining the system transfer function from the stimulus–response spectra, we consider the following study on the catfish retina. The system input is light covering the retina uniformly in space and modulated in time by a broadband random signal. The system response is the evoked ERG (electroretinogram) recorded by a gross electrode. We seek to determine the transfer function of this light → ERG system.

Figure 3.14 shows a portion of the light stimulus signal and the corresponding ERG response. It also shows the spectra of the stimulus, $\Phi_{xx}(\omega)$ and of the response, $\Phi_{yy}(\omega)$. From these two spectra, by employing Eq. (3.81), we can estimate the magnitude of the system transfer function $H(\omega)$. Its plot is also shown in Fig. 3.14. We note that (a) the plot of $|H(\omega)|$ has two prominent corner frequencies, one around 5 Hz and the other around 11 Hz; (b) its high-frequency asymptote is 24 db/octave; and (c) its low-frequency asymptote is about 1 db/octave (i.e., much less than the minimum 6 db/octave required if a zero were present). From these observations and under the assumption of minimum phase shift (and linearity), we can estimate the system transfer function as

$$H(s) \simeq K\left[\left(\frac{s^2}{\omega_a^2} + \frac{2\zeta_a}{\omega_a}s + 1\right)\left(\frac{s^2}{\omega_b^2} + \frac{2\zeta_b}{\omega_b}s + 1\right)\right]^{-1} \tag{3.85}$$

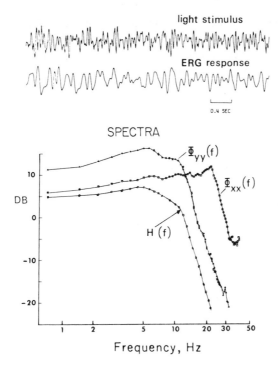

Fig. 3.14. Determination of transfer function from stimulus and response spectra for system light → ERG.

where $K \simeq 2.5$, $\omega_a \cong 2\pi(5)$, $\zeta_a \simeq 0.5$, $\omega_b \simeq 2\pi(11)$, and $\zeta_b \simeq 0.5$. Of course, this is not the only representation for the $H(\omega)$ of Fig. 3.14. Others are also plausible, depending on the degree of accuracy with which we wish to describe the curve resulting from these data. However, a word of caution is in order: Obviously an analytical curve for $H(s)$ can be found that will go through every single point of the data; this $H(s)$ will be of the form $N(s)/D(s)$, where the degree of the polynomial $N(s)$ is n and that of $D(s)$ is $(n+4)$ for this example. However, a lot of the terms in the numerator $N(s)$ and in the denominator $D(s)$ will be due to the presence of error (or noise) in the data and will not reflect the underlying mechanisms. (This is similar to fitting $N+1$ data points with a polynomial of degree N.) Therefore, we must keep the degree of $N(s)$ and $D(s)$ much smaller than the number of data points, the exact number being determined by experience or additional information about the system.

The transfer function $H(s)$ of Eq. (3.85) (assuming it is correct) suggests certain things about the light → ERG system. For example, it suggests that perhaps the system is a concatenation of two subsystems or a sum of two parallel subsystems, one with parameters (ω_a, ζ_a) and the other with (ω_b, ζ_b). For example, the slower subsystem, (ω_a, ζ_a), may be reflecting the rod contribution to the ERG signal while the faster one, (ω_b, ζ_b), the contribution of the cones and other retinal neurons. If this hypothesis is true, then Eq. (3.85) gives us directly the complete dynamics of these two retinal subsystems.

3.4. Coherence Function

As we saw in the previous section, the measured power spectra, such as $\Phi_{x_m x_m}(\omega)$, $\Phi_{y_m y_m}(\omega)$, are contaminated by noise. Therefore, the system equation

$$\Phi_{yx}(\omega) = H(\omega)\Phi_{xx}(\omega) \tag{3.86}$$

given such assumptions as $\Phi_{x\varepsilon_1}(\omega) = 0$ becomes

$$\Phi_{y_m x_m}(\omega) = H(\omega)[\Phi_{x_m x_m}(\omega) - \Phi_{\varepsilon_1 \varepsilon_1}(\omega)] \tag{3.87}$$

In addition, the system may be somewhat nonlinear, further invalidating Eq. (3.87). It is desirable to have a measure (an index) of the extent to which the response is due to the stimulus (is "coherent" with the stimulus) and not to extraneous sources of noise. To achieve this, we define the following quantity, which is called the *coherence function*:

$$\gamma^2(\omega) = \frac{|\Phi_{y_m x_m}(\omega)|^2}{\Phi_{x_m x_m}(\omega)\Phi_{y_m y_m}(\omega)} \tag{3.88}$$

where $x_m(t)$ and $y_m(t)$ are the measured signals. We note that this quantity, $\gamma^2(\omega)$, is real. If the system is linear and there is no measurement noise, then

$$\Phi_{y_m x_m}(\omega) = H(\omega)\Phi_{x_m x_m}(\omega) \tag{3.89}$$

and

$$|\Phi_{y_m x_m}(\omega)|^2 = |H(\omega)|^2\Phi_{x_m x_m}(\omega) = \Phi_{y_m y_m}(\omega)\Phi_{x_m x_m}(\omega) \tag{3.90}$$

Therefore, when the system is linear and noise is absent,

$$\gamma^2(\omega) = 1 \tag{3.91}$$

However, if the stimulus and response signals are contaminated by measurement noise, $\varepsilon_1(t)$ and $\varepsilon_2(t)$, respectively, then the *measured* spectra (assuming ε_1 and ε_2 are independent and have zero means) are as follows:

cross spectrum: $\Phi_{yx}(\omega) = \Phi_{y_m x_m}(\omega)$ (3.92)

response spectrum: $\Phi_{yy}(\omega) + \Phi_{\varepsilon_2 \varepsilon_2}(\omega) = \Phi_{y_m y_m}(\omega)$ (3.93)

stimulus spectrum:
$$\Phi_{xx}(\omega) + \Phi_{\varepsilon_1\varepsilon_1}(\omega) = \Phi_{x_m x_m}(\omega) \qquad (3.94)$$

Therefore, in this case

$$\gamma^2(\omega) = \frac{|\Phi_{yx}(\omega)|^2}{[\Phi_{xx}(\omega) + \Phi_{\varepsilon_1\varepsilon_1}(\omega)][\Phi_{yy}(\omega) + \Phi_{\varsigma_2\varepsilon_2}(\omega)]} \qquad (3.95)$$

a quantity clearly less than unity since the power spectrum is a positive definite function. Therefore, in the presence of contaminating noise the coherence function becomes less than unity. Also, from Eq. (3.88), the coherence function is a positive quantity, and is *always* less than or equal to unity. This can be shown as follows: Consider any input–output pair of signals $x(t)$ and $y(t)$. Then we have

$$E[[x(t-\tau) + ay(t)]^2] = \phi_{xx}(0) + 2a\phi_{yx}(\tau) + a^2\phi_{yy}(0) \geq 0 \qquad (3.96)$$

This is a non-negative quadratic in a. Therefore, its discriminant must be

$$4\phi_{yx}^2(\tau) - 4\phi_{yy}(0)\phi_{xx}(0) \leq 0 \qquad (3.97)$$

and, therefore,

$$\phi_{yx}^2(\tau) \leq \phi_{yy}(0)\phi_{xx}(0) \qquad (3.98)$$

Then, of course,

$$\phi_{yx}^2(0) \leq \phi_{yy}(0)\phi_{xx}(0) \qquad (3.99)$$

Substituting in terms of the power spectra,

$$\phi_{yy}(0) = \frac{1}{2\pi} \int_{-\infty}^{\infty} \Phi_{yy}(\omega)\, d\omega \qquad (3.100)$$

$$\phi_{xx}(0) = \frac{1}{2\pi} \int_{-\infty}^{\infty} \Phi_{xx}(\omega)\, d\omega \qquad (3.101)$$

$$\phi_{yx}(0) = \frac{1}{2\pi} \int_{-\infty}^{\infty} \Phi_{yx}(\omega)\, d\omega \qquad (3.102)$$

we obtain

$$\int\int_{-\infty}^{\infty} [\Phi_{yx}(\omega)\Phi_{yx}^*(\omega') - \Phi_{xx}(\omega)\Phi_{yy}(\omega')]\, d\omega\, d\omega' \leq 0 \qquad (3.103)$$

which holds for any $x(t)$ and $y(t)$ and consequently for any $\Phi_{xx}(\omega)$, $\Phi_{yy}(\omega)$ and resulting $\Phi_{yx}(\omega)$. If we choose $x(t)$ and $y(t)$ as ideal narrow-band signals at some *arbitrary* frequency ω_1, i.e.,

$$\left.\begin{array}{l} \Phi_{xx}(\omega) \neq 0 \\ \Phi_{yy}(\omega) \neq 0 \\ \Phi_{yx}(\omega) \neq 0 \end{array}\right\} \text{ only for } \omega_1 - \Delta\omega < \omega < \omega_1 + \Delta\omega \qquad (3.104)$$

then we easily see from (3.103) that

$$|\Phi_{yx}(\omega_1)|^2 \le \Phi_{yy}(\omega_1)\Phi_{xx}(\omega_1) \qquad (3.105)$$

This says that, indeed, the coherence function is

$$0 \le \gamma^2(\omega) \le 1 \qquad (3.106)$$

It should be noted that between the relations (3.98) and (3.105), relation (3.105) is the more powerful since $\Phi_{yx}(\omega)$ is bounded at ω in terms of the values of $\Phi_{xx}(\omega)$ and $\Phi_{yy}(\omega)$ at ω, while $\phi_{yx}(\tau)$ is bounded at τ in terms of the values of $\phi_{yy}(0)$ and $\phi_{xx}(0)$, i.e., at $\tau = 0$.

Returning to Eq. (3.95) we also have, assuming $\Phi_{\varepsilon_1\varepsilon_1}(\omega) = 0$,

$$\gamma^2(\omega) = \frac{|H(\omega)|^2 \Phi_{xx}(\omega)}{|H(\omega)|^2 \Phi_{xx}(\omega) + \Phi_{\varepsilon_2\varepsilon_2}(\omega)} \qquad (3.107)$$

Therefore, at any frequency ω, the coherence function $\gamma^2(\omega)$ gives the fraction of power at the response that is due to the input. In any case, whenever $\gamma^2(\omega)$ is less than unity, either the system is nonlinear, the signals do not have a *"causal"* relationship (i.e., the signals are contaminated by noise), or both. The deviation of $\gamma^2(\omega)$ from unity is a quantitative measure of these conditions. Since physiological systems are both nonlinear *and* have high noise content, it is expected that the coherence function should be widely used in their study; however, this has not been the case in the past, with few exceptions (cf. Stein *et al.*, 1972).

Finally, it should be noted that the utility of the coherence function derives from the fact that it indicates directly the "incoherence" between stimulus and response, the effect of the transfer relationship having been compensated for by normalization.

Let us consider as an example a physiological system whose input is a broadband random signal and whose output is corrupted by noise. Figure 3.15 shows the resulting coherence function for this system. We note that at low frequencies the coherence is small (about 0.5). Also, at high frequencies the coherence decreases somewhat. This indicates the frequency regions where the signal-to-noise ratio may be low or where nonlinear effects are large.

3.5. Multi-Input Linear Systems

Physiological systems, because of their complexity, often need to be studied as systems with multiple inputs. In practice, the effect of most inputs is usually ignored—we call them "unwanted" noise and we simply forget about them—while we concentrate on a small number of them, usually one, and their causal relationships to the responses under study. In

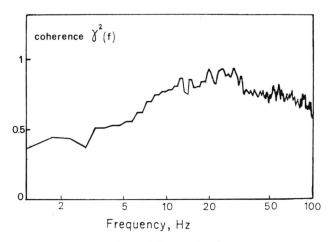

Fig. 3.15. Coherence function.

this section we consider only linear systems in which the effects of the various input stimuli on the response are simply additive, the simplest but rather unrealistic form of interaction. Physiological systems are almost always nonlinear, and the effects of the various natural stimuli (e.g., light, temperature, motion, etc.) are nonlinear in their interactions. The non-linear, multi-input systems and interactions between them are examined in a later chapter, through the white-noise analysis technique.

3.5.1. Two-Input Systems

For a linear two-input system, as shown in Fig. 3.16, the input-output relationship can be written as

$$y(t) = \int_0^\infty h_x(\tau)x(t-\tau)\,d\tau + \int_0^\infty h_u(\tau)u(t-\tau)\,d\tau \qquad (3.108)$$

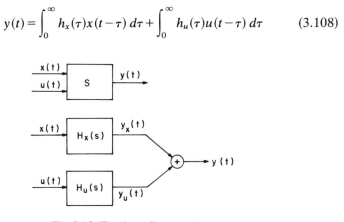

Fig. 3.16. Two-input linear system.

In the frequency domain it is

$$Y(s) = H_x(s)X(s) + H_u(s)X(s) \qquad (3.109)$$

From Eq. (3.108) we can easily find the correlation relationships for a linear two-input system:

$$\phi_{yy}(\tau) = \int\int_0^\infty h_x(\mu)h_x(\nu)\phi_{xx}(\tau + \mu - \nu)\, d\mu\, d\nu$$

$$+ \int\int_0^\infty h_u(\mu)h_u(\nu)\phi_{uu}(\tau + \mu - \nu)\, d\mu\, d\nu$$

$$+ \int\int_0^\infty h_x(\mu)h_u(\nu)\phi_{xu}(\tau + \mu - \nu)\, d\mu\, d\nu$$

$$+ \int\int_0^\infty h_x(\nu)h_u(\mu)\phi_{ux}(\tau + \mu - \nu)\, d\mu\, d\nu \qquad (3.110)$$

In case the two input signals are statistically independent and at least one of them has zero mean, $\phi_{xu}(\tau) = \phi_{ux}(\tau) = 0$; then,

$$\phi_{yy}(\tau) = \int\int_0^\infty h_x(\mu)h_x(\nu)\phi_{xx}(\tau + \mu - \nu)\, d\mu\, d\nu$$

$$+ \int\int_0^\infty h_u(\mu)h_u(\nu)\phi_{uu}(\tau + \mu - \nu)\, d\mu\, d\nu \qquad (3.111)$$

Taking the FT of Eqs. (3.110) and (3.111) we can find these systems relationships in terms of the stimulus–response power spectra. From Eq. (3.110) we obtain easily, after some manipulation,

$$\Phi_{yy}(\omega) = |H_x(\omega)|^2\Phi_{xx}(\omega) + H_x^*(\omega)H_u(\omega)\Phi_{xu}(\omega)$$

$$+ |H_u(\omega)|^2\Phi_{uu}(\omega) + H_x(\omega)H_u^*(\omega)\Phi_{ux}(\omega) \qquad (3.112)$$

and, from Eq. (3.111) we have

$$\Phi_{yy}(\omega) = |H_x(\omega)|^2\Phi_{xx}(\omega) + |H_u(\omega)|^2\Phi_{uu}(\omega) \qquad (3.113)$$

In a similar fashion, we can find system expressions, for the two-input case, that involve the crosscorrelations of the response with each of the inputs. Thus, assuming that the system and its inputs are stationary, we have

$$\phi_{yx}(\tau) = \int_0^\infty h_x(\mu)\phi_{xx}(\tau-\mu)d\mu + \int_0^\infty h_u(\mu)\phi_{ux}(\tau-\mu)\,d\mu \qquad (3.114)$$

Of course, in case $u(t)$ and $x(t)$ are independent and at least one of them has zero mean $\phi_{ux}(\tau) = 0$, and

$$\phi_{yx}(\tau) = \int_0^\infty h_x(\mu)\phi_{xx}(\tau-\mu)\,d\mu \qquad (3.115)$$

Taking the FT of Eq. (3.114) we have

$$\Phi_{yx}(\omega) = H_x(\omega)\Phi_{xx}(\omega) + H_u(\omega)\Phi_{ux}(\omega) \qquad (3.116)$$

and analogously

$$\Phi_{yu}(\omega) = H_x(\omega)\Phi_{xu}(\omega) + H_u(\omega)\Phi_{uu}(\omega) \qquad (3.117)$$

Taking the FT of Eq. (3.115) we obtain

$$\Phi_{yx}(\omega) = H_x(\omega)\Phi_{xx}(\omega) \qquad (3.118)$$

and analogously,

$$\Phi_{yu}(\omega) = H_u(\omega)\Phi_{uu}(\omega) \qquad (3.119)$$

In practice, therefore, if we wish to measure $H_x(\omega)$ and $H_u(\omega)$ it is convenient to use as input stimuli, if we have such freedom, signals that are broadband (covering the system bandwidth, such as white noise) *and* statistically independent. If the latter condition is satisfied, then the system transfer characteristics can be readily found from Eqs. (3.118) and (3.119) as

$$H_x(\omega) = \Phi_{yx}(\omega)/\Phi_{xx}(\omega) \qquad (3.120)$$

$$H_u(\omega) = \Phi_{yu}(\omega)/\Phi_{uu}(\omega) \qquad (3.121)$$

If we cannot control the input signals so that the independence requirement is satisfied, Eqs. (3.116) and (3.117) must be used to find $H_x(\omega)$ and $H_u(\omega)$. These are two equations that are linear in the two unknowns $H_x(\omega)$, $H_u(\omega)$. By solving them we find

$$H_x(\omega) = \frac{\Phi_{yx}(\omega)\Phi_{uu}(\omega) - \Phi_{yu}(\omega)\Phi_{ux}(\omega)}{\Phi_{xx}(\omega)\Phi_{uu}(\omega) - |\Phi_{xu}(\omega)|^2} \qquad (3.122)$$

$$H_u(\omega) = \frac{\Phi_{yu}(\omega)\Phi_{xx}(\omega) - \Phi_{yx}(\omega)\Phi_{xu}(\omega)}{\Phi_{xx}(\omega)\Phi_{uu}(\omega) - |\Phi_{ux}(\omega)|^2} \qquad (3.123)$$

Note that $\Phi_{ux}(\omega) = \Phi_{xu}^*(\omega)$ and therefore

$$\Phi_{ux}(\omega)\Phi_{xu}(\omega) = |\Phi_{ux}(\omega)|^2 = |\Phi_{xu}(\omega)|^2 \qquad (3.124)$$

Recall that the coherence function between two signals $x(t)$ and $u(t)$ is defined by

$$\gamma^2(\omega) = \frac{|\Phi_{ux}(\omega)|^2}{\Phi_{uu}(\omega)\Phi_{xx}(\omega)} \tag{3.125}$$

Therefore, the denominator in Eqs. (3.122) and (3.123) is

$$\Phi_{xx}(\omega)\Phi_{uu}(\omega)[1 - \gamma^2(\omega)] \geq 0 \tag{3.126}$$

i.e., a real, nonnegative quantity. The question arises: What happens if $\gamma^2(\omega) = 1$? This is the case in which $x(t)$ and $u(t)$ are related as input and output of a linear system, without any noise or nonlinearity present. Obviously, in this case Eqs. (3.122) and (3.123) do not hold. However, $x(t)$ and $u(t)$ are related by

$$U(\omega) = G(\omega)X(\omega) \tag{3.127}$$

where $G(\omega)$ is the transfer function of a linear system. Then the two-input system virtually collapses into a one-input system. In this case, we first find $G(\omega)$ by

$$G(\omega) = \Phi_{ux}(\omega)/\Phi_{xx}(\omega) \tag{3.128}$$

Then, the two equations (3.116) and (3.117) become, respectively,

$$\Phi_{yx}(\omega) = [H_x(\omega) + H_u(\omega)G(\omega)]\Phi_{xx}(\omega) \tag{3.129}$$

$$\Phi_{yu}(\omega) = [H_x(\omega) + H_u(\omega)G(\omega)]G^*(\omega)\Phi_{xx}(\omega) \tag{3.130}$$

But also,

$$\Phi_{yu}(\omega) = Y(\omega)U^*(\omega)$$
$$= Y(\omega)G^*(\omega)X^*(\omega) \tag{3.131}$$

and since

$$\Phi_{yx}(\omega) = Y(\omega)X^*(\omega) \tag{3.132}$$

we have

$$\Phi_{yu}(\omega) = \Phi_{yx}(\omega)G^*(\omega) \tag{3.133}$$

Thus Eq. (3.130) becomes identical to Eq. (3.129). Therefore, in this case the two equations (3.129) and (3.130) collapse into one equation. It should be noted that in this case we can measure the transfer quantities

$$G(\omega) \quad \text{and} \quad [H_u(\omega)G(\omega) + H_x(\omega)]$$

but we are not able to measure $H_x(\omega)$ and $H_u(\omega)$ separately.

For example, consider the system shown in Fig. 3.17. If input 2 is not activated we simply observe $u(t)$ as the output of system $G(\omega)$, i.e., as the

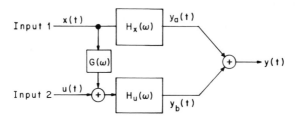

Fig. 3.17. System with two related inputs.

input to system $H_u(\omega)$, and record it. In this case the coherence function between $x(t)$ and $u(t)$ is unity and we can measure the following transfer quantities:

$$G(\omega) = \Phi_{ux}(\omega)/\Phi_{xx}(\omega) \qquad (3.134)$$

and

$$H_x(\omega) + H_u(\omega)G(\omega) = \Phi_{yx}(\omega)/\Phi_{xx}(\omega) \qquad (3.135)$$

Suppose now that we force a stimulus at input 2. Then, the coherence between $x(t)$ and $u(t)$ will, in general, be less than unity. To simplify matters further and make the measurement problem easier we can choose $u(t)$ to be independent of $x(t)$ and with zero mean. Then, $\phi_{ux}(\tau) = 0$. We have, in this case,

$$Y(\omega) = [H_x(\omega) + G(\omega)H_u(\omega)]X(\omega) + H_u(\omega)U(\omega) \qquad (3.136)$$

and from this, multiplying by $X^*(\omega)$ or $U^*(\omega)$, and taking into account that $\Phi_{xu}(\omega) = 0$, we have

$$\Phi_{yx}(\omega) = [H_x(\omega) + G(\omega)H_u(\omega)]\Phi_{xx}(\omega) \qquad (3.137)$$

$$\Phi_{yu}(\omega) = H_u(\omega)\Phi_{uu}(\omega) \qquad (3.138)$$

Therefore, in this case, we can measure by an appropriate experiment the following transfer quantities:

$$H_u(\omega) = \Phi_{yu}(\omega)/\Phi_{uu}(\omega) \qquad (3.139)$$

$$H_x(\omega) + G(\omega)H_u(\omega) = \Phi_{yu}(\omega)/\Phi_{xx}(\omega) \qquad (3.140)$$

Combining these results with those of the previous measurements, in which no stimulus was applied at input 2, we see that we can measure the transfer characteristics of all subsystems: $H_x(\omega)$, $H_u(\omega)$, $G(\omega)$. Equation (3.134) gives $G(\omega)$, Eq. (3.139) gives $H_u(\omega)$, and then Eq. (3.140) can be used to find $H_x(\omega)$.

Figure 3.18 shows the results of an experiment on a two-input linear system. The two subsystems of this system, $H_x(\omega)$ and $H_u(\omega)$, are known to

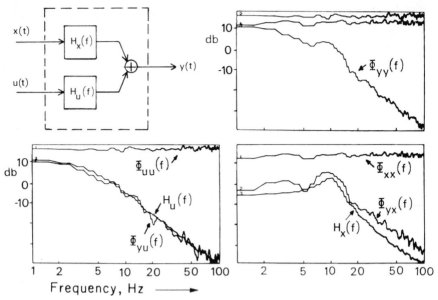

Fig. 3.18. Identification of two-input linear system from power spectra.

be linear. The stimulus signals $x(t)$, $u(t)$ are broadband, of zero mean, and statistically independent. They are recorded along with the response $y(t)$. From these data, the following spectra are computed: $\Phi_{xx}(\omega)$, $\Phi_{uu}(\omega)$, $\Phi_{yy}(\omega)$, $\Phi_{yx}(\omega)$, and $\Phi_{yu}(\omega)$, as shown in Fig. 3.18. Our objective is to determine the system transfer functions $H_x(\omega)$, $H_u(\omega)$. To this end we employ Eqs. (3.120) and (3.121), and the results are shown in Fig. 3.18. We note that the x-input path is a second-order underdamped system with a peak frequency around 10 Hz, while the u-input path is second-order overdamped system with a corner frequency around 5 Hz.

3.5.2. Application to a Two-Input Neural System

The neural system of the catfish retina was analyzed using two lights as stimuli. The light intensities of the two stimuli were modulated in random fashion. The first light source consisted of a spot area (0.3 mm in diameter), the second of a concentric annulus area (inner diameter of 0.35 mm and outer diameter of 5 mm) focused on the retina; the response was the intracellular potential changes of a bipolar cell, recorded with a micro-electrode (Fig. 3.19). The spot and annulus areas were roughly chosen to correspond to the "center" and "surround" components of the receptive field of this cell. From these stimulus–response data the power spectra $\Phi_{xx}(f)$, $\Phi_{uu}(f)$, $\Phi_{yx}(f)$, $\Phi_{yu}(f)$ were computed. Then, using Eqs. (3.118)

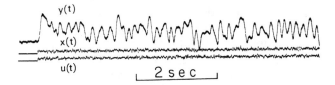

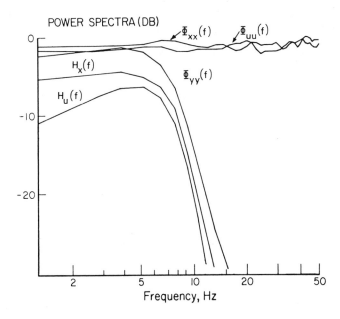

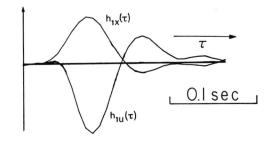

Fig. 3.19. Identification of a two-input physiological system from stimulus–response spectra.

and (3.119) the transfer functions of each input—spot $x(t)$ and annulus $u(t)$—to the output were estimated and are shown in Fig. 3.19. Taking the inverse FT of $H_x(\omega)$ and $H_u(\omega)$ the impulse responses $h_{1x}(t)$ and $h_{1u}(t)$ can be found (shown in Fig. 3.19).

The underlying assumption in this identification of the light → bipolar cell system is that the system is linear. The question arises: How do we check this assumption? How valid is the system characterization as found above? Fortunately, we can give an *a posteriori* answer to these questions. First, we note that the broadband random signals used as stimuli are quite *rich* in the sense that they contain a great variety of waveforms; therefore they provide a fairly exhaustive test of the system. Second, we may compute the system response to these signals, $u(t)$ and $x(t)$, as it would be predicted by the estimated transfer functions, and compare it to the one observed experimentally. If the actual and predicted responses to waveform-rich stimuli $x(t)$ and $u(t)$ are close, then our assumption of linearity is justified. A final assumption, implicitly made here, is that $u(t)$ and $x(t)$ are independent [so that Eq. (3.118) can be used rather than Eq. (3.116)].

In this application both these assumptions were checked, as described above, and found to be valid.

3.5.3. n-Input Systems

Similar results and relationships can be formulated for linear systems with n inputs.

Consider the inputs to be

$$x_1(t), x_2(t), \ldots, x_n(t)$$

and the output $y(t)$. Then, it can be shown, much in the same way as for a two-input system, that

$$\phi_{yy}(\tau) = \sum_{i=1}^{n} \sum_{j=1}^{n} \int_0^\infty h_i(\mu) \int_0^\infty h_j(\nu) \phi_{x_i x_j}(\tau + \mu - \nu) \, d\nu \, d\mu \quad (3.141)$$

and hence

$$\Phi_{yy}(\omega) = \sum_{i=1}^{n} |H_i(\omega)|^2 \Phi_{x_i x_i}(\omega) + \sum_{\substack{i \neq j \\ i,j=1}}^{n} H_i^*(\omega) H_j(\omega) \Phi_{x_i x_j}(\omega) \quad (3.142)$$

Similarly, we obtain for the stimulus–response cross-spectra relationships

$$\phi_{yx_k}(\tau) = \int_0^\infty \sum_{i=1}^{n} h_i(\nu) \phi_{x_i x_k}(\tau - \nu) \, d\nu \quad (3.143)$$

and hence

$$\Phi_{yx_k}(\omega) = \sum_{i=1}^{n} H_i(\omega) \Phi_{x_i x_k}(\omega) \quad (3.144)$$

As for the two-input system case, if all possible pairs of stimuli are statistically independent with zero means—a condition that may be very desirable in practice if we have the freedom to control the inputs in this manner—then the above equations are significantly simplified. For example, Eq. (3.142) becomes

$$\Phi_{yy}(\omega) = \sum_{i=1}^{n} |H_i(\omega)|^2 \Phi_{x_i x_i}(\omega) \tag{3.145}$$

and Eq. (3.144) becomes

$$\Phi_{y x_k}(\omega) = H_k(\omega) \Phi_{x_k x_k}(\omega) \tag{3.146}$$

The latter relationship allows us to measure the system transfer characteristic directly and independently of the presence of the other inputs. For example, in practice if we choose $\{x_i(t)\}$ to be independent white-noise signals, then we have

$$\Phi_{x_k x_k}(\omega) = P_k \tag{3.147}$$

where P_k is a constant, and therefore the $H_k(\omega)$ are directly found from the cross spectra,

$$H_k(\omega) = \Phi_{y x_k}(\omega)/P_k \tag{3.148}$$

Of course, in practice, for reasons discussed in Section 3.3, it is preferable, if the extra computation is not objectionable and increased accuracy is desired, to use

$$H_k(\omega) = \Phi_{y x_k}(\omega)/\Phi_{x_k x_k}(\omega) \tag{3.149}$$

in order to measure $H_k(\omega)$, so as to account for any deviations of the "white-noise" source from whiteness.

3.6. Nonlinear Systems: Identification Using "Describing Functions"

Thus far we have considered analytical tools to study linear, time-invariant systems. We saw that these tools are quite powerful and complete. Unfortunately from the point of view of analysis—and fortunately from the point of view of optimal functioning and hence survival—physiological systems are almost always nonlinear. As we have discussed, a nonlinear system is one that does not obey the *principle of superposition* and hence its analysis becomes greatly complicated, if not practically impossible in some cases. The beauty and completeness of linear analysis should not, however, lure us towards unrealistic idealizations of the physiological systems under study. For it is in the *nonlinear* nature of these systems that most of the *information* about their behavior lies. It is in the *richness* of the various nonlinear behaviors that we stand to gain the most knowledge about our systems. In this same sense, a *linear* system idealization is nothing more than a "proportionality" relationship, and therefore it offers us little insight. On the other hand, the *diversity* of nonlinear behavior offers us the opportunity of matching the complexity of nonlinear description with the realistic complexity of living organisms. In addition, nonlinearities are often necessary for the optimal functioning of biological systems. The examples abound: logarithmic transformations of sensory input in order to accommodate large ranges, threshold mechanisms to increase the reliability of information transmission, directional sensing, and so forth.

Aside from the white-noise stimulation technique described in this book, there are very few nonlinear analysis techniques, and these are very restricted as to the specific types of system to which they are applicable. They are known under the name of "describing functions." We briefly examine them here, primarily to complete our background before starting with the white-noise nonlinear approach in the next chapter.

3.6.1. Describing Functions

Consider the nonlinear system shown in Fig. 3.20. If the stimulus to this nonlinear system is sinusoidal, $A \sin \omega t$, the response is, in general, not sinusoidal but still a periodic function that can be represented by a Fourier series. The describing function analysis is based on the assumption that only the fundamental component of the output is significant. The response of the system contains components at the fundamental frequency, and, in general, at all higher harmonic frequencies, since

$$y(t) = B_0 + B_1 \sin (\omega t + \phi_1) + B_2 \sin (2\omega t + \phi_2) + \cdots \qquad (3.150)$$

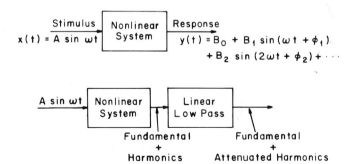

Fig. 3.20. Response of a nonlinear system to a sine wave stimulus.

Two facts make plausible the basic assumption of describing-function analysis: (a) For most types of nonlinearities encountered in practice, the harmonics of the response are of rapidly decreasing amplitude, with the fundamental being the largest component; and (b) often the nonlinear subsystem is followed by a low-pass subsystem—all physical systems are in a sense low pass—which greatly attenuates the high frequencies at which the harmonics are found. If these two conditions are satisfied in a system, its study by describing functions can be meaningful. That is, we have reduced the problem to a quasilinear one since we only consider the stimulus–response relationship at the *same* frequency, i.e., the frequency of the stimulus. In a very natural manner, therefore, we can define the *describing function* (DF) as follows:

$$Q(A, \omega) = (B_1/A)\, e^{i\phi_1} \tag{3.151}$$

i.e., as a complex quantity giving the "gain" at the fundamental frequency and the phase difference.

It should be noted that although the describing function is defined as the ratio of amplitudes of two sinusoidal signals at the same frequency, it is not a linear transfer function. In fact, in general, Q is a function of the stimulus amplitude or the frequency (or both). A few examples will show this point and clarify the use of the describing-function technique.

Consider a nonlinear system that has a transfer characteristic such as that shown in Fig. 3.21. Let us compute its DF $Q(A, \omega)$. Figure 3.21 shows the response when a sinusoidal input $x(t) = A \sin \omega t$ is applied to this nonlinear subsystem. We easily find, since the nonlinearity is an odd

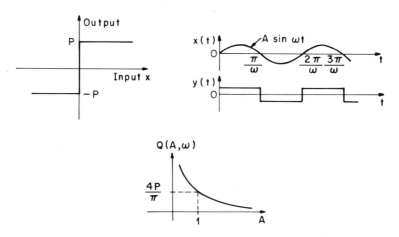

Fig. 3.21. Describing function for relay (bang-bang) nonlinearity.

function, that

$$y(t) = \sum_{k=1}^{\infty} B_k \sin k\omega t \qquad (k = 1, 3, 5, \ldots) \qquad (3.152)$$

where the B_k's attenuate as

$$1, \tfrac{1}{3}, \tfrac{1}{5}, \ldots$$

at harmonics

$$\omega, 3\omega, 5\omega, \ldots$$

We have for the fundamental

$$B_1 = \frac{2}{T} \int_0^T y(t) \sin \omega t \, dt = 4P/\pi$$

$$\phi_1 = 0 \qquad (3.153)$$

Therefore, the describing function, in this case, is

$$Q(A, \omega) = 4P/\pi A \qquad (3.154)$$

i.e., it has zero phase for all frequencies and it is independent of frequency. It is shown in Fig. 3.21.

Let us now consider how this describing function is changed, if, in addition, the nonlinear subsystem has a "dead zone"; Fig. 3.22 shows the transfer characteristic in this case. The same figure also shows the response waveform to a sinusoidal stimulus. Obviously if the stimulus amplitude A is less than a then the response is zero. For a nonzero response we must have $A > a$. Again, by Fourier series analysis we find the fundamental frequency

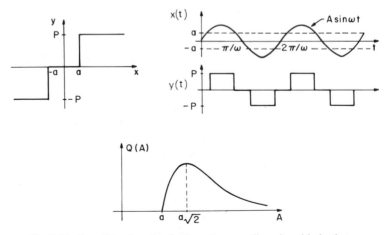

Fig. 3.22. Describing function for bang-bang nonlinearity with dead zone.

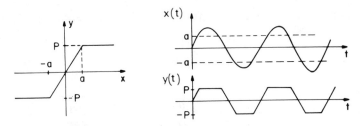

Fig. 3.23. Saturating nonlinearity.

response component to be

amplitude:

$$B_1 = \frac{4P}{\pi}\left[1-\left(\frac{a}{A}\right)^2\right]^{1/2}$$

phase:

$$\phi_1 = 0$$

(3.155)

and therefore the describing function for this nonlinearity is

$$Q(A, \omega) = \frac{B_1}{A} = \frac{4P}{\pi A}\left[1-\left(\frac{a}{A}\right)^2\right]^{1/2}$$

(3.156)

This is plotted in Fig. 3.22. We note that $Q(\ )$ is a function only of the input amplitude and not its frequency. In addition, its phase is zero for all frequencies. Note that as the ratio (a/A) becomes small, by making A very large compared to a, the describing function of this nonlinearity approaches that of the previous case—as it should.

However, a more realistic nonlinearity, often encountered in physiological systems, is the one shown in Fig. 3.23. Following a similar procedure we find that

$$Q(A, \omega) = \begin{cases} P/a & \text{if } A < a \\ (2P/a\pi)(\theta + \frac{1}{2}\sin 2\theta) & \text{if } A > a \end{cases}$$

(3.157)

where

$$\theta = \sin^{-1}(P/A)$$

and where the phase ϕ_1 is again zero and there is no variation with the stimulus frequency ω.

We consider one last example in which the describing function has nonzero phase shift. This is also a type of nonlinearity encountered in biological systems, that of hysteresis (Fig. 3.24). Fourier analysis gives us the magnitude and phase of the fundamental component of the response:

$$B_1 = (A_1^2 + A_2^2)^{1/2}$$

$$\phi_1 = -\tan^{-1}(A_2/A_1) \tag{3.158}$$

where

$$A_1 = A\left[1 - \frac{\theta}{\pi} + \frac{2}{\pi}\left(1 - 2\frac{a}{A}\right)\sin\theta - \frac{1}{2\pi}\sin 2\theta\right]$$

$$A_2 = A\left[\frac{1}{\pi} - \frac{2}{\pi}\left(1 - 2\frac{a}{A}\right)\cos\theta + \frac{1}{\pi}\cos 2\theta\right] \qquad (\text{for } A > \alpha)$$

and

$$\theta = \cos^{-1}(1 - 2a/A)$$

Figure 3.25 shows plots for both the magnitude and phase of the describing function

$$Q(A, \omega) = \begin{cases} 0, & A \leqslant a \\ (B_1/A)\,e^{i\phi_1}, & A > a \end{cases} \tag{3.159}$$

Thus, this type of nonlinearity has a describing function $Q(\ )$ dependent on stimulus amplitude and exhibiting also a phase lag dependent upon stimulus amplitude. However, it is still independent of the stimulus frequency.

In order to have a describing function dependent upon frequency, the nonlinearity must have a dynamic response with nonzero memory, i.e., it must contain energy-storing elements. In all previous examples the nonlinearity had no "memory," hence the describing function $Q(\ )$ was independent of stimulus frequency. With reference to Fig. 3.26, we note that if the no-memory nonlinearity is followed, or preceded (or both), by a nonzero-memory linear system, then the describing function would be dependent upon the frequency of the stimulus (since attenuation for the linear system is a function of frequency). For example, consider the system shown in Fig. 3.26. We find that in this case the describing function is a

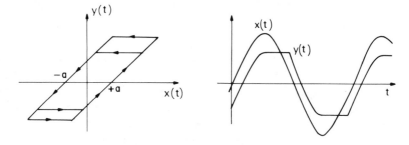

Fig. 3.24. Hysteresis.

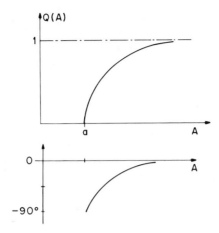

Fig. 3.25. Describing function (both magnitude and phase) for hysteresis.

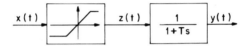

Fig. 3.26. Nonlinear system with memory.

function of frequency

$$Q'(A, \omega) = Q(A, \omega)[1/(1+\omega^2 T^2)^{1/2}] \tag{3.160}$$

where $Q(A, \omega)$ is given by Eq. (3.157) and is independent of ω.

3.6.2. Use of Describing Functions for Identification of Systems

We can now see how this technique can be used to identify systems. First, we have to build a library (catalog) of various nonlinearities and their describing functions. Then, we excite the system with sinusoidal stimuli with various amplitudes and frequencies. From a single period of the response obtained we compute the amplitude and phase of the fundamental component, and the results of these computations are used to plot $Q(A, \omega)$. From the shape of $Q(A, \omega)$ we can then go to the library of $Q(A, \omega)$'s and see to which type of nonlinearity the measured $Q(A, \omega)$ corresponds. Thus, the system nonlinearity is identified. However, it should be noted that the assumptions underlying the validity of this approach must be satisfied.

3.6.3. A Linearization Technique

A modified version of the describing function technique has been used to identify certain physiological systems (cf. Spekreijse, 1969). This is based on the fact that the harmonic content of the response of a zero-memory nonlinear system depends not only on the nature of the non-linearity, but also on the signal-to-noise ratio at the input. This is illus-trated graphically in Fig. 3.27 for three types of nonlinearity that are commonly encountered in physiological systems. They show the effect on the response if noise is added to the output and the sinusoidal input stimulus. It is noted that the effect of the noise is to round off the sharp corners of the response that are caused by the nonlinearity, i.e., the added noise has a *linearizing* effect on the nonlinear nature of the response. Assuming that the added linearizing noise signal is ergodic, low-pass filter-ing of the response tends to produce a sine wave of the same frequency, ω, as the stimulus

$$y(t) = B \sin \omega t$$

as the signal-to-noise ratio is decreased further and further. Moreover, it can be shown that this "linearizing" effect can be obtained if the added periodic signal is of almost any type (sinusoidal, square, triangular, etc.).

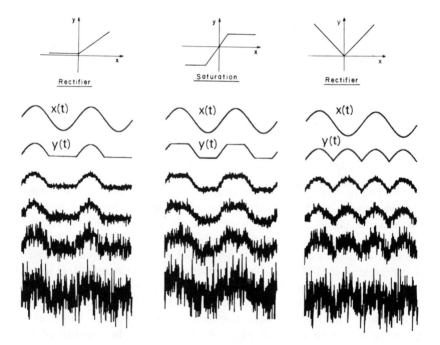

Fig. 3.27. Linearizing effect of noise on three types of nonlinearity.

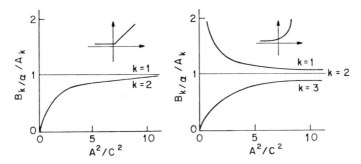

Fig. 3.28. Harmonic content as a function of signal-to-noise ratio for two nonlinearities (after Spekreijse, 1969).

It can be shown (Rice, 1945; Spekreijse and Oosting, 1970) that the amplitude of the kth harmonic in the response, for a given zero-memory nonlinearity $y = f(x)$ and an added linearizing signal $\alpha(t)$ is given by

$$B_{k/\alpha} = \frac{\varepsilon_k}{2\pi i} \int_{\sigma-i\infty}^{\sigma+i\infty} F(s)I_k(As)M_\alpha(s)\, ds, \qquad k = 0, 1, 2, \ldots$$

(3.161)

where ε_k is the Neumann factor, $\varepsilon_0 = 1$, $\varepsilon_k = 2$ for $k = 1, 2, 3, \ldots$; I_k is the modified Bessel function of the first kind; A is the amplitude of the input sine wave; $F(s)$ is the Laplace transform of $f(x)$; and $M_\alpha(s)$ is the first-order characteristic function of the auxiliary signal $\alpha(t)$, i.e.,

$$M_\alpha(s) = E[\![e^{s\alpha(t)}]\!] \cong \frac{1}{T} \int_0^T e^{s\alpha(t)}\, dt$$

(3.162)

Note that if $\alpha(t) = 0$, then $M_\alpha(s) = 1$ and then the above equation (3.161) simply gives the amplitude of the kth harmonic in the response to the sine wave stimulus.

Spekreijse has calculated the effect of various input-added "noise" signals upon the amplitudes of the response harmonics for a wide class of nonlinearities. This method is based upon the fact that the variation in the amplitudes of the harmonics as a function of the changes in the signal-to-noise ratio is dependent on the characteristics of the nonlinearity. For example, reduction of the added "noise" does not affect the amplitude of the fundamental component in the response of a linear rectifier, but in a quadratic rectifier the amplitude of this component decreases. However, the amplitude of the second harmonic remains constant in a quadratic rectifier (see Fig. 3.28).

Therefore, to use this technique as a tool for identifying physiological systems, the following procedure should be used. The system is tested with

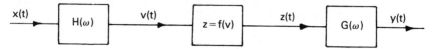

Fig. 3.29. System cascade.

sine waves to which an added "noise" signal is introduced at the input. The response is analyzed for its harmonic content, i.e., for the amplitude of each response harmonic. The procedure is repeated by varying the signal-to-noise ratio at the input and again performing Fourier analysis on the response signal. Thus, graphs can be obtained for the content of each harmonic as a function of the signal-to-noise ratio at the input, such as those shown in Fig. 3.28 for rectifiers. Once these graphs have been obtained a "reference search" is made in the catalog of nonlinearities $f(x)$ and their characteristics in terms of these functions (of harmonic amplitude versus signal-to-noise ratio). This "reference search" may then identify the type of nonlinearity that the system under study exhibits, simply by seeing which nonlinearity in the catalog matches the characteristics measured. If the system has memory, as is usually the case in practice, then we would need to vary, in addition, the frequency of the stimulus sine wave to discover the "dynamics."

The method can be used to identify the various subsystems in a system having the configuration shown in Fig. 3.29: a cascade combination of a linear system with transfer function $H(\omega)$, a nonlinear zero-memory system given by $z = f(v)$, and a linear system with transfer function $G(\omega)$.

The main idea of this approach is the following: For a sinusoidal input $x(t) = A \sin \omega t$, the output, $v(t)$, of the first linear system, which is the input to the nonlinearity, is also sinusoidal.

The amplitude and phase of $v(t)$ depend on the transfer function $H(\omega)$. However, as we saw previously, the response of a zero-memory nonlinearity depends only upon the *amplitude* of the sine wave stimulus; therefore, $z(t)$ depends only upon the amplitude of $v(t)$ but not upon its frequency. Therefore, by varying separately the amplitude and frequency of the input stimulus it should be possible, in principle, to determine separately the linear transfer functions $H(\omega)$, $G(\omega)$ and the nonlinear zero-memory characteristic $z = f(v)$.

For this argument to be valid, the nonlinearity must have zero memory and be single valued, e.g., zero-memory nonlinearities like hysteresis are excluded.

Note that the zero-memory nonlinearity can be described to an arbitrary degree of accuracy for large enough M by

$$z(t) = \sum_{m=0}^{M} a_m v^m(t) \tag{3.163}$$

[provided that $f(v)$ is analytic]. For the subsystems shown in Fig. 3.29, we have

$$v(t) = \int_0^\infty h(\tau)x(t-\tau)\,d\tau \tag{3.164}$$

$$y(t) = \int_0^\infty g(\tau)z(t-\tau)\,d\tau \tag{3.165}$$

From Eqs. (3.163), (3.164), and (3.165) it can be shown (cf. Sec. 9.1) that, if the stimulus $x(t)$ is Gaussian white noise, then

$$\phi_{yx}(\tau) = C\int_0^\infty g(\mu)h(\tau-\mu)\,d\mu \tag{3.166}$$

where C is a constant. Taking the FT we have

$$\Phi_{yx}(\omega) = CG(\omega)H(\omega) \tag{3.167}$$

Thus, from the cross spectrum $\Phi_{yx}(\omega)$ of the stimulus and response we obtain, up to a proportionality constant, the product of transfer functions of the two linear subsystems. Therefore, if we can determine one of them independently, we can find the other one from Eq. (3.167).

Spekreijse and his colleagues (Spekreijse, 1969; Spekreijse and Oosting, 1970) have shown how to measure the transfer characteristic $H(\omega)$ by repeated applications of an "auxiliary" sinusoidal signal whose frequency is changed. Then, from Eq. (3.167) the transfer function of $G(\omega)$ can also be determined. Finally, the transfer characteristic of the zero-memory nonlinearity can be determined by the following approach: The amplitudes of the response harmonics are measured as the signal-to-"noise" ratio at the input of the system is varied. This gives a measure of the nonlinear characteristic, since this effect of the signal-to-"noise" ratio on the harmonic content depends on the nature of the nonlinearity.

This method of identifying physiological systems has two disadvantages. First, it requires repeated applications of stimuli while varying two parameters, the signal-to-noise ratio of the input and the frequency of the auxiliary signal, in order to identify the subsystems in Fig. 3.29. Since experimental times on physiological systems are very limited, this procedure can become undesirably long. In a later chapter it is shown how the same results, viz., identification of components $H(\omega)$, $G(\omega)$, can be obtained much more easily from a single application of a short burst of a white-noise stimulus. Second, this method, in its present form, is applicable only to systems having the fixed configuration of Fig. 3.29 and containing a single zero-memory nonlinearity. Biological systems usually have dynamic (nonzero-memory) nonlinearities, which cannot be treated by such describing-function techniques. However, the white-noise approach is perfectly suited to describing systems with both zero- and nonzero-memory nonlinearities in arbitrary configurations with other linear or nonlinear systems (cf. Chapter 9).

3.7. Effects of Feedback in Physiological Systems

Most physiological systems can be conceptualized as having feedback paths. Some of the reasons why this might be desirable from the functional point of view will be apparent from the discussion below. The concept of feedback is familiar even though an exact definition of it is rather difficult. Moreover, many systems that we usually think of as nonfeedback could be formulated so that they do exhibit a feedback mechanism.

From the point of view of physiological system identification this discussion on the effects of feedback is valuable in interpreting the results of the identification, e.g., detecting the presence and identifying the dynamics of feedback mechanisms. It should be noted that such mechanisms abound in living organisms, e.g., as homeostatic mechanisms that regulate vital body functions (body temperature, respiration, hormone level, etc.) or as body mechanisms attuned to environmental stimuli "feeding back" this information in order to control the position of the body in this environment. In any case, the existence of feedback is ubiquitous and vital for the survival and well-being of an organism.

Besides these general reasons for the existence of feedback mechanisms in living organisms, the employment of feedback in physiological systems improves their performance as "systems." Specifically, physiological systems exhibit (a) imprecise components even though signals are processed with high reliability, (b) high-noise content but "low-noise" performance, (c) higher bandwidths than those afforded by their components, and (d) an abundance of intrinsic oscillators (biological clocks), e.g., endocrine systems. We examine below how these common characteristics could be explained in terms of systems with feedback.

3.7.1. On the System Gain

Figure 3.30 shows a simple feedback system (employing negative feedback). In general the *forward gain* G and the feedback gain α are functions of frequency as given by the transfer functions of the system components they represent and reflecting the "dynamics" of these components. To simplify our discussion here we will take G and α to be constants, independent of frequency; this will not change our conclusions. For the system of Fig. 3.30 we have then

$$A = \frac{y(t)}{x(t)} = \frac{G}{1 + \alpha G} \tag{3.168}$$

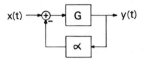

Fig. 3.30. Feedback system.

We note, first, that the overall gain A of the system is reduced from G (in the case of no feedback) to $G/(1+\alpha G)$ in the case of feedback α. Thus, negative feedback tends to decrease the gain of the system.

However, if α and G are functions of frequency (which is the case in practice), then it is possible that for certain ranges of frequency the gain of the system decreases with feedback and for certain others it increases; in the former case we have *degenerative feedback*, while in the latter we have *regenerative feedback*.

3.7.2. On Reliability of Processing Signals

Components of physiological systems are often imprecise, i.e., exhibit great variability in their characteristics. How is it then that organisms seem to process signals with high reliability? There are probably many reasons for this performance (such as redundant, "parallel" design, in some cases); however, feedback can certainly contribute to this high reliability of organisms in processing signals. Continuing with the previous above simple example of a feedback system, let us see what is the effect of a variation in the forward gain G. Let G change by ΔG. Then, in the absence of feedback, the overall gain A will change by the same amount:

$$\Delta A = \Delta G \tag{3.169}$$

or

$$\Delta A/A = \Delta G/G \tag{3.170}$$

i.e., the percentage change is the same. If feedback α is employed in the system then

$$\Delta A \cong \frac{\partial A}{\partial G} \Delta G = \frac{1}{(1+\alpha G)^2} \Delta G \tag{3.171}$$

and

$$\frac{\Delta A}{A} \cong \frac{1}{1+\alpha G} \frac{\Delta G}{G} \tag{3.172}$$

We note that in this case (where we have feedback) the percentage change $\Delta A/A$ in the overall gain is much less than the percentage change in the gain of component G. In fact, if the value of G is large and the feedback α

is also large then the factor $1/(1+\alpha G)$ can become very small and the change in the overall system gain would be negligible.

What happens if the components in the feedback path α are imprecise? To answer we need to examine the effect of a change $\Delta\alpha$. We have

$$\Delta A \cong \frac{\partial A}{\partial \alpha} \Delta\alpha = -\frac{G^2}{(1+\alpha G)^2} \Delta\alpha \tag{3.173}$$

and

$$\frac{\Delta A}{A} \cong -\frac{\alpha G}{1+\alpha G} \frac{\Delta\alpha}{\alpha} \tag{3.174}$$

We note that if $\alpha G \gg 1$ (as is often the case) then

$$\Delta A/A \cong -\Delta\alpha/\alpha \tag{3.175}$$

and the percentage change of the overall system gain is of the same magnitude as that of the imprecise feedback component α. Thus, no increase in reliability takes place in the case where the components in the feedback path are unreliable.

In conclusion, we see that in order to have reliable physiological systems made up of unreliable components by utilizing feedback, we need to have precise components in the feedback path, while the components of the forward path can be imprecise. This is a plausible requirement since the feedback components need be only "sensors" of the response, which, in general, would be of *low energy*; on the other hand, the components of the forward path, which are usually of *high energy*, can be sluggish in their performance.

3.7.3. On Signal-to-Noise Ratio

Physiological signals are often plagued with a high noise content (low signal-to-noise ratios). Let us consider here the effect of feedback on the signal-to-noise ratio. In much the same way as the effect of feedback on system performance in the case of an unreliable component depended upon the location of this component in the system, the effect of feedback on the signal-to-noise ratio depends upon the location of this noise signal in the system.

Figure 3.31 shows a simple system in which the contaminating noise $\varepsilon(t)$ is added somewhere in the forward path. If there is no feedback, i.e., $\alpha = 0$, then

$$y_m = G_1 G_2 x + G_2 \varepsilon \tag{3.176}$$

Thus, the measured response y_m consists of two components, one given by $G_1 G_2 x = y$ due to the pure signal x and the other given by $G_2 \varepsilon = y_\varepsilon$ due to

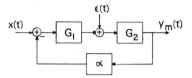

Fig. 3.31. Effect of feedback on signal-to-noise ratio.

the contaminating noise ε. Therefore, the signal-to-noise ratio at the output is

$$\frac{y}{y_\varepsilon} = \frac{G_1 G_2 x}{G_2 \varepsilon} = \frac{G_1 x}{\varepsilon} \qquad (3.177)$$

From this relation, it is obvious that the gain G_2 has no effect on the signal-to-noise ratio but G_1 does. If feedback α is employed, then the measured response is

$$y_m = \underbrace{\frac{G_1 G_2}{1 + \alpha G_1 G_2} x}_{y} + \underbrace{\frac{G_2}{1 + \alpha G_1 G_2} \varepsilon}_{y_\varepsilon} \qquad (3.178)$$

and we note that the signal-to-noise ratio is still $G_1 x / \varepsilon$. Therefore no advantage results. However, if the gain G_1 is increased so that the response is of the same magnitude as in the open-loop case, then a substantial advantage results. To achieve this, i.e., to bring the response up to the level of the open-loop case, we must increase G_1. But if G_1 is increased, then we note from Eq. (3.178) that the error component y_ε is decreased but the signal component y stays approximately the same. Thus, the signal-to-noise ratio improves. In fact, it can easily be shown that, under these conditions,

$$(y/y_\varepsilon)_{\text{feedback}} \cong (y/y_\varepsilon)_{\text{no feedback}}(1 + \alpha G_1' G_2) \qquad (3.179)$$

where G_1' is the new (increased) value of G_1. Thus, under the assumption that the response level stays the same in the presence of feedback, the signal-to-noise ratio improves.

3.7.4. On System Bandwidth

The bandwidth of a system is a measure of the frequency range to which the system responds. Figure 3.32 shows the bandwidth of some typical systems. It is an important indicator of how well the system responds to very low or high frequencies as well as the ranges in which it rejects noise. To illustrate the effect of feedback on the system bandwidth

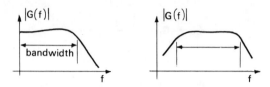

Fig. 3.32. System bandwidth.

let us consider a simple first-order linear system (as in Fig. 3.30):

$$G = G(s) = \frac{1}{1 + Ts} \qquad (3.180)$$

In the absence of feedback ($\alpha = 0$), the bandwidth of this system is

$$(\text{bandwidth})_{\text{no feedback}} = \frac{1}{2\pi T} \quad \text{Hz} \qquad (3.181)$$

If feedback α is added to the system, then the transfer function becomes

$$A(s) = \frac{G(s)}{1 + \alpha G(s)} = \frac{1}{1 + Ts + \alpha} \qquad (3.182)$$

thus making the system bandwidth

$$(\text{bandwidth})_{\text{feedback}} = \frac{1 + \alpha}{2\pi T} \quad \text{Hz} \qquad (3.183)$$

i.e., greater than in the no-feedback case by $(1 + \alpha)$ (see Fig. 3.33). Of course, α itself may be a function of frequency (reflecting the dynamics in the feedback path), which would further modify the frequency response of the system. We conclude that feedback increases the bandwidth of the system, thus allowing it to follow higher (and lower) frequencies than in the no-feedback case.

This effect of feedback on bandwidth is illustrated on a physiological system later in this section.

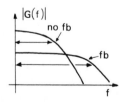

Fig. 3.33. Effect of feedback on system bandwidth.

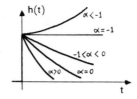

Fig. 3.34. Effect of feedback on system stability.

3.7.5. On System Response and Stability

Directly related to bandwidth is, of course, the behavior of the system response. Continuing the above example we find that the system impulse response is

$$h(t) = \frac{1}{T} \exp\left(-\frac{t}{T}\right) \qquad \text{(no feedback)} \qquad (3.184)$$

$$h(t) = \frac{1}{T} \exp\left[-\frac{1+\alpha}{T}t\right] \qquad \text{(feedback)} \qquad (3.185)$$

i.e., in the presence of feedback the system response becomes faster. Figure 3.34 shows the effect of feedback on the system impulse response for various values of α. We note that for α negative (i.e., positive feedback) and less than -1 the system becomes unstable.

3.7.6. On Sustained Physiological Oscillations

There has always been great interest in the origin and mechanism of physiological oscillators (e.g., certain endocrine systems, brain waves, circadian rhythms, etc.). We examine briefly how feedback and nonlinearities can be used to study these oscillations—their origin and reason for existence.

Consider the three-stage system shown in Fig. 3.35. Note that the third stage, while it has a gain k_3, has a bounded output between $\pm E_b$ (e.g., the dc supply voltage of the amplifiers). Therefore, it effectively has the

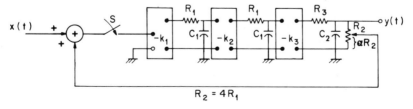

Fig. 3.35. Three-stage amplifier with feedback.

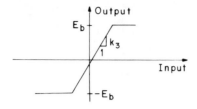

Fig. 3.36. Nonlinear saturation characteristic curve.

characteristic shown in Fig. 3.36, viz., of a zero-memory nonlinear system. Therefore, it has a describing function such as the one given by Eq. (3.157). From this equation we note that as the input amplitude to such a nonlinearity increases (beyond the value E_b/k_3) the gain of it decreases.

To analyze the system we need to utilize the tool of *root locus*. This is a plot of the poles of the closed-loop system as a certain percentage "gain" of the loop is varied. The system can be put in the form shown in Fig. 3.37, in terms of the transfer function of its component subsystems. Then the root locus plot of the system can be shown to be as in Fig. 3.38. When the switch is closed, putting the feedback around the system, any small noise

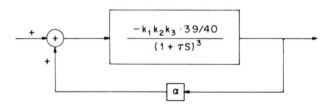

Fig. 3.37. Equivalent system of amplifier with feedback.

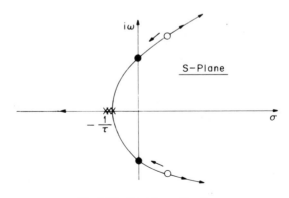

Fig. 3.38. Root-locus diagram.

anywhere in the loop will get amplified increasingly with time *if* the overall gain

$$k = -k_1 k_2 k_3 (39/40) \qquad (3.186)$$

is such as to place the system (closed-loop) poles in the right half-plane—the unstable region in which responses grow exponentially. However, note that if the poles are indeed in the right half of this complex plane, then, since the response grows with time, it will eventually saturate the third amplifier. When this saturation occurs, the "effective" gain of this element is decreased as shown by the describing function of Eq. (3.157). But, since the gain decreases, the (closed-loop) system poles effectively "travel" (although not rigorously in mathematical terms) toward the imaginary axis where they settle! Then the system simply oscillates! In fact this is a stable position for the system poles; for, if the gain tends to increase and hence push the poles into the right half-plane, the nonlinearity reduces the loop gain and causes the poles to travel back toward the $i\omega$ axis; on the other hand, if the gain tends to decrease and move the poles into the left half-plane, where the oscillation amplitude would be reduced and eventually simply die out, the describing function shows that the nonlinear element "effective" gain would be increased and push the poles back toward the right and onto the $i\omega$ axis. Thus, we see how a *nonlinearity* in a feedback situation—abundantly found in physiological systems—can cause *stable* oscillations in the system. Finally we note that the fact that we see something, at the output, that looks like a sine wave is due to the low-pass characteristic of the elements following the nonlinear (saturating) stage—i.e., they filter out the higher harmonics. If at the $i\omega$ axis the gain has been decreased sufficiently for the third stage to go out of saturation and into a linear range of operation, then this position of the roots—on the $i\omega$ axis—is no longer stable.

The transfer function of the overall system in the linear range is

$$A(s) = \frac{G(s)}{1 - G(s)H(s)} \qquad (3.187)$$

where

$$G(s) = \frac{k}{(1 + T_1 s)^3} \qquad (3.188)$$

and

$$H(s) = \alpha \qquad (3.189)$$

Then, application of the Routh–Hurwitz criterion (cf. Elgerd, 1967) gives the relationship between the frequency of oscillations ω_0 and the various parameters of the system:

$$\omega_0 = \frac{1}{T_1}\left(\frac{13}{40}\alpha k_1 k_2 k_3 + \frac{1}{3}\right)^{1/2} \tag{3.190}$$

In conclusion, we note that the describing-function technique can be used, along with some basic tools from linear feedback control theory, to identify oscillations in systems. In particular, since stable oscillations exist in many physiological systems we note two sufficient requirements for their existence: the existence of a *feedback* mechanism and of a saturating *nonlinearity*.

3.8. Feedback Analysis in a Neurosensory System

The effects of feedback discussed above can be illustrated in a physiological system. Experiments were performed on the retinal system, whose input is light and whose output is the intracellular response of the horizontal cell. There is evidence that this system, at high mean light levels, acts as a feedback system (the feedback is from the horizontal cells back to the photoreceptors), while at low mean light levels the feedback path is inactive. Thus, we can study both the open-loop (no feedback) and the closed-loop (feedback) configurations of this system. The transfer functions of this system were measured under both these conditions and are shown in Fig. 3.39. The figure shows both the impulse response of the linear system representation and the gain plot as a function of frequency. From these we note the following: (a) The gain decreases at the high mean light level, i.e.,

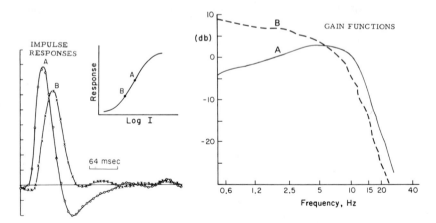

Fig. 3.39. Transfer characteristics of system light → horizontal cell in the catfish retina under high mean level (A) and low mean level (B) stimulation.

when the feedback is active, (b) the bandwidth increases as the feedback becomes active, from about 5 Hz to about 11 Hz, (c) the impulse response of the system becomes faster when the feedback is active.

A consequence of these feedback effects is the improvement of the performance of the initial stages in the processing of the visual signal as it is able, at higher light levels, to respond to a greater range of frequencies (cf. P. Z. Marmarelis and Naka, 1973b,d).

From the data of Fig. 3.39 we can find the dynamics (transfer function) of the postulated feedback mechanism from the horizontal cells back to the receptors. Under the assumption of linearity (a somewhat strenuous assumption, since we indicated that the feedback is inactive at low mean light levels) we have, letting the transfer function of the feedback be $F(s)$,

$$A(s) = \frac{B(s)}{1 + F(s)B(s)} \qquad (3.191)$$

where $A(s)$ and $B(s)$ can be estimated from the data of Fig. 3.39 by the methods discussed in Sec. 3.2. We have approximately

$$B(s) \simeq \frac{K_B}{(1 + Ts)^4} \qquad (3.192)$$

where $K_B \simeq 4$ and $T \simeq 1/(2\pi \cdot 7)$, and

$$A(s) = K_A \left[\left(\frac{s^2}{\omega_1^2} + \frac{2\zeta_1}{\omega_1} s + 1 \right) \left(\frac{s^2}{\omega_2^2} + \frac{2\zeta_2}{\omega_2} s + 1 \right) \right]^{-1} \qquad (3.193)$$

where $K_A \simeq 0.8$, $\omega_1 \simeq 2\pi \cdot 5$, $\omega_2 \simeq 2\pi \cdot 10$, $\zeta_1 \simeq 0.4$, $\zeta_2 \simeq 0.7$.

From these results we can solve Eq. (3.191) for the desired $F(s)$:

$$F(s) = \frac{1}{A(s)} - \frac{1}{B(s)} \qquad (3.194)$$

The White-Noise Method in System Identification

"... besides, what is a linear description of a system but a proportionality relationship! ... not very interesting or informative ... It's in the richness and versatility of *nonlinear* behavior that we stand to gain more insight into the workings of the system ... I love it when it (the system I study in the lab) is exotically nonlinear!" *From a conversation with a good friend and noted physiologist.*

Introduction

Early in the study of the dynamics of a physiological system the bioscientist is faced with the task of recognizing the domains of linearity and of nonlinearity of the stimulus–response transformation that the system performs and how these domains compare with the dominant natural variation of the stimuli in the system's environment. As we saw in the previous chapter, the analytical advantages of linear systems are many, and, therefore, they justify the search for a linear domain in the system's operational range (if such exists). However, the bioscientist must resist the temptation of being carried away by a natural desire for beautiful and explicit solutions since they often tend to be unrealistic idealizations. We cannot but bow to the evidence that nonlinear system characteristics are abundant in nature and go far beyond the trite admission that every physical system is in some way nonlinear. In much the same way that nonlinearities optimize the design of artificial systems, nonlinearities seem to be necessary for the optimal functioning of physiological systems from the behavioral point of view. There are many such examples: the logarithmic transformation of sensory input in order to accommodate large stimulus ranges, dynamic asymmetries arising from such physiological necessities as sensing direction, and many others.

Faced, therefore, with *nonlinear* physiological systems, for which the principle of superposition does not hold, the question naturally arises as to which types of test stimuli should be applied, so that from the resulting responses the bioscientist is able to deduce (or learn as much as possible

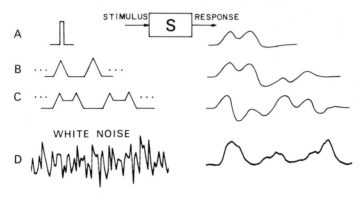

Fig. 4.1. Various stimulus–response pairs.

about) the functional relationship between the stimulus and response of the system. The application of sinusoidal stimuli is certainly unpromising since the response of the system to two such stimuli of different frequencies is different, in general, from the sum of the responses due to each stimulus separately—so no additional information is gained besides the sinusoidal behavior. In general, the same will hold true for other types of stimulus such as steps, pulses, etc. Figure 4.1 illustrates the situation. If a pulse stimulus is applied, we learn the response of the system to this pulse and have little notion of the response of the system to any other type of stimulus. If the stimulus consists of two triangular pulses as shown in the figure, then we know the response of the system to these two triangular pulses and little else. The same applies for any other specific waveform, such as the one shown in part C of the same figure. Therefore, faced with a *nonlinear* system it appears that we can do nothing less than test it with a great variety of stimuli and *catalog* the responses to them. This is exactly what a white-noise stimulus accomplishes in an efficient manner.

Provided that the system is subjected to a Gaussian white-noise stimulus for a long enough time, there is a finite probability that any given stimulus waveform will be represented arbitrarily closely (over a finite time interval) by some sample of this white-noise signal. Thus, the system is tested with every possible stimulus (or a great variety of them depending on the length of the white-noise signal and experiment). This is accomplished because the Gaussian white-noise signal contains every possible frequency and all amplitudes within the Gaussian distribution of signal amplitude. In short, a white-noise stimulus is a very rich stimulus.

Following this line of reasoning, it is easy to see that two systems are equivalent if and only if they respond identically to a white-noise signal, because then they will respond identically to any other input also. The objective of the functional identification of the system, then, is to find a mathematical description (model) that responds to white noise in the same way that the physical system responds to white noise. This is one justification for characterizing physiological systems by testing them with white-noise stimuli. In a sense, one may say that the white-noise testing of the system allows us to nearly maximize the information-gathering rate about the stimulus–response behavior of the system.

It should be emphasized that the white-noise method, developed for the analysis of nonlinear systems, is also perfectly suited to the analysis of linear (or nearly linear) systems. In fact, as we will see in the next few chapters, even in the case of a linear system, the white-noise approach of testing has definite advantages over the traditional approach of testing such systems with pulse and sine wave stimuli. Specifically, it will be shown that the identification of a physiological system through white-noise stimulation is largely unaffected by the types of contaminating noise usually present in such systems, and it is achieved over a much shorter period of experimental testing. Both of these advantages are crucially important in the study of physiological systems (such as neural systems), which usually are plagued with low signal-to-noise ratios and whose experimental preparations have short stable and viable lives. In addition, in the case of a linear or nearly linear system, the method can readily recognize them as such, apart from permitting a substantial decrease in the effort required for data analysis.

The white-noise method is applicable to a very large class of physiological systems. This is the class of systems that are time invariant and have a finite memory (or settling time: the time it takes for the system response to die out for any instantaneous input at time t). Excluded, therefore, are systems whose characteristics change with time and systems such as oscillators, which have infinite memory. Neither of these two restrictions, however is severe. If the system characteristics change with time rather slowly compared to the system time constants, the method can still be applied very usefully. Also, if the system does act as an oscillator (such as a neural pacemaker), it can still be studied usefully by an appropriate change of variable for the input and output signals. Therefore, compared with other methods of nonlinear system analysis such as the phase-plane technique or the describing-function technique (which have serious limitations and are applicable to narrow classes of physiological systems), clearly the white-noise approach has a much greater range of applicability and can describe nearly all physiological systems.

Recently, experimental studies of certain visual systems have been carried out with satisfactory results (cf. P. Z. Marmarelis and Naka, 1973*a,b,c,d*, 1974*a,b,c,d*; P. Z. Marmarelis and McCann, 1973; McCann, 1974; Naka *et al.*, 1975; V. Z. Marmarelis and McCann, 1975, 1977). In these studies the experimental applicability of the white-noise method to biological systems has been shown to be well suited for the treatment of such common idiosyncratic features of neural systems as nonlinearities, short experimental lifetimes, and high noise content.

4.1. Linear and Nonlinear Systems—The Volterra Series

We are faced with a physiological system S, which over reasonably long periods of time can be considered stationary, i.e., its characteristics do not change rapidly with time and the system response remains the same to identical stimuli.

The stimulus $x(t)$ and response $y(t)$ are functions of time t (Fig. 4.2). For example, the input $x(t)$ is light intensity uniformly distributed in space and the output $y(t)$ is the potential of a photoreceptor cell in the eye recorded by a microelectrode. The system S, in this case, is comprised by the chain of processes that transform light intensity (varying in time) to the photoreceptor potential (varying in time) evoked by this light.

4.1.1. Linear Systems

Figure 4.2 shows the stimulus and response of the system for three separate experiments. Stimulus $x_a(t)$, a short rectangular pulse, produces a response $y_a(t)$, stimulus $x_b(t)$ produces response $y_b(t)$, and stimulus $x_c(t)$ [which is the sum of $x_a(t)$ and $x_b(t)$] produces a response $y_c(t)$. If the system is *linear*, then response $y_c(t)$ is

$$y_c(t) = y_a(t) + y_b(t) \qquad (4.1)$$

i.e., the response is equal to the sum of responses due to the two stimuli (x_a and x_b) separately. This result is even more general for linear systems. Specifically, if we multiply stimuli x_1 and x_2 by arbitrary constants a_1 and

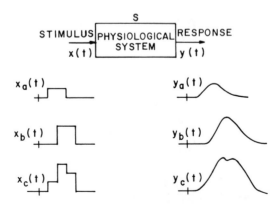

Fig. 4.2. Stimulus and response signals.

a_2 (i.e., amplify, invert, or attenuate them), then stimulus

$$a_1x_1(t)+a_2x_2(t)$$

would produce a response

$$a_1y_1(t)+a_2y_2(t)$$

where $y_1(t)$ and $y_2(t)$ are the responses elicited by $x_1(t)$ and $x_2(t)$ when they are given alone. Of course, the same holds true if, instead of two, any number of stimuli $(x_1, x_2, x_3, \ldots, x_n)$ are considered, so that stimulus

$$a_1x_1(t)+a_2x_2(t)+\cdots+a_nx_n(t)$$

would produce a response

$$a_1y_1(t)+a_2y_2(t)+\cdots+a_ny_n(t)$$

This is the so-called *superposition principle* obeyed by linear systems.

If the stimulus is a very narrow pulse of unit area [i.e., a delta function, $\delta(t)$] the system response to it is called the "impulse response," $h(t)$. The unit impulse $\delta(t)$ has the property that

$$\int_{-\infty}^{\infty} f(t)\delta(t-t_0)\, dt = f(t_0) \tag{4.2}$$

In practice it is approximated by a very narrow (compared to the system time constants) pulse of height a and duration d such that

$$ad = 1 \qquad \text{(in the chosen units)} \tag{4.3}$$

We say, then, that a signal $x(t) = A\delta(t)$ has strength A. The "impulse response" $h(t)$ of a linear system has special significance for the following reasons. Suppose that the stimulus consists of a train of such impulses, each multiplied by a constant a_k, and occurring at time $t_1, t_2, t_3, \ldots$

$$x(t)=\sum_k a_k\delta(t-t_k), \qquad k=1, 2, \ldots \tag{4.4}$$

Then, because the principle of superposition holds for linear systems, the corresponding response is

$$y(t)=\sum_k a_kh(t-t_k), \qquad k=1, 2, \ldots \tag{4.5}$$

This is shown in Fig. 4.3. An arbitrary signal $x(t)$ may be considered as the sum of a great number of such rectangular impulses, each of duration Δt and height $x(t)$, placed next to each other as shown in Fig. 4.3. Then the stimulus signal from time zero to any time $t = N\Delta t$ can be represented by

$$x(t) = x(N\Delta t) = \sum_{k=0}^{N} \Delta tx(k\Delta t)\delta(t-k\Delta t) \tag{4.6}$$

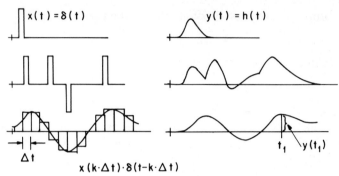

$$x(k \cdot \Delta t) \cdot \delta(t - k \cdot \Delta t)$$

Fig. 4.3. Superposition of responses.

and the response therefore at any time t is (using superposition)

$$y(t) = y(N\Delta t) = \sum_{k=0}^{N} \Delta t x(k\Delta t) h(t - k\Delta t) \tag{4.7}$$

In the limit, as Δt becomes very small, this sum becomes an integral. Letting $k\Delta t = \tau$, we have

$$y(t) = \int_0^t x(\tau) h(t - \tau) \, d\tau \tag{4.8}$$

This has the simple interpretation that the response at time t is equal to the sum of responses to impulses of strength $x(\tau) \, d\tau$ that make up the input signal $x(t)$. This is the so-called *convolution integral*, which can also be written, after a simple change of variable, as

$$y(t) = \int_0^t h(\tau) x(t - \tau) \, d\tau \qquad \text{if } x(t) = 0 \text{ for } t < 0 \tag{4.9}$$

Otherwise, if $x(t) \neq 0$ for $t < 0$,

$$y(t) = \int_0^{\infty} h(\tau) x(t - \tau) \, d\tau \tag{4.10}$$

For all physical systems obeying the principle of causality

$$h(\tau) = 0, \qquad \tau < 0 \tag{4.11}$$

i.e., the response must follow the stimulus in a cause–effect relationship. It should be noted that if we know $h(\tau)$ for a particular linear system, then we can predict its response to any stimulus by using Eq. (4.10). That is, we have complete knowledge of the dynamic stimulus–response transfer characteristics of the system. Therefore, in the case of linear systems, the measurement of $h(\tau)$ (or any function equivalent to it such as its Fourier transform) becomes the objective of the identification procedure.

4.1.2. Nonlinear Systems

If the system is *nonlinear*, then the principle of superposition does not hold. As shown in Fig. 4.4, an impulse stimulus at time t_1 [i.e., $x_a(t) = \delta(t-t_1)$] produces a response $y_a(t)$, and a stimulus impulse at time t_2 [i.e., $x_b(t) = \delta(t-t_2)$] produces a response $y_b(t)$. Since the system is time invariant, $y_b(t)$ is exactly the same as $y_a(t)$ but occurring (t_2-t_1) sec later in time. The system is now stimulated by a stimulus consisting of two impulses, one at time t_1 and the other at time t_2, as shown in Fig. 4.4. Thus the stimulus is

$$x_c(t) = x_a(t) + x_b(t) \tag{4.12}$$

and produces a response $y_c(t)$ such that, in general,

$$y_c(t) \neq y_a(t) + y_b(t) \tag{4.13}$$

that is, superposition of responses is no longer valid. It should be noted that the deviation of $y_c(t)$ from the sum of $y_a(t)$ and $y_b(t)$ can only occur, in this case, for $t \geq t_2$, i.e., only after the occurrence of the second impulse. This is depicted in Fig. 4.4. Therefore, we can write that

$$y_c(t) = y_a(t) + y_b(t) + \theta_{t_1t_2}(t) \tag{4.14}$$

where

$$\theta_{t_1t_2}(t) = 0, \qquad t < t_2 \tag{4.15}$$

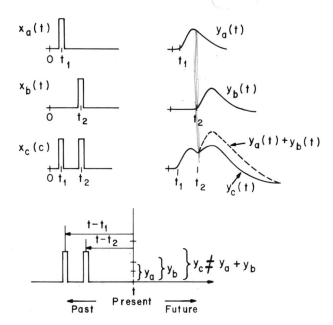

Fig. 4.4. Nonlinear interaction.

Since $\theta_{t_1 t_2}(t)$ is nonzero only for $t \geqslant t_2$ *and* $t \geqslant t_1$ and its value depends, in general, on t_1 and t_2, we can write it as

$$\theta_{t_1 t_2}(t) = f_2(t - t_1, t - t_2) \tag{4.16}$$

where f_2 is zero if $t < \max\{t_1, t_2\}$. Therefore, this function f_2 denotes the amount by which the response deviates from superposition of the responses $y_a(t)$ and $y_b(t)$ to impulses at time t_1 and t_2, respectively.

We may now approximate a continuous stimulus $x(t)$ by a train of closely spaced impulses whose strength (amplitude) is modulated by $x(t)$, as we did above (Fig. 4.3). Then we may be tempted to write the response at any time t by taking the superposed responses due to each impulse

$$y_1(t) = \sum_k f_1(t - k\Delta t) \tag{4.17}$$

and adding to it the nonlinear corrections described by $f_2(t - t_1, t - t_2)$,

$$y_2(t) = \sum_n \sum_m f_2(t - m\Delta t, t - n\Delta t) \tag{4.18}$$

which describes the nonlinear "cross talk" between all possible pairs of impulses that constitute $x(t)$. This appears plausible, at first, but since the system is a general nonlinear system, there may also be a cross-talk effect between three impulses, and so on. This contribution to the response would similarly be given by a term

$$y_3(t) = \sum_m \sum_n \sum_l f_3(t - m\Delta t, t - n\Delta t, t - l\Delta t) \tag{4.19}$$

Of course, this can be generalized to four impulses, five impulses, etc., giving the total response $y(t)$ as

$$y(t) = y_1(t) + y_2(t) + y_3(t) + \cdots \tag{4.20}$$

Volterra showed that, in general, for a system that is nonlinear, time invariant, has finite memory, and is analytic, the relationship between input $x(t)$ and output $y(t)$ can be written as

$$y(t) = k_0 + \int_0^\infty k_1(\tau)x(t - \tau)\, d\tau$$

$$+ \int_0^\infty \int_0^\infty k_2(\tau_1, \tau_2)x(t - \tau_1)x(t - \tau_2)\, d\tau_1\, d\tau_2$$

$$+ \int_0^\infty \int_0^\infty \int_0^\infty k_3(\tau_1, \tau_2, \tau_3)\, x(t - \tau_1)x(t - \tau_2)x(t - \tau_3)\, d\tau_1\, d\tau_2\, d\tau_3 \cdots$$

$$\tag{4.21}$$

where $k_0, k_1(\tau), k_2(\tau_1, \tau_2), k_3(\tau_1, \tau_2, \tau_3), \ldots$ are called the kernels of the system and they are symmetric functions of their arguments. Notice that the zeroth-order kernel k_0, a constant, can be taken to be zero without loss of generality [for input $x(t) \equiv 0$ we simply define $y(t)$ to be zero]. The first-order term is exactly the convolution integral for a linear system. In fact, if $k_2 = k_3 = \cdots = 0$, then

$$y(t) = \int_0^\infty k_1(\tau) x(t - \tau) \, d\tau \qquad (4.22)$$

and the system is linear with impulse response $h(\tau) = k_1(\tau)$.

4.1.3. Analogy between Volterra and Taylor Series

It would be expedient at this point to elaborate a little on the mathematical constituency of the Volterra series. The Volterra series may be thought of as a generalization of the Taylor series of a function of multiple arguments. Recall that the Taylor series of such a function is

$$F(x_1, x_2, \ldots, x_n) = \sum a_{i_1 i_2 \cdots i_n} x_1^{i_1} x_2^{i_2} \cdots x_n^{i_n} \qquad (4.23)$$

where the coefficients $a_{i_1 \cdots i_n}$ are the values of multiple partial derivatives of the function F at the origin, i.e., where all the arguments are zero. Now consider the situation where the arguments $x_1, \ldots, x_n$ are taken to be all the values of a continuous function $x(t)$ in some interval. Then, the number of arguments becomes infinite and F becomes a "functional." It is evident that, in this case, the Taylor series, shown above, becomes the Volterra series and the coefficients $\{a\}$ become the kernels $\{k(\ )\}$ and the sum of discrete quantities becomes a sum of integrals. We must also point out that a Taylor expansion can be written around any other point besides the origin as long as the function is analytic at this point. The same is true for a Volterra expansion of a functional. Therefore, the Volterra series can be written around any function as long as the functional remains analytic. One such function is a constant, an observation that is of importance in practical cases where the physical measure, described by the stimulus $x(t)$, cannot assume negative values, for example when $x(t)$ is light intensity. In these cases, since, as we will see later, the white-noise approach requires random fluctuations around a *zero* mean value, we consider the Volterra expansion around some proper positive value C and we compute the kernels by naming C our "computational zero." On the basis of the argument that was given above in connection with the reference function of the functional expansion, we assert that the computational reference to a conventional zero level is completely legitimate, as long as we stay within the region of analyticity of the functional at hand.

Of course, the kernels of the functional series depend on the chosen reference level (which is here the average level of the stimulus), in the same way that the derivatives of a function depend on the specific value of the independent variable that is used as a reference point in the Taylor-series expansion. Thus, the kernels depend on the functional derivatives at the chosen reference level. It is interesting to see the analytical relations between the Volterra kernels of a system corresponding to a nonzero reference level $C\{k_n^c\}$ and the ones corresponding to the zero reference level $\{k_n\}$. Since

$$y(t) = \sum_{n=0}^{\infty} \int_0^{\infty} \cdots \int_0^{\infty} k_n^c(\tau_1, \ldots, \tau_n) \prod_{i=1}^{n} x(t-\tau_i) \, d\tau_i$$

$$= \sum_{n=0}^{\infty} \int_0^{\infty} \cdots \int_0^{\infty} k_n(\tau_1, \ldots, \tau_n) \prod_{i=1}^{n} [x(t-\tau_i) + C] \, d\tau_i \qquad (4.24)$$

it follows that

$$k_n^c(\tau_1, \ldots, \tau_n)$$
$$= \sum_{l=n}^{\infty} \binom{l}{n} C^{l-n} \underbrace{\int_0^{\infty} \cdots \int_0^{\infty}}_{(l-n)} k_l(\tau_1, \ldots, \tau_n, \tau_{n+1}, \ldots, \tau_l) \, d\tau_{n+1} \cdots d\tau_l \qquad (4.25)$$

The important point is that the resulting kernels and their description of the system are still valid, but they are strictly associated with the value C. To illustrate this, let us consider two zero-memory systems:

$$(1) \quad y = e^x$$
$$(2) \quad y = \log |x|$$

The first function is analytic everywhere, while the second is not analytic at $x = 0$. Therefore, a Volterra-series expansion for the second one is not valid wherever the stimulus $x(t)$ becomes zero, and thus we have to consider for this case a Volterra series around some constant function $C \neq 0$. It can easily be found that the Volterra kernels of the first system, for expansion around the origin, are

$$k_0 = 1$$
$$k_1(\tau) = \delta(\tau)$$
$$k_2(\tau_1, \tau_2) = \tfrac{1}{2}\delta(\tau_1)\delta(\tau_2) \qquad (4.26)$$
$$\vdots$$
$$k_n(\tau_1, \tau_2, \ldots, \tau_n) = (1/n!)\delta(\tau_1)\delta(\tau_2) \cdots \delta(\tau_n)$$
$$\vdots$$

Or, for expansion around $C \neq 0$,

$$k_0^c = e^c$$

$$k_1^c(\tau) = e^c \delta(\tau)$$

$$k_2^c(\tau_1, \tau_2) = (e^c/2)\delta(\tau_1)\delta(\tau_2) \tag{4.27}$$

$$\vdots$$

$$k_n^c(\tau_1, \tau_2, \ldots, \tau_n) = (e^c/n!)\delta(\tau_1)\delta(\tau_2) \cdots \delta(\tau_n)$$

$$\vdots$$

For the second system and expansion around $C = 1$ we have

$$k_0^1 = 0$$

$$k_1^1(\tau) = \delta(\tau)$$

$$k_2^1(\tau_1, \tau_2) = \tfrac{1}{2}\delta(\tau_1)\delta(\tau_2) \tag{4.28}$$

$$\vdots$$

$$k_n^1(\tau_1, \tau_2, \ldots, \tau_n) = (1/n)\delta(\tau_1)\delta(\tau_2) \cdots \delta(\tau_n)$$

$$\vdots$$

Of course, all these arguments can be easily extended to cover the non-zero-memory systems, too. For example, consider the cascade of a linear system with impulse response $g(\tau)$ and the zero-memory nonlinear system $y = e^x$. Then, the kernels of the Volterra expansion around the origin are

$$k_0 = 1$$

$$k_1(\tau) = g(\tau)$$

$$k_2(\tau_1, \tau_2) = \tfrac{1}{2}g(\tau_1)g(\tau_2) \tag{4.29}$$

$$\vdots$$

$$k_n(\tau_1, \tau_2, \ldots, \tau_n) = (1/n!)g(\tau_1)g(\tau_2) \cdots g(\tau_n)$$

$$\vdots$$

and similarly for all the other cases discussed above.

4.1.4. Functional Meaning of the Volterra Kernels

The question naturally arises as to what the kernels $k_1(\tau)$, $k_2(\tau_1, \tau_2) \cdots$ represent. The previous discussion about the system response to one, two, or more impulses makes a loose association between the Volterra kernels and the "cross talk" among the several impulses. Recalling also the functional meaning of the first-order kernel, which was explained above to be the pattern in which the past values of the stimulus affect the present value of the system response, we can form the following understanding of the higher-order Volterra kernels: The nth-order Volterra kernel is the pattern of interaction among n pieces of the stimulus past with regard to the effect that this interaction has upon the system response.

Notice, however, that the nth-order interaction is not exclusively described by the nth-order Volterra kernel but also by all kernels of order higher than nth. This can be easily illustrated in the case of the system impulse response. From the Volterra series [Eq. (4.21)] we see that the impulse response of a nonlinear system is, in general,

$$y(t) = k_0 + k_1(t) + k_2(t, t) + k_3(t, t, t) + \cdots \tag{4.30}$$

That is, the impulse response of a nonlinear system includes the main diagonal points of all kernels.

This is an interesting remark in view of the fact that the impulse response of a nonlinear system is often confused with its first-order kernel, something that is apparently true only in the case of a linear system.

Because of the participation of all kernels in the system response to a set of impulses, the evaluation of the Volterra kernels using impulses as stimuli becomes a burdensome task in the general case. This must not be confused with the use of Poisson pulse trains in connection with the Wiener method for system identification (cf. Sec. 10.6). We simply point out that the use of finite sets of impulses for nonlinear system identification encounters great problems because of the effect of higher-order Volterra kernels on the system response, the limited time available for experimentation on physiological systems, and the high content of contaminating noise that is usually present. It is desirable, therefore, that each kernel be measured independently. This can be accomplished if each term in the series becomes orthogonal *for a certain stimulus* to all other terms. This is achieved by Wiener's formulation of the Volterra series.

4.2. The Wiener Theory

A main theoretical concern in the analysis-synthesis problem of a nonlinear system is that of finding a proper mathematical representation of the system. This representation must be such that it is convenient to handle algebraically and computationally and it must reveal certain basic functional characteristics of the system under study. Without elaborating on the representation problem for nonlinear systems we note that, for these purposes, the concept of a *functional* representation has been well established by a series of investigators (cf. Bose, 1956; Brilliant, 1958; George, 1959; Barrett, 1963).

4.2.1. System Representation by Functionals

A functional is a function of a function, i.e., a function whose argument is a function and whose value is a number. We may write it as

$$y = F[x(t); \quad a \le t \le b] \tag{4.31}$$

where F is the functional, the function $x(t)$ over the interval $[a, b]$ is the argument, and y is the value of the functional.

Example. A definite integral is a functional whose argument is the integrand and whose value is the value of the definite integral. Specifically, such an example is

$$y = F[x(t); \quad a \le t \le b] = \int_a^b x(t)\, dt \tag{4.32}$$

and we would have for $a = 0$, $b = 1$,

Argument, $x(t)$	$3t$	$4t^2$	1.5	e^t	$\cdots$
Value of functional, y	$\frac{3}{2}$	$\frac{4}{3}$	1.5	1.72	$\cdots$

Example. A functional may only be a "rule" with no simple mathematical representation. For example, the value of the functional is unity if, within the interval $[a, b]$, the argument $x(t)$ exceeds the value θ, and otherwise it is zero. Let us take $a = 0$, $b = 1$, and $\theta = 2$. Then, we would have

Argument, $x(t)$	$3t$	t^2	1.5	e^t	$\cdots$
Value of functional, y	1	0	0	1	$\cdots$

Realizing that the system output, at any fixed time t, is a number—the value of the output at this time—which depends on the past history of the input signal (a function), we can see how the concept of a *functional* can be used to describe the stimulus–response behavior of a system. Consider a system S with input $x(t)$ and output $y(t)$. Then we have

$$y(t) = F_S[x(t'); \quad -\infty < t' \le t] \tag{4.33}$$

where t is the *present time* and $x(t')$ describes the whole past history of the input. If the system characteristics vary with time (i.e., the system is time variant) then obviously the response at any time t depends also on t, so that we can write

$$y(t) = F_S[t, x(t'); \quad -\infty < t' \le t] \tag{4.34}$$

However, we consider here only time-invariant systems, and, therefore, the relationship between stimulus and response is given by Eq. (4.33).

The memory, μ, of a system is the length of time it takes for the effect of the stimulus on the response to die out, i.e., become negligibly small. For example, consider the simple system of Fig. 4.5. An impulse stimulus at time t produces a response that decreases with time (depending on the RC time constant). We may consider this response negligible after five time constants. Thus, the memory of this system is $\mu = 5RC$ sec. Clearly,

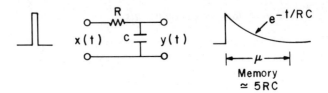

Fig. 4.5. System memory.

then, the response of a system at any time t depends only on the portion of the past history of the stimulus signal that extends to μ sec before t. Therefore, if the system is time invariant and it has finite memory μ, its stimulus–response functional relationship becomes

$$y(t) = F_S[x(t'); \quad t - \mu \le t' \le t] \tag{4.35}$$

Figure 4.6 shows a system S with input $x(t)$ and output $y(t)$. The input (and the output) are zero for $t < 0$. For the fixed times t_1, t_2, t_k, t, the output values, which are the numbers $y(t_1)$, $y(t_2)$, $y(t_k)$, $y(t)$, respectively, depend on the past history of the input extending μ sec before these times. This figure gives a graphical statement of the functional correspondence

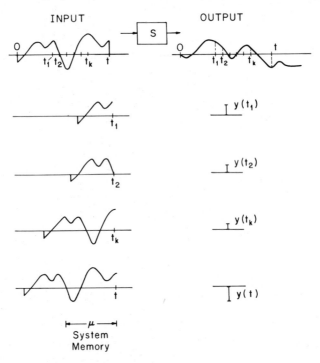

Fig. 4.6. Output dependence on the input past.

between input and output. If the system is linear, then the input past is weighted linearly and the *convolution integral*

$$y(t) = \int_{-\infty}^{t} h(t-\tau)x(\tau)\,d\tau \qquad (4.36)$$

is an example of a functional representation of a system.

Volterra is credited with originally applying the concept of a functional to expand the input–output relationship of a *nonlinear* system in a "power series" with functionals as terms, as discussed in the previous sections.

In fact, Volterra's functional series in terms of the input $x(t)$

$$y(t) = \sum_{n=0}^{\infty} \int_{-\infty}^{\infty} \cdots \int_{-\infty}^{\infty} k_n(\tau_1, \ldots, \tau_n) x(t-\tau_1) \cdots x(t-\tau_n)\,d\tau_1 \cdots d\tau_n$$

$$(4.37)$$

is simply a generalization of the convolution integral representation of a linear system.

The Volterra kernels $k_1(\tau_1)$, $k_2(\tau_1, \tau_2)$, ..., are zero for any of their arguments being less than zero since a physical system must satisfy the causality principle. That is, simply stated, the "effect" of a "cause" cannot precede the stimulus that causes it. From Eq. (4.37) it is easily seen that the first term (neglecting the constant term) describes the linear behavior and that the higher-order terms are generalizations of the linear convolution integral.

In the previous section we concluded that a convenient scheme for measuring the system kernels (since knowledge of them is equivalent to knowledge of the system function) could result from making the terms of the Volterra series orthogonal to each other for a certain specific stimulus $x(t)$. This is exactly what Wiener accomplished. He showed that if the input is a *Gaussian white-noise signal* then a simple change of the Volterra series results in a series whose terms are mutually orthogonal. A Gaussian white-noise signal is a random signal whose power spectrum is constant for all frequencies and whose amplitude is distributed in a Gaussian fashion (Fig. 4.7). In practice, of course, the power density decreases at high frequencies because of finite energy requirements, and also decreases at low frequencies because of the finite length of a signal. However, the bandwidth of the white-noise signal is chosen to be considerably greater than the bandwidth of the system under study.

4.2.2. The Wiener Series

Specifically, Wiener constructed a hierarchy of functionals of increasing order that are orthogonal to each other with respect to a Gaussian

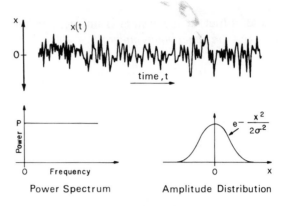

Fig. 4.7. Gaussian white noise.

white-noise input and whose sum characterizes the system. Wiener's approach is approximately as follows: The functional of zero order is h_0. The functional of first order is

$$\int_0^\infty h_1(\tau)x(t-\tau)\,d\tau + K_1$$

where $x(t)$ is a Gaussian white-noise signal of zero mean. He then makes this functional orthogonal to the zero-order functional. We easily see that this is so if $K_1 = 0$ for $x(t)$ a Gaussian variable of zero mean, since

$$E\left[h_0\int_0^\infty h_1(\tau)x(t-\tau)\,d\tau + h_0K_1\right] = 0 \qquad \text{if } K_1 = 0$$

Then, he uses a method very similar to the Gram–Schmidt orthogonalization procedure to make the functional of the second order orthogonal to all functionals of zero order and first order that are homogeneous with respect to $x(t)$. Then he makes the functional of third order orthogonal to all homogeneous functionals of second, first, and zero orders and so on.

Finally, Wiener showed that the relationship between the input $x(t)$ and the output $y(t)$ of a system S can be written as

$$y(t) = \sum_{m=0}^\infty G_m[h_m(\tau_1, \ldots, \tau_m); x(t'), t' \leq t] \qquad (4.38)$$

where the G_i are orthogonal functionals if $x(t)$ is a Guassian white-noise signal with zero mean and $\{h_i\}$ is the set of *Wiener kernels*. Each $h_m(\tau_1, \tau_2, \ldots, \tau_m)$ is a symmetrical function with respect to its arguments. The first four Wiener functionals are

$$G_0[h_0; x(t)] = h_0 \qquad (4.39)$$

$$G_1[h_1; x(t)] = \int_0^\infty h_1(\tau) x(t-\tau) \, d\tau \tag{4.40}$$

$$G_2[h_2; x(t)] = \int_0^\infty \!\!\! \int h_2(\tau_1, \tau_2) x(t-\tau_1) x(t-\tau_2) \, d\tau_1 \, d\tau_2 - P \int_0^\infty h_2(\tau_1, \tau_1) \, d\tau_1 \tag{4.41}$$

$$G_3[h_3; x(t)] = \int_0^\infty \!\!\! \int \!\! \int h_3(\tau_1, \tau_2, \tau_3) x(t-\tau_1) x(t-\tau_2) x(t-\tau_3) \, d\tau_1 \, d\tau_2 \, d\tau_3$$

$$- 3P \int_0^\infty \!\!\! \int h_3(\tau_1, \tau_2, \tau_2) x(t-\tau_1) \, d\tau_1 \, d\tau_2 \tag{4.42}$$

where the power density spectrum of the white noise $x(t)$ is $\Phi_{xx}(f) = P$.

Orthogonality of the G functionals means that the expected value (time average) of the product of any two of them is zero. Indeed, for example,

$$E[[G_1[h_1; x(t)] G_2[h_2; x(t)]]]$$

$$= E\left[\left[\int h_1(\tau) x(t-\tau) \, d\tau \cdot \int\!\!\int h_2(\tau_1, \tau_2) x(t-\tau_1) x(t-\tau_2) \, d\tau_1 \, d\tau_2\right]\right]$$

$$- E\left[\left[\int h_1(\tau) x(t-\tau) \, d\tau \cdot P \int h_2(\tau_1, \tau_1) \, d\tau_1\right]\right]$$

$$= \int\!\!\int\!\!\int h_1(\tau) h_2(\tau_1, \tau_2) E[[x(t-\tau) x(t-\tau_1) x(t-\tau_2)]] \, d\tau \, d\tau_1 \, d\tau_2$$

$$- P \int\!\!\int h_1(\tau) h_2(\tau_1, \tau_1) E[[x(t-\tau)]] \, d\tau \, d\tau_1$$

$$= 0$$

since $x(t)$ is a Gaussian signal of zero mean and the average of the product of an odd number of Gaussian signals (of zero mean) is zero. Similarly,

$$E[[G_0[h_0; x(t)] G_2[h_2; x(t)]]]$$

$$= h_0 \int\!\!\int h_2(\tau_1, \tau_2) E[[x(t-\tau_1) x(t-\tau_2)]] \, d\tau_1 \, d\tau_2 - h_0 P \int h_2(\tau_1, \tau_1) \, d\tau_1$$

But since $x(t)$ is a white-noise signal $E[[x(t-\tau_1) x(t-\tau_2)]] = P\delta(\tau_1 - \tau_2)$ and we then have

$$h_0 \int\!\!\int h_2(\tau_1, \tau_2) P\delta(\tau_1 - \tau_2) \, d\tau_1 \, d\tau_2 - h_0 P \int h_2(\tau_1, \tau_1) \, d\tau_1 = 0$$

4.2.3. Comparison of Wiener and Volterra Representations

The set of Wiener kernels $\{h_i\}$ characterizes the system; that is, knowledge of these kernels allows the prediction of the system response to a given stimulus, by use of the Wiener series. Clearly, the knowledge of the power level of the white noise, with which the Wiener kernels are estimated, is also required since the Wiener functionals of order higher than first depend explicitly on this power level. Furthermore, the Wiener kernels themselves depend on that power level, as becomes evident later from the discussion about Wiener kernel estimation. In this respect, the Wiener kernels are different from the Volterra kernels since the Volterra kernels are invariant characteristics of a system. It should be noted that if the system kernels are zero for order higher than the second, then the Wiener kernels $h_1(\tau)$ and $h_2(\tau_1, \tau_2)$ are equal to the Volterra kernels $k_1(\tau)$ and $k_2(\tau_1, \tau_2)$. This is illustrated in the following example.

Figure 4.8A shows an example of a nonlinear system. This system consists of the cascade combination of a linear system, with impulse response function $g(\tau)$, followed by an instantaneous zero-memory nonlinear transformation, $aw(t) + bw^2(t)$, of the linear system output $w(t)$. We have

$$y(t) = aw(t) + bw^2(t)$$

$$= \int_0^\infty ag(\tau)x(t-\tau)\,d\tau + \int_0^\infty \int_0^\infty bg(\tau_1)g(\tau_2)x(t-\tau_1)x(t-\tau_2)\,d\tau_1\,d\tau_2$$

$$(4.43)$$

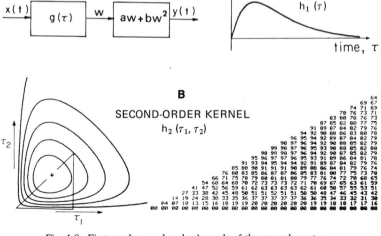

Fig. 4.8. First- and second-order kernels of the cascade system.

Therefore, the Volterra kernels for this system are

$$k_1(\tau) = ag(\tau) \tag{4.44}$$

$$k_2(\tau_1, \tau_2) = bg(\tau_1)g(\tau_2) \tag{4.45}$$

shown plotted in Fig. 4.8B. The second-order kernel is exhibited in two different ways: (i) as a map of constant-elevation contours in the (τ_1, τ_2) plane and (ii) as a matrix of values for various discrete values of the independent variables τ_1, τ_2. These values have been normalized so that the maximum corresponds to 99. The range of (τ_1, τ_2) for which k_2 is shown here as a matrix of values corresponds to the triangular area indicated on the contour map of k_2.

If $x(t)$ is Gaussian white noise, then the Wiener kernels of the system are found through the crosscorrelation technique (see Sec. 4.3.2):

$$h_0 = E[y(t)]$$

$$= \int_0^\infty ag(\tau)E[x(t-\tau)]\,d\tau$$

$$+ \int_0^\infty \int_0^\infty bg(\tau_1)g(\tau_2)E[x(t-\tau_1)x(t-\tau_2)]\,d\tau_1\,d\tau_2$$

$$= P\int_0^\infty bg^2(\tau_1)\,d\tau_1 \tag{4.46}$$

$$h_1(\lambda) = \frac{1}{P}E[y(t)x(t-\lambda)]$$

$$= \frac{1}{P}\int_0^\infty ag(\tau)\,E[x(t-\tau)x(t-\lambda)]\,d\tau$$

$$+ \frac{1}{P}\int_0^\infty \int_0^\infty bg(\tau_1)g(\tau_2)E[x(t-\tau_1)x(t-\tau_2)x(t-\lambda)]\,d\tau_1\,d\tau_2$$

$$= ag(\lambda) \tag{4.47}$$

$$h_2(\lambda_1, \lambda_2) = \frac{1}{2P^2}E[[y(t)-h_0]x(t-\lambda_1)x(t-\lambda_2)]$$

$$= \frac{1}{2P^2}\int_0^\infty ag(\tau)\,E[x(t-\tau)x(t-\lambda_1)x(t-\lambda_2)]\,d\tau$$

$$+ \frac{1}{2P^2}\int_0^\infty \int_0^\infty bg(\tau_1)g(\tau_2)\,E[x(t-\tau_1)x(t-\tau_2)x(t-\lambda_1)x(t-\lambda_2)]\,d\tau_1\,d\tau_2$$

$$- \frac{1}{2P^2}h_0\,E[x(t-\lambda_1)x(t-\lambda_2)]$$

$$= bg(\lambda_1)g(\lambda_2) \tag{4.48}$$

$$h_n(\lambda_1, \lambda_2, \ldots, \lambda_n) = 0 \qquad \text{for any } n > 2 \qquad (4.49)$$

Therefore the first- and second-order Wiener kernels of the system are the same as the respective Volterra kernels. Of course, if the system had higher than second-order kernels then the Wiener kernels would be, in general, different from the Volterra kernels, as demonstrated below.

Clearly, the Wiener series is equivalent to the Volterra series since they are both constructed from linear expressions of the same mathematical structures (the multiple convolution integrals) and they are both expansions of the same function [the system response $y(t)$]. Consequently, there is a unique analytical relation between the Volterra and the Wiener kernels of a system, which represents the transformation of the functional expansion basis. The explicit analytical relations between the Wiener kernels $\{h\}$ and the Volterra kernels $\{k\}$ of a system are

$$h_{2n}(\sigma_1, \ldots, \sigma_{2n})$$

$$= \sum_{m=n}^{\infty} \frac{2m! P^{m-n}}{2n!(m-n)!2^{m-n}}$$

$$\times \int_0^{\infty} \cdots \int_0^{\infty} k_{2m}(\tau_1, \tau_1, \ldots, \tau_{m-n}, \tau_{m-n}, \sigma_1, \ldots, \sigma_{2n}) \, d\tau_1 \cdots d\tau_{m-n}$$

$$\qquad (4.50)$$

$$h_{2n+1}(\sigma_1, \ldots, \sigma_{2n+1})$$

$$= \sum_{m=n}^{\infty} \frac{(2m+1)! P^{m-n}}{(2n+1)!(m-n)!2^{m-n}}$$

$$\times \int_0^{\infty} \cdots \int_0^{\infty} k_{2m+1}(\tau_1, \tau_1, \ldots, \tau_{m-n}, \tau_{m-n}, \sigma_1, \ldots, \sigma_{2n+1}) \, d\tau_1 \cdots d\tau_{m-n}$$

Clearly, the even- (odd-) order Wiener kernels are polynomials in P with coefficients depending on all the higher even- (odd-) order Volterra kernels.

The expressions (4.50) clearly state the fact of the dependence of the Wiener kernels and the G functionals on P. Similar expressions can be derived for the Volterra kernels of the system in terms of the Wiener kernels and the respective power level P by collecting the appropriate terms from the G functionals.

One interesting implication of the derived relation between the Volterra and the Wiener kernels of the system is that the first-order Wiener functional of a nonlinear system is, in general, different from the linear part of the system (first-order Volterra functional), and it is actually dependent on higher-order Volterra kernels, i.e., has some of the system nonlinearities. This demonstrates the efficiency of the Wiener representation, where even the first-order functional term reflects some of the nonlinear characteristics of the system.

Notice that the Wiener series involves one more parameter, in addition to the system kernels: the power level P. This is because the Wiener series is so constructed as to possess the special feature of orthogonality with respect to Gaussian white noise, and the power level P determines the range of validity of this orthogonality in function space, in much the same way that the domain of the independent variable determines the range of validity of the orthogonality of two functions. Why is orthogonality so insistently pursued? There are three main reasons. The first reason is that an orthogonal basis spans the space within the range of its validity most efficiently. Therefore, the Wiener series is expected to have stronger convergence than the Volterra series, for an arbitrarily chosen stimulus signal; and consequently, it can be expected to provide (i.e., over a large number of signals) a better truncated model of the system. (This does not exclude the possibility of a special case where the opposite is true; recall, however, that Gaussian white noise is an exhaustive input, i.e., it tests the system with a great variety of stimuli.) The second reason is that if the expansion basis is orthogonal then the truncated model can be extended to include higher-order terms without affecting the terms already estimated. The third reason is that the orthogonality enables us to estimate the system kernels in a relatively simple way (discussed below), in the same way that the determination of the coordinates of a given vector is greatly simplified if the vector basis is orthogonal (diagonalization of the coefficient matrix).

This last advantage that orthogonality provides is especially important in the actual identification of nonlinear systems, since the determination (or estimation) of the Volterra kernels in the general case of a nonlinear system is an impossible task with present analytical and computational means. Nonetheless, as shown below, exploitation of the orthogonality property of the G functionals allows relatively simple estimation of the system Wiener kernels.

It must be noted that the Gaussian white noise is not the only signal with respect to which the functional series can be orthogonalized. The orthogonalization can be achieved for any other signal that possesses suitable autocorrelation properties. For each such signal a corresponding set of kernels can be estimated (as discussed in Chapter 5).

4.2.4. Meaning of Wiener Kernels

We noted above that the terms of the Wiener series are orthogonal with respect to a stimulus that is Gaussian white noise. This implies that if the series is truncated after the nth-order term (as it must be, in practice), then the resulting approximation in terms of kernels $\{h_0, h_1, \ldots, h_n\}$ is the best in the mean-square-error sense. That is, the approximation

$$y_n(t) = \sum_{k=0}^{n} G_k[h_k(\ ); x(t)] \tag{4.51}$$

where $x(t)$ is Gaussian white noise, minimizes the mean-square error (MSE) between the measured system response $y(t)$ and $y_n(t)$ for a given number of kernels $\{h_0, h_1, \ldots, h_n\}$, as would be obtained for any other set of n kernels. That is, the Wiener series gives, because of orthogonality, the best system representation in MSE at each stage of truncation (e.g., $\{h_0, h_1\}$ is the best linear representation, $\{h_0, h_1, h_2\}$ is the best second-order non-linear representation, etc.). Since, as we argued before, a system's performance is best judged by its response to a Gaussian white-noise stimulus (because such a stimulus tests a system with all possible inputs), *and* the Wiener series gives the best representation at any state of truncation with respect to a Gaussian white-noise stimulus, we see that our objective of system identification is well served by measuring the system Wiener kernels. Accordingly, it should be noted that the Volterra series, since it is not orthogonal with respect to a Gaussian white noise, will not give the best (in the least MSE sense) system representation for a Gaussian white-noise stimulus. This is another reason why, in applications, we seek to measure the Wiener kernels rather than the Volterra kernels of the system.

The set of kernels $\{h_i\}$, under certain conditions, can be considered as generalized "combined impulse responses" of the system much in the way that $h(t)$ is the impulse response of a linear system. To see this and also to get an insight as to the meaning of the kernels, let us consider a system S that is completely described by the linear and quadratic terms of the series, that is,

$$y(t) = \int_0^{\infty} h_1(\tau)x(t-\tau)\, d\tau + \int\int_0^{\infty} h_2(\tau_1, \tau_2)x(t-\tau_1)x(t-\tau_2)\, d\tau_1\, d\tau_2 \tag{4.52}$$

The response of S to an impulse of strength A at $t = 0$, i.e., $x_a(t) = A\delta(t)$, is

$$y_a(t) = Ah_1(t) + A^2h_2(t, t) \tag{4.53}$$

Similarly, the response of S to an impulse of strength B at $t = t_0$, i.e., $x_b(t) = B\delta(t-t_0)$, is

$$y_b(t) = Bh_1(t-t_0) + B^2h_2(t-t_0, t-t_0) \tag{4.54}$$

The response of S to a stimulus consisting of an impulse of strength A at $t = 0$ and an impulse of strength B at $t = t_0$, i.e., $x_c(t) = A\delta(t) + B\delta(t-t_0)$, is

$$y_c(t) = Ah_1(t) + Bh_1(t-t_0) + A^2h_2(t, t) + ABh_2(t, t-t_0) + BAh_2(t-t_0, t)$$
$$+ B^2h_2(t-t_0, t-t_0) \tag{4.55}$$

If we subtract algebraically from the response to the two impulses (response y_c) the contributions of each impulse when each alone acted upon the system (responses y_a and y_b), we have left

$$ABh_2(t, t-t_0) + BAh_2(t-t_0, t)$$

which, since $h_2(\tau_1, \tau_2)$ is a symmetric function, reduces to

$$2ABh_2(t, t-t_0)$$

Therefore, it is seen that, under the condition that the system kernels of order higher than the second are zero [i.e., $h_i(\ )=0$ for $i \geqslant 3$], the second-order kernel $h_2(\tau_1, \tau_2)$ gives a quantitative measure of the nonlinear "cross talk" between the two impulse stimuli, as a function of time t for each separation t_0, between the impulses. As seen, this "cross-talk" effect also depends on the product AB of the strengths of the two impulse stimuli.

It should be noted that even if the two impulses coincide in time (i.e., $t_0 = 0$), the deviation of the system response to the two-impulse stimulus from the sum (superposition) of the responses to each stimulus impulse alone is given by

$$2ABh_2(t, t)$$

proportional to the quantity represented by the diagonal of $h_2(\tau_1, \tau_2)$. This latter, therefore, manifests any amplitude-dependent nonlinearities. Therefore, the term $2ABh_2(t, t-t_0)$ represents deviation from "time superposition." That is, the value of $h_2(\tau_1, \tau_2)$ gives a quantitative measure of the nonlinear deviation from superposition due to interaction between portions of the stimulus signal that are τ_1 and τ_2 sec in the past, in affecting the system response at the present (see Fig. 4.9). Or if $\tau_1 = \tau_2$, it denotes the amplitude-dependent nonlinearities.

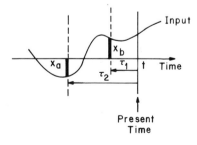

Fig. 4.9. Second-order interaction of input past values.

4.2.5. Kernels of System Cascades

Consider the system shown in Fig. 4.10A. It consists of the two subsystems in cascade. The first subsystem is a zero-memory nonlinear system—a squarer. That is, the output of this system is exactly the square of the input without any phase or gain dependence on frequency of the input (i.e., the transformation is instantaneous and algebraic). The second subsystem is a linear system with memory whose impulse response function is $g(\tau)$. We wish to find the kernels of the overall system—obviously, a nonlinear system. We have for the input–output relationships of the two subsystems

$$z(t) = x^2(t) \tag{4.56}$$

$$y(t) = \int_0^\infty g(\tau)z(t-\tau)\,d\tau \tag{4.57}$$

Therefore

$$y(t) = \int_0^\infty g(\tau)x^2(t-\tau)\,d\tau$$

$$= \int\!\!\int_0^\infty g(\tau_1)\delta(\tau_1-\tau_2)x(t-\tau_1)x(t-\tau_2)\,d\tau_1\,d\tau_2 \tag{4.58}$$

Since the Wiener representation is *unique* for a given system, it follows that for this system

$$h_1(\tau) = 0 \tag{4.59}$$

$$h_2(\tau_1, \tau_2) = g(\tau_1)\delta(\tau_1-\tau_2) \tag{4.60}$$

$$h_k(\tau_1, \ldots, \tau_k) = 0 \qquad \text{for } k \geq 3 \tag{4.61}$$

We note that the second-order kernel for this system consists of a wall of impulses along the diagonal whose strength is modulated by $g(\tau)$ as shown in Fig. 4.11; the kernel is zero everywhere else. It should be noted that, if

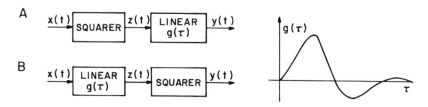

Fig. 4.10. Alternate cascades.

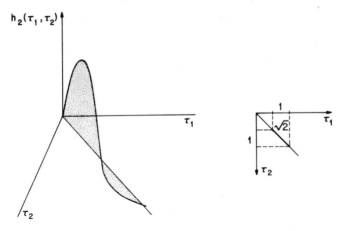

Fig. 4.11. Second-order kernel of cascade A in Fig. 4.10.

we just look along the diagonal, the waveform is like $g(\tau)$ except "elongated" by $2^{1/2}$. That is, going a distance of one unit along the τ_1 and τ_2 axes corresponds to going $2^{1/2}$ units along the diagonal.

Using Eq. (4.53), the response of this system to an impulse stimulus at $t = 0$, i.e., $x_a(t) = A\delta(t)$, is

$$y_a(t) = A^2 h_2(t, t)$$
$$= A^2 g(t)\delta(0) \tag{4.62}$$

where we may think of $\delta(0)$ from the approximation of the delta function by a rectangular pulse of height $\delta(0)$ and width Δt (Fig. 4.12), i.e., $\delta(0) = 1/\Delta t$. Using Eq. (4.54) the response of this system to $x_b(t) = B\delta(t - t_0)$ is

$$y_b(t) = B^2 g(t - t_0)\delta(0) \tag{4.63}$$

and finally the response to $x_c(t) = A\delta(t) + B\delta(t - t_0)$ is [see Eq. (4.55)]

$$y_c(t) = A^2 g(t)\delta(0) + B^2 g(t - t_0)\delta(0) + 2ABg(t)\delta(t_0) \tag{4.64}$$

The nonlinear deviation from superposition is

$$y_c(t) - y_a(t) - y_b(t) = 2ABg(t)\delta(t_0) \tag{4.65}$$

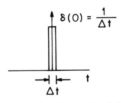

Fig. 4.12. Approximation to the delta function.

If $t_0 \neq 0$, i.e., if the two impulses do not coincide, this term is zero since $\delta(t_0) = 0$. This should have been obvious since $h_2(\tau_1, \tau_2)$ for $\tau_1 \neq \tau_2$ is zero for this system. However, if $t_0 = 0$, i.e., if the two impulses coincide, then the nonlinear deviation for this system is obviously nonzero and equal to

$$2ABg(t)\delta(0)$$

Consider now the same two subsystems as in the previous case [the squarer and the linear system $g(\tau)$] but connected in reverse, i.e., the linear system precedes the nonlinear squarer (Fig. 4.10B). Then we have

$$z(t) = \int_0^\infty g(\tau)x(t-\tau)\,d\tau \tag{4.66}$$

$$y(t) = z^2(t) \tag{4.67}$$

and therefore

$$y(t) = \left[\int_0^\infty g(\tau)x(t-\tau)\,d\tau\right]^2$$

$$= \int\int_0^\infty g(\tau_1)g(\tau_2)x(t-\tau_1)x(t-\tau_2)\,d\tau_1\,d\tau_2 \tag{4.68}$$

Thus, the kernels of this system are

$$h_1(\tau) = 0 \tag{4.69}$$

$$h_2(\tau_1, \tau_2) = g(\tau_1)g(\tau_2) \tag{4.70}$$

$$h_k(\tau_1, \ldots, \tau_k) = 0 \qquad \text{for } k \geqslant 3 \tag{4.71}$$

The second-order kernel is now nonzero everywhere and its value at each point (τ_1, τ_2) is $g(\tau_1)g(\tau_2)$. Its maximum peak is obviously at the point on the diagonal $(\tau_1 = \tau_2)$ for which $g(\tau)$ is maximum.

Using Eqs. (4.53), (4.54), and (4.55) we find the following:

(a) stimulus: $x_a(t) = A\delta(t)$

     response: $y_a(t) = A^2 g^2(t)$ (4.72)

(b) stimulus: $x_b(t) = B\delta(t-t_0)$

     response: $y_b(t) = B^2 g^2(t-t_0)$ (4.73)

(c) stimulus: $x_c(t) = A\delta(t) + B\delta(t-t_0)$

     response: $y_c(t) = A^2 g^2(t) + B^2 g^2(t-t_0) + 2ABg(t)g(t-t_0)$ (4.74)

Therefore the deviation from superposition of the two responses at any time t is

$$y_c(t) - y_a(t) - y_b(t) = 2ABg(t)g(t-t_0) \tag{4.75}$$

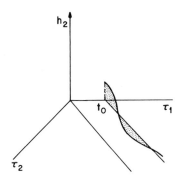

Fig. 4.13. "Cross talk" for cascade B in Fig. 4.10.

which is nothing else but a scaled version of the second-order kernel $h_2(\tau_1, \tau_2)$ of this system and therefore can be simply read off the plot of this kernel by noting that $t = \tau_1$ and $t_0 = t - \tau_2$. For a given t_0, the deviation from superposition, i.e., the nonlinear "cross talk," can be simply found from the plot of $h(\tau_1, \tau_2)$ as follows: For $t < t_0$, this deviation is zero. For $t \geq t_0$, the time history of the deviation is found by drawing a line parallel to the diagonal and starting at the point $\tau_1 = t_0$ along the τ_1 axis (Fig. 4.13). It should be noted that this procedure of finding the nonlinear cross talk due to two impulse stimuli is not peculiar to this example but is quite general for all nonlinear systems that have only the first two kernels.

In the previous two examples, if the nonlinear system (the squarer) is of a different form, e.g.,

$$r(t) = C_1 s(t) + C_2 s^2(t) \tag{4.76}$$

where $r(t)$ is its output and $s(t)$ is its input, then it can easily be shown that the kernels would be, for the system of Fig. 4.10A,

$$h_1(\tau) = C_1 g(\tau) \tag{4.77}$$

$$h_2(\tau_1, \tau_2) = C_2 g(\tau_1) \delta(\tau_1 - \tau_2) \tag{4.78}$$

$$h_k(\tau_1, \ldots, \tau_k) = 0, \qquad k \geq 3 \tag{4.79}$$

and, for the system of Fig. 4.10B,

$$h_1(\tau) = C_1 g(\tau) \tag{4.80}$$

$$h_2(\tau_1, \tau_2) = C_2 g(\tau_1) g(\tau_2) \tag{4.81}$$

$$h_k(\tau_1, \ldots, \tau_k) = 0, \qquad k \geq 3 \tag{4.82}$$

We note that the first-order kernels are the same in both cases but the second-order kernels are quite different. Therefore, conceivably, if we do not know how these two systems are connected—that is, which one comes first because they are inside a "black box"—it is possible to determine the sequence by estimating the kernels of the overall system and examining the second-order kernel. This is so provided we have *a priori* information that the overall system consists of two subsystems, one of which is a zero-memory nonlinear system and the other of which is a linear system. Notice that we do not need any other *a priori* information since the measured first-order kernel of the overall system reveals directly (except for a scalar multiplier) the impulse response $g(\tau)$ of the linear subsystem. Moreover, even if we do not have any *a priori* information, we can always make this as a hypothesis and then check to see if the measured $h_1(\tau)$ and $h_2(\tau_1, \tau_2)$ of the overall system are related by any of the equations (4.78) or (4.81). This procedure can be used readily in the case of biological systems since we usually have little information about the underlying substructure of these systems and the functional characteristics of their subsystems. This is one of the cases where examination of *function* can reveal information about the system *structure*. This approach has been used successfully in studying the sequence of processing nerve signals in a vertebrate retina (Marmarelis and Naka, 1973*a,b,c,d*).

The latter point is important since, in addition to the "functional" identification of a system, the bioscientist is concerned with its "structural" identification, wanting to answer primarily the following questions: Having found the complete dynamic description, $y = F[x]$, of the system, how is F realized physically by components inside the "black box"? How do changes in the characteristics of a particular component affect the system function F? Paradoxically, a complete solution to this problem may be nearly impossible if the system is linear, while plausible solutions are often obtainable if the system is nonlinear. We explain this apparently perverse viewpoint by noting that in a nonlinear system it is sometimes possible to determine the sequence of underlying events because nonlinear operators do not in general commute, while such a determination is impossible if the system is linear, since linear operators commute.

4.3. Schemes for the Estimation of the System Kernels

A system is completely characterized once its set of kernels $\{h_i\}$ is determined. Therefore, the objective of the identification procedure is to measure (estimate) the kernels of a system.

4.3.1. The Wiener–Bose Approach

As we discussed in Sec. 4.1, given a time-invariant system S with input $x(t)$ and output $y(t)$, the output at time t is a function of the present value and past values of the input, i.e.,

$$y(t) = F_s[x(\tau); \ \tau \leq t] \tag{4.83}$$

The function $[x(\tau), \tau \leq t]$ can be expanded into a series of orthonormal functions, like the family of Laguerre functions $\{\Psi_i(\tau)\}$:

$$x(-\tau) = \sum_{n=0}^{\infty} c_n \Psi_n(\tau), \qquad \tau \geq 0 \tag{4.84}$$

The set of coefficients $\{c_i\}$ completely describes the stimulus up to the present $[x(\tau), \tau \leq t]$, the present being considered as $t = 0$ with time going backwards. The Laguerre functions form a complete orthonormal basis in the interval $(0, \infty)$. That is,

$$\int_0^{\infty} \Psi_i(\tau)\Psi_j(\tau) \, d\tau = \begin{cases} 0, & i \neq j \\ 1, & i = j \end{cases} \tag{4.85}$$

Therefore, we can easily obtain the coefficients $\{c_i\}$ by

$$c_n = \int_0^{\infty} x(-\tau)\Psi_n(\tau) \, d\tau \tag{4.86}$$

Wiener chose the Laguerre family of functions to expand the past of the input because these functions have certain desirable mathematical properties (which we will describe briefly later), and, in addition, they can be easily generated by linear analog circuits.

In practice we would use a finite number $n + 1$ of coefficients c_i to describe the past of the input, a valid approximation for a system with finite memory. Then Eq. (4.83) becomes

$$y(t) = F_s[c_0(t), c_1(t), \ldots, c_n(t)] \tag{4.87}$$

where $[c_0(t), c_1(t), \ldots, c_n(t)]$ describes the stimulus past at each instant t. Note that the past of the input $[x(\tau), \tau \leq t]$ changes with t. The coefficients $c_0, c_1, \ldots, c_n$, then, change at each instant t and assume both positive and negative values.

The functional F_s can now be considered as a function of $n + 1$ variables and it can be expanded in terms of the class of Hermite functions which constitute an orthonormal function family over the interval $(-\infty, \infty)$. Wiener chose the class of Hermite functions for this purpose because they have some convenient mathematical properties if the coefficients $c_0, c_1, \ldots, c_n$ are the Laguerre coefficients of a white-noise signal (which they are). The result of this expansion can be shown to be (cf. Bose, 1956)

$$y(t) = \sum_{i=0}^{\infty} \sum_{j=0}^{\infty} \cdots \sum_{k=0}^{\infty} a_{ij\cdots k}\eta_i(c_0)\eta_j(c_1) \cdots \eta_k(c_n) \exp\left[-\tfrac{1}{2}(c_0^2 + \cdots + c_n^2)\right] \tag{4.88}$$

where η are the Hermite polynomials.

The coefficients $a_{ij\cdots k}$ characterize the system S completely and the identification problem reduces to the problem of determining these coefficients. That is, knowing the set of these coefficients for a particular system we can compute the response of this system to any input by use of Eq. (4.88). It can be shown that the characterizing coefficients are given by

$$a_{ij\cdots k} = (2\pi)^{n/2} E[y(t)\eta_i(c_0)\eta_j(c_1)\cdots \eta_k(c_n)] \qquad (4.89)$$

where $y(t)$ is the response of the system to a white-noise input $x(t)$ and $\{c_0, c_1, \ldots, c_n\}$ is the set of coefficients that characterize $x(t)$ at each time. Equation (4.89) is obtained by performing a least mean-square-error fit between the actual response of the system, $y(t)$, and the response as given by Eq. (4.88) over the entire range of the input–output record [where the input $x(t)$ is Gaussian white noise].

After the system has been tested with white noise for a sufficiently long time and both the input $x(t)$ and the output $y(t)$ have been recorded, we proceed as shown in Fig. 4.14 to determine the set of characterizing coefficients $\{a_{ij\cdots k}\}$. In this analysis procedure the coefficients are evaluated serially, and each time the whole length of the records has to be used. Once these coefficients have been determined they can be used to synthesize the nonlinear model of the system in terms of Eq. (4.88). The synthesis procedure is shown diagrammatically in Fig. 4.14.

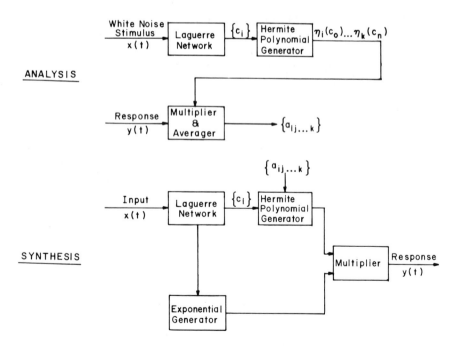

Fig. 4.14. Analysis and synthesis procedure of Wiener method.

This formulation is impractical and difficult to apply to physiological systems in an experimental situation for the following reasons:

(a) The number of coefficients needed to characterize almost any system, linear or nonlinear, is extremely large. If n coefficients are used in the Laguerre expansion to describe the past of the input at any time and p coefficients are used to expand the system functional in terms of Hermite functions, then the number of coefficients needed to characterize the system is p^n. Exploratory calculations showed that even for a simple nonlinear system such as a system with only a second-order nonlinearity the number of characterizing coefficients has to be as large as 10^{10}.

(b) The computing time required for the evaluation of the characterizing coefficients is extremely long, especially since the computation has to be performed serially. In the synthesis phase, when the response to a particular input is desired, the computation is again very long because of the multitude of the coefficients and the repeated Laguerre and Hermite expansions.

(c) It is difficult to assign some meaning to the characterizing coefficients that would reveal some functional and structural features of the system under this formulation of the theory. The coefficients of the expansion are purely formal mathematical quantities, and it appears futile to attempt to draw an analogy between them and properties of the system that they characterize.

(d) The method is basically a curve-fitting procedure and not a descriptive algebra of systems from which we are able to manipulate systems as building blocks for more and more complicated structures. This point is very crucial for the study of biological systems and especially for the ambitious undertaking of the study of the very complicated structure of the central nervous system.

(e) Even a linear system, which is characterized very simply by the classical linear theory, is characterized in a very cumbersome way by this method. A vast number of coefficients are needed to identify a linear system. This is due to the fact that a very large number of Hermite functions is needed to represent a linear transformation.

(f) It is very difficult to incorporate into Wiener's method any *a priori* information about the system so as to plan the computation for shorter length and to reduce the number of the characterizing coefficients. Point (e) is an example of this serious shortcoming of this very general method: The method, in being so very general, fails to recognize a simple situation and treat it accordingly.

(g) The derived nonlinear model is too cumbersome to use for prediction or comparison with experimental results even if a digital computer is available.

All these reasons point to the need for alternative schemes of measuring the system kernels if the white-noise method is to become a working tool for identifying physiological systems. There are other schemes where the kernels are expanded in terms of families of functions, but all tend to suffer from at least some of these difficulties (cf. Bose, 1956; Brandstetter and Amorocho, 1970; French and Butz, 1974).

4.3.2. The Lee–Schetzen Approach (Crosscorrelation Technique)

Lee and Schetzen (1965) starting with the Wiener functional series, showed how the set of kernels h_i can be evaluated by use of crosscorrelation techniques.

An experiment is performed on a system S with $x(t)$ the white-noise input signal and $y(t)$ the response of S to it. The kernels can then be estimated by the following procedures.

Measurement of h_0. The average value of each $G_k[h_k; x(t)]$ (for $k \geq 1$) is zero if $x(t)$ is Gaussian white noise with zero mean, since they are constructed orthogonal to the constant h_0, i.e., $E[h_0 G_k] = h_0 E[G_k] = 0$. For example,

$$E[G_2[h_2; x(t)]]$$

$$= E\left[\iint h_2(\tau_1, \tau_2)x(t-\tau_1)x(t-\tau_2)\, d\tau_1\, d\tau_2\right] - E\left[P\int h_2(\tau_1, \tau_1)\, d\tau_1\right]$$

$$= \iint h_2(\tau_1, \tau_2)E[x(t-\tau_1)x(t-\tau_2)]\, d\tau_1\, d\tau_2 - P\int h_2(\tau_1, \tau_1)\, d\tau_1$$

$$= \iint h_2(\tau_1, \tau_2)P\delta(\tau_1-\tau_2)\, d\tau_1\, d\tau_2 - P\int h_2(\tau_1, \tau_1)\, d\tau_1 = 0 \qquad (4.90)$$

Therefore, taking the average of the response $y(t)$ to Gaussian white-noise input $x(t)$ results in

$$E[y(t)] = h_0 \qquad (4.91)$$

Thus, the zero-order kernel h_0 is simply the average of the system response to a Gaussian white-noise input.

Measurement of $h_1(\tau)$. Wiener constructed each functional $G_k[h_k; x(t)]$ such that it is orthogonal to *all* homogeneous functionals of $x(t)$ whose degree is less than k. With this in mind, we multiply both sides of Eq. (4.38) by $x(t-\sigma)$ and take their average value. Since $x(t-\sigma)$ is a homogeneous functional of degree 1, all G functionals of order higher than 1 vanish. Also

$$E[x(t-\sigma)h_0] = 0 \qquad (4.92)$$

since $x(t)$ is a Gaussian signal of zero mean. Then, all that remains is

$$E[y(t)x(t-\sigma)] = E\left[x(t-\sigma)\int_0^\infty h_1(\tau)x(t-\tau)\, d\tau\right] \qquad (4.93)$$

or

$$\phi_{yx}(\sigma) = \int_0^\infty h_1(\tau)E[x(t-\sigma)x(t-\tau)] \, d\tau \tag{4.94}$$

Since $x(t)$ is Gaussian white noise we have

$$E[x(t-\sigma)x(t-\tau)] = \phi_{xx}(\tau-\sigma) = P\delta(\tau-\sigma) \tag{4.95}$$

and then

$$\phi_{yx}(\sigma) = \int_0^\infty h_1(\tau)P\delta(\tau-\sigma) \, d\tau$$

$$= Ph_1(\sigma) \tag{4.96}$$

Thus, the first-order kernel is given by the crosscorrelation function between the input white-noise stimulus and the resulting response

$$h_1(\sigma) = (1/P)\phi_{yx}(\sigma) \tag{4.97}$$

Measurement of $h_2(\tau_1, \tau_2)$. To measure $h_2(\tau_1, \tau_2)$ we multiply both sides of Eq. (4.38) by $x(t-\sigma_1)x(t-\sigma_2)$ and take the average. Terms of degree higher than the second vanish since $x(t-\sigma_1)x(t-\sigma_2)$ is a homogeneous functional of $x(t)$ of degree 2. The zero-order functional gives

$$E[G_0 x(t-\sigma_1)x(t-\sigma_2)] = h_0 P\delta(\sigma_1-\sigma_2) \tag{4.98}$$

The first-order functional gives

$$E[G_1(t)x(t-\sigma_1)x(t-\sigma_2)] = \int h_1(\tau)E[x(t-\sigma_1)x(t-\sigma_2)x(t-\tau)] \, d\tau$$

$$= 0 \tag{4.99}$$

since the average of an odd number of Gaussian variables of zero mean is zero. Proceeding, we have for the second-order functional

$$E[G_2(t)x(t-\sigma_1)x(t-\sigma_2)]$$

$$= E\left[x(t-\sigma_1)x(t-\sigma_2)\int\int h_2(\tau_1, \tau_2)x(t-\tau_1)x(t-\tau_2) \, d\tau_1 \, d\tau_2\right]$$

$$- E\left[x(t-\sigma_1)x(t-\sigma_2)P\int h_2(\tau_1, \tau_1) \, d\tau_1\right] \tag{4.100}$$

Recalling that for Gaussian variables x_1, x_2, x_3 and x_4 we have

$$E[x_1 x_2 x_3 x_4] = E[x_1 x_2]E[x_3 x_4] + E[x_1 x_3]E[x_2 x_4] + E[x_1 x_4]E[x_2 x_3]$$

$$\tag{4.101}$$

Since $x(t)$ is both Gaussian and white, the expression (4.100) becomes

$$P^2 \iint h_2(\tau_1, \tau_2)[\delta(\tau_1 - \tau_2)\delta(\sigma_1 - \sigma_2) + \delta(\tau_1 - \sigma_1)\delta(\tau_2 - \sigma_2)$$

$$+ \delta(\tau_2 - \sigma_1)\delta(\tau_1 - \sigma_2)] \, d\tau_1 \, d\tau_2$$

$$- P^2\delta(\sigma_1 - \sigma_2) \int h_2(\tau_1, \tau_1) \, d\tau_1$$

$$= P^2\left[\int h_2(\tau_1, \tau_1)\delta(\sigma_1 - \sigma_2) \, d\tau_1 + h_2(\sigma_1, \sigma_2) + h_2(\sigma_2, \sigma_1)\right]$$

$$- P^2\delta(\sigma_1 - \sigma_2) \int h_2(\tau_1, \tau_1) \, d\tau_1$$

$$= 2P^2 h_2(\sigma_1, \sigma_2) \tag{4.102}$$

Thus, finally collecting the terms due to G_0, G_1, and G_2 we have

$$\phi_{yxx}(\sigma_1, \sigma_2) = Ph_0\delta(\sigma_1 - \sigma_2) + 2P^2 h_2(\sigma_1, \sigma_2) \tag{4.103}$$

In order to eliminate the first term on the right-hand side it is desirable to subtract from $y(t)$ its average value (i.e., h_0) and then perform the second-order crosscorrelation with the resulting function, which we may call $y_0(t)$. That is,

$$y_0(t) = y(t) - h_0 = y(t) - E[\![y(t)]\!] \tag{4.104}$$

Then,

$$\phi_{y_0xx}(\sigma_1, \sigma_2) = 2P^2 h_2(\sigma_1, \sigma_2) \tag{4.105}$$

and

$$h_2(\sigma_1, \sigma_2) = (1/2P^2)\phi_{y_0xx}(\sigma_1, \sigma_2) \tag{4.106}$$

Suppose now that besides subtracting h_0 [the average value of $y(t)$] we also subtract the part of the response due to the linear kernel $h_1(\tau)$, i.e.,

$$y_1(t) = y(t) - h_0 - \int_0^\infty h_1(\tau)x(t - \tau) \, d\tau \tag{4.107}$$

where $x(t)$ is the white-noise signal used in the experiment. Then it is easily shown that we still have

$$\phi_{y_1xx}(\sigma_1, \sigma_2) = 2P^2 h_2(\sigma_1, \sigma_2) \tag{4.108}$$

In fact, in practice, it is usually desirable to subtract both the average value of the response and its "linear component" due to $h_1(\tau)$ before performing the second-order crosscorrelation that gives $h_2(\tau_1, \tau_2)$. This is due to the fact that in practice we deal with finite-length signals for which the averages may deviate somewhat (statistical variance) from the ones obtained in theory. In the present example, the average of $x(t-\sigma_1)x(t-\sigma_2)$ multiplied by $G_1[h_1; x(t)]$ might be a small number rather than zero, introducing an error that may be reduced if we use Eq. (4.108) rather than Eq. (4.106).

Figure 4.15 shows all the computational steps necessary for the estimation of the first- and second-order kernels of a given nonlinear system. Segments of the stimulus and response signals and how these are processed during this procedure are shown.

Measurement of $h_3(\tau_1, \tau_2, \tau_3)$. To measure $h_3(\tau_1, \tau_2, \tau_3)$ we multiply both sides of Eq. (4.38) by $x(t-\sigma_1)x(t-\sigma_2)x(t-\sigma_3)$ and take the average. Then G functionals of order higher than the third vanish since they are orthogonal to this functional. Using the properties of the autocorrelation functions of Gaussian signals discussed in Sec. 2.5, we can easily show that

$$E[\![G_0 x(t-\sigma_1)x(t-\sigma_2)x(t-\sigma_3)]\!] = 0 \tag{4.109}$$

$$E[\![G_1(t)x(t-\sigma_1)x(t-\sigma_2)x(t-\sigma_3)]\!]$$
$$= P^2[h_1(\sigma_1)\delta(\sigma_2-\sigma_3)+h_1(\sigma_2)\delta(\sigma_1-\sigma_3)+h_1(\sigma_3)\delta(\sigma_1-\sigma_2)] \tag{4.110}$$

$$E[\![G_2(t)x(t-\sigma_1)x(t-\sigma_2)x(t-\sigma_3)]\!] = 0 \tag{4.111}$$

$$E[\![G_3(t)x(t-\sigma_1)x(t-\sigma_2)x(t-\sigma_3)]\!] = 6P^3 h_3(\sigma_1, \sigma_2, \sigma_3) \tag{4.112}$$

Equation (4.110) suggests that before doing the third-order crosscorrelation [which leads us to the estimation of $h_3(\tau_1, \tau_2, \tau_3)$] one should subtract from the response $y(t)$ the contribution of functional $G_1(t)$. Since $h_1(\tau)$ has already been estimated, this can be done easily. Further, the subtraction of the estimated zero- and second-order G functionals will improve the accuracy of the third-order kernel estimate, even though it is not theoretically required. Therefore, we first compute the second-order response residual $y_2(t)$:

$$y_2(t) = y(t) - G_2(t) - G_1(t) - G_0 \tag{4.113}$$

and then we estimate the third-order kernel by computing the third-order crosscorrelation ϕ_{y_2xxx}. Then

$$h_3(\sigma_1, \sigma_2, \sigma_3) = (1/6P^3)E[\![y_2(t)x(t-\sigma_1)x(t-\sigma_2)x(t-\sigma_3)]\!] \tag{4.114}$$

Similarly, we can show that for the estimation of the nth-order kernel we need to obtain the nth-order crosscorrelation

$$h_n(\sigma_1, \sigma_2, \ldots, \sigma_n)$$
$$= \frac{1}{n!P^n} E\left[\!\left[\left(y(t) - \sum_{k=0}^{n-1} G_k(t)\right) x(t-\sigma_1)x(t-\sigma_2) \cdots x(t-\sigma_n)\right]\!\right] \tag{4.115}$$

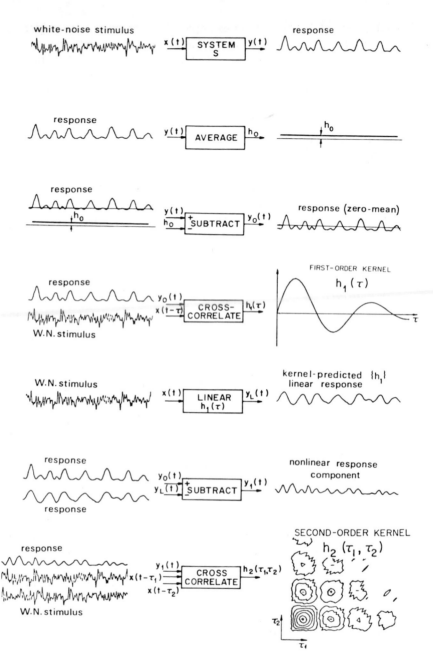

Fig. 4.15. Successive steps of first- and second-order kernel estimation.

between the stimulus $x(t)$ and the response, which is unaccounted for by the previous $(n-1)$ G functionals.

The approach of estimating the kernels through crosscorrelation has several advantages over the Wiener formulation and it makes it feasible (with some restrictions) to identify a physical nonlinear system by subjecting it to a white-noise stimulus.

First, it directly estimates the kernels, which, as described earlier, have a definite functional meaning; they can reveal interesting properties and provide an insight to the structure of the system under study.

Second, the crosscorrelation method is much simpler computationally because it does not involve the cumbersome Laguerre and Hermite transformations.

Third, a linear system is easily recognized by the crosscorrelation method, because the derived model takes a simple form and therefore the computational burden is reduced while insight into the nature of the system is increased.

Fourth, the synthesis problem is very simple. Estimating the response to a particular input involves only a few integrations.

Fifth, once the kernels are known, it is not difficult to construct alternative mathematical models such as structures consisting of linear filters (for which powerful theories exist) and static nonlinearities.

Sixth, truncation error does not occur in the crosscorrelation method, whereas in the Wiener formulation the expansion of the stimulus in the orthogonal family of Laguerre functions, which for any practical application has to be truncated, induces an inherent approximation error.

Seventh, *a priori* information about the system can be utilized to reduce the identification effort by reducing the computational burden.

4.3.3. A Paradigm: White-Noise Analysis of a Physiological System

To illustrate some of the ideas so far presented, we give here an example of applying the Gaussian white-noise method to a specific physiological system. This system is the one that transforms light intensity variations, impinging upon the vertebrate retina, into a variable ganglion cell discharge rate (Fig. 4.16). The stimulus, therefore, consists of light intensity modulated in Gaussian white-noise fashion around a nonzero mean. The response is the extracellularly recorded neural spikes train, which has been transformed in time to produce a quasicontinuous waveform reflecting the instantaneous spike frequency of the cell. Once the Gaussian white-noise experiment is performed, the stimulus–response data are processed to estimate the first- and second-order kernels of the system, as was illustrated in Fig. 4.15. Figure 4.17 shows the results for this particular experiment.

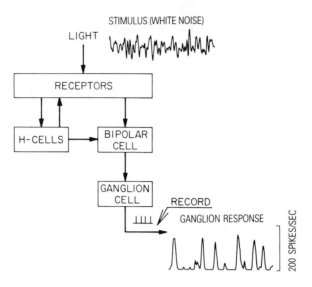

Fig. 4.16. Experiment diagram.

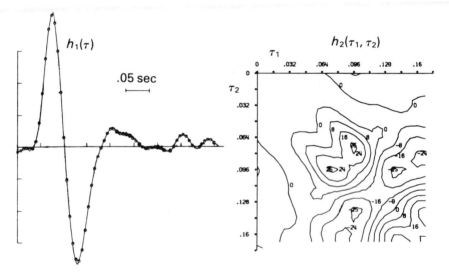

Fig. 4.17. First- and second-order kernels for field light → ganglion cell.

The linear kernel h_1 is strongly underdamped; in fact, it seems that the system acts as a differentiator. The same figure also shows the estimated second-order kernel. As discussed in Sec. 4.2, this denotes the nonlinear interaction between portions of the stimulus past, as they affect the system response at the present. For example, with reference to the second-order kernel shown, we note that a positive stimulus impulse given 100 msec in the past followed by another positive impulse given 80 msec in the past will produce at the present a strong additional component to the response beyond that already predicted by the first-order kernel. On the other hand, depression of the response will occur for an impulse given 150 msec in the past followed by one given 100 msec in the past. All this information is exhibited in the contour map figure of the second-order kernel.

Using these kernels, one can predict the system response to any input. Of course, the question arises as to how good the characterization of the system in terms of these two kernels is. Wiener has argued that the most stringent test to which a system characterization (model) can be subjected is to obtain the system response, as predicted by this characterization, to Gaussian white-noise stimulus and compare it to the actual system response to the same stimulus. The rationale behind this argument is, of course, that with white-noise input one tests the system and also its characterization exhaustively with almost all possible stimuli.

Accordingly, we indicate the goodness of the present characterization of the light → ganglion system as shown in Fig. 4.18. We consider a portion of the white-noise stimulus and corresponding experimental response, and then compute the linear model response, that is, the response predicted by the first-order kernel to this same white-noise stimulus (shown in the figure). In addition, we compute the nonlinear model response as predicted by both the first- and second-order kernels (also shown in the figure). We note that while the linear model does behave somewhat as the experimental response, the nonlinear model is a considerable improvement, especially in reproducing the high frequencies in the system response and nonlinearities manifested by the cutoff.

A convenient quantitative way to measure the agreement of the characterization with the experimental response is in terms of the mean-

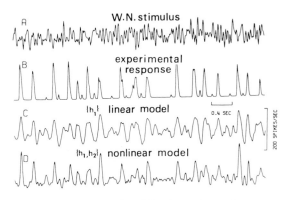

Fig. 4.18. Comparison of model and experimental responses.

square-error reduction. This process is approximately the following: A straight line, as given by the zero-order kernel, is least-squares-error fitted to the experimental response. The mean-square deviation of the response waveform from this straight line is measured and normalized to 100 units. Subsequently, the model response as predicted by the first-order kernel $\{h_1\}$ (e.g., shown in trace C in Fig. 4.18) is estimated and its mean-square deviation from the experimental response is measured. This error is normalized to the same units as before, and, of course, in general it should be a number less than 100 (note that, because of the orthogonality of the Wiener functionals, this is the minimum mean-square error achievable with a linear model). Subsequently the deviation of the nonlinear model response, as predicted by kernels $\{h_1, h_2\}$, is measured and normalized to the same units. For the system at hand, these reductions were found to be

Characterization	$\{h_0\}$	$\{h_0, h_1\}$	$\{h_0, h_1, h_2\}$
Mean-square error	100	46	21

From the mean-square-error reduction we can see that the system is quite nonlinear and that the nonlinear second-order kernel introduces a substantial improvement.

4.4. Multi-Input, Multi-Output Systems

The white-noise method can readily be extended to systems with more than one input and output. As will be discussed below, such an extension is very desirable in the case of biological systems, which, as a rule, have short experimental lifetimes over which the identification process (white-noise test) can be carried out. This shortness of the testing period is often a result of the technical difficulty in measuring the system responses or a result of nonstationarity of physiological systems, which forces us to complete the experiment within time intervals over which the system characteristics do not change appreciably. A multi-input white-noise test, as extended here, allows us to maximize the rate of information gathering on the stimulus–response behavior of the system, because, as will be shown, it allows us—by its nature—to separate the effect of each input on the response. Thus, a two-input white-noise experiment provides the information of two one-input experiments plus additional information (about the interaction between the two input stimuli).

Consider, for instance, a system with two inputs $x(t)$ and $u(t)$ and one output, $y(t)$ (Fig. 4.19). For example, input $x(t)$ may be light intensity of a visual stimulus, $u(t)$ may be an acoustic signal, and $y(t)$ the measured evoked response from an electrode on the cortex (an EEG). Or, $x(t)$ may be current injected into one neuron and $u(t)$ may be the current injected

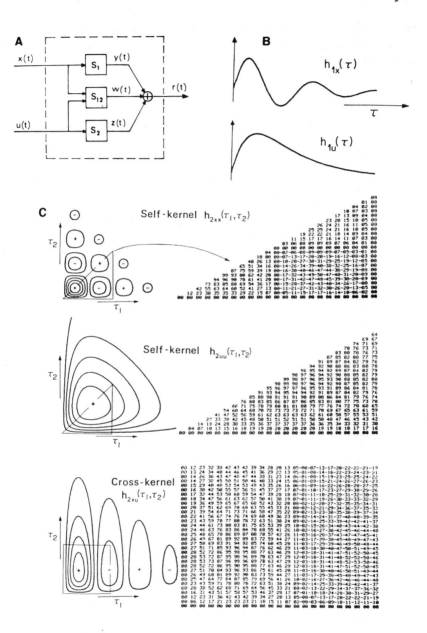

Fig. 4.19. (A) Two-input system characterizing (B) first- and (C) second-order kernels.

into a second neuron, while $y(t)$ is the response of a neuron further up in the signal-processing chain. Then, proceeding in a manner analogous to the one-input case, we have

$$y(t) = \sum_{n=0}^{\infty} G_n[\{h\}_n; x(t), u(t)] \tag{4.116}$$

where $\{h\}_n$ is the set of nth-order kernels arising from homogeneous functionals in both $x(t)$ and $u(t)$. The G functionals are again constructed orthogonal for $x(t)$ and $u(t)$ being statistically independent Gaussian white-noise signals. The orthogonalization procedure is similar to the one followed in the single-input case. Notice that terms depending on both inputs appear in this case. These terms represent the nonlinear interaction between the two inputs.

The first three terms of this series are given by

$$G_0[\{h\}_0; x(t), u(t)] = h_{0x} + h_{0u} \tag{4.117}$$

$$G_1[\{h\}_1; x(t), u(t)] = \int_0^{\infty} h_{1x}(\tau)x(t-\tau)\, d\tau + \int_0^{\infty} h_{1u}(\tau)u(t-\tau)\, d\tau \tag{4.118}$$

$$G_2[\{h\}_2; x(t), u(t)]$$

$$= \int\!\!\int_0^{\infty} h_{2xx}(\tau_1, \tau_2)x(t-\tau_1)x(t-\tau_2)\, d\tau_1\, d\tau_2 - P_x \int_0^{\infty} h_{2xx}(\tau, \tau)\, d\tau$$

$$+ \int\!\!\int_0^{\infty} h_{2uu}(\tau_1, \tau_2)u(t-\tau_1)u(t-\tau_2)\, d\tau_1\, d\tau_2 - P_u \int_0^{\infty} h_{2uu}(\tau, \tau)\, d\tau$$

$$+ \int\!\!\int_0^{\infty} h_{2xu}(\tau_1, \tau_2)x(t-\tau_1)u(t-\tau_2)\, d\tau_1\, d\tau_2 \tag{4.119}$$

where P_x, P_u are the power levels of the independent white-noise inputs $x(t)$ and $u(t)$, respectively. That is,

$$E[x(t)x(t-\tau)] = \phi_{xx}(\tau) = P_x \delta(\tau) \tag{4.120}$$

$$E[u(t)u(t-\tau)] = \phi_{uu}(\tau) = P_u \delta(\tau) \tag{4.121}$$

Kernels h_{0x}, h_{1x}, h_{2xx} (along with h_{0u}, h_{1u}, h_{2uu}) are called "*self-kernels*" since they describe the effect of each input by itself (notice that the self-kernels are not affected by the other input for a second-order system). The self-kernels are symmetric functions of their arguments. Kernel $h_{2xu}(\tau_1, \tau_2)$ is called a "*cross-kernel*," and it is, in general, an asymmetric function of its arguments (notice that the term arising from it depends on

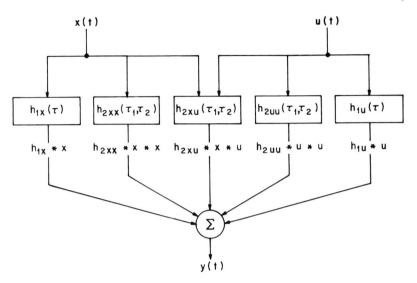

Fig. 4.20. Kernel diagram for two-input–one-output second-order system.

both $x(t)$ and $u(t)$). The cross-kernel describes the (second-order) *non-linear interaction* of the two inputs as it affects the system response, while the self-kernels describe the individual contribution of each input to the response. Figure 4.19 shows a nonlinear system with two inputs and one output along with the first- and second-order self- and cross-kernels characterizing it. A schematic diagram is shown in Fig. 4.20.

These kernels can be estimated through the use of crosscorrelation techniques on the stimulus–response data (as shown below) in a way similar to the one of the single-input case.

Estimation of Multi-Input System Kernels

Measurement of h_{0x} or h_{0u}. Each G functional of order higher than zero has zero average value if $x(t)$ and $u(t)$ are independent Gaussian white-noise signals of zero mean. Thus

$$E[y(t)] = h_{0x} + h_{0u} \qquad (4.122)$$

It may be desirable to know h_{0x} and h_{0u} separately. Assuming that all kernels of order higher than the second are zero, we can find each of h_{0x} and h_{0u}. If we let $x(t) = 0$ in Eq. (4.116), the resulting expression should be the same as for the single-input $[u(t)$ only$]$ case. Thus, we must have

$$h_{0x} = P_x \int_0^\infty h_{2xx}(\tau, \tau)\, d\tau \qquad (4.123)$$

Similarly

$$h_{0u} = P_u \int_0^\infty h_{2uu}(\tau, \tau) \, d\tau \qquad (4.124)$$

Thus we can find h_{0x} and h_{0u} separately once the second-order self-kernels h_{2xx} and h_{2uu} have been measured.

Also, h_{0x}, and h_{0u} can *always* be found separately by performing separate single-input white-noise experiments, regardless of the number of functional terms in the series.

Measurements of $h_{1x}(\tau)$ or $h_{1u}(\tau)$. To estimate $h_{1x}(\sigma)$ we multiply each side of Eq. (4.116) by $x(t-\sigma)$ and take the average. It should be noted that all the G_k functionals of order other than the first are by construction orthogonal to $x(t-\sigma)$ (a homogeneous functional of first order). Thus we obtain

$$\phi_{yx}(\sigma) = E[\![y(t)x(t-\sigma)]\!]$$

$$= E\left[\!\left[\int h_{1x}(\tau)x(t-\tau) \, d\tau x(t-\sigma) \right]\!\right]$$

$$+ E\left[\!\left[\int h_{1u}(\tau)u(t-\tau) \, d\tau x(t-\sigma) \right]\!\right] \qquad (4.125)$$

and since $x(t)$ and $u(t)$ are statistically independent

$$E[\![x(t-\sigma)u(t-\tau)]\!] = 0 \qquad (4.126)$$

and

$$\phi_{yx}(\sigma) = \int h_{1x}(\tau)\phi_{xx}(\tau-\sigma) \, d\tau$$

$$= P_x h_{1x}(\sigma) \qquad (4.127)$$

Therefore

$$h_{1x}(\sigma) = (1/P_x)\phi_{yx}(\sigma) \qquad (4.128)$$

and, similarly

$$h_{1u}(\sigma) = (1/P_u)\phi_{yu}(\sigma) \qquad (4.129)$$

Measurement of $h_{2xx}(\tau_1, \tau_2)$ or $h_{2uu}(\tau_1, \tau_2)$. We proceed in a similar fashion, multiplying both sides by $x(t-\sigma_1)x(t-\sigma_2)$ in order to estimate $h_{2xx}(\sigma_1, \sigma_2)$. Again, taking into account that $x(t)$ and $u(t)$ are statistically independent Gaussian white-noise signals, we find

$$h_{2xx}(\sigma_1, \sigma_2) = (1/2P_x^2)\phi_{yoxx}(\sigma_1, \sigma_2) \qquad (4.130)$$

and

$$h_{2uu}(\sigma_1, \sigma_2) = (1/2P_u^2)\phi_{youu}(\sigma_1, \sigma_2) \qquad (4.131)$$

where

$$y_0(t) = y(t) - G_0 \qquad (G_0 = h_{0x} + h_{0u}) \qquad (4.132)$$

Measurement of $h_{2xu}(\tau_1, \tau_2)$. To estimate the cross-kernel $h_{2xu}(\sigma_1, \sigma_2)$ at (σ_1, σ_2) we multiply both sides of Eq. (4.116) by $x(t-\sigma_1)u(t-\sigma_2)$ and take the expected value to get (considering each term separately) the following:

$$E[G_0 x(t-\sigma_1)u(t-\sigma_2)] = 0 \tag{4.133}$$

Since $x(t)$ and $u(t)$ are independent, i.e.,

$$\phi_{xu}(\sigma_1 - \sigma_2) = E[x(t-\sigma_1)u(t-\sigma_2)] = 0 \tag{4.134}$$

The G_1 functional gives rise to terms of the form

$$E\left[\int h_{1x}(\tau)x(t-\tau)\,d\tau x(t-\sigma_1)u(t-\sigma_2)\right]$$

$$= \int h_{1x}(\tau)E[x(t-\tau)x(t-\sigma_1)u(t-\sigma_2)]\,d\tau = 0 \tag{4.135}$$

since the average of the product of three Gaussian variables with zero mean is zero. Similarly for the term that involves $h_{1u}(\tau)$. The G_2 functional gives rise to terms of the form

$$E\left[\int h_{2xx}(\tau_1, \tau_2)x(t-\tau_1)x(t-\tau_2)\,d\tau_1\,d\tau_2 x(t-\sigma_1)u(t-\sigma_2)\right]$$

$$= \int h_{2xx}(\tau_1, \tau_2)E[x(t-\tau_1)x(t-\tau_2)x(t-\sigma_1)u(t-\sigma_2)]\,d\tau_1\,d\tau_2 \tag{4.136}$$

Since $x(t)$ and $u(t)$ are independent and have zero mean, we have

$$E[x(t-\tau_1)x(t-\tau_2)x(t-\sigma_1)u(t-\sigma_2)]$$

$$= E[x(t-\tau_1)x(t-\tau_2)x(t-\sigma_1)]E[u(t-\sigma_2)]$$

$$= 0 \tag{4.137}$$

Similarly for the term that involves $h_{2uu}(\tau_1, \tau_2)$.

Further, the G functionals of order higher than the second are also orthogonal to $x(t-\sigma_1)u(t-\sigma_2)$. Thus the crosscorrelation ϕ_{yxu} reduces to

$$\phi_{yxu}(\sigma_1, \sigma_2) = E[y(t)x(t-\sigma_1)u(t-\sigma_2)]$$

$$= E\left[\int\int\int_0^\infty h_{2xu}(\tau_1, \tau_2)x(t-\tau_1)u(t-\tau_2)\,d\tau_1\,d\tau_2 x(t-\sigma_1)u(t-\sigma_2)\right]$$

$$= \int\int_0^\infty h_{2xu}(\tau_1, \tau_2)E[x(t-\tau_1)x(t-\sigma_1)]$$

$$\times E[u(t-\tau_2 u(t-\sigma_2)]\,d\tau_1\,d\tau_2$$

$$= \int\int_0^\infty h_{2xu}(\tau_1, \tau_2)P_x\delta(\tau_1-\sigma_1)P_u\delta(\tau_2-\sigma_2)\,d\tau_1\,d\tau_2$$

$$= P_x P_u h_{2xu}(\sigma_1, \sigma_2) \tag{4.138}$$

Therefore the cross-kernel h_{2xu} is estimated as

$$h_{2xu}(\sigma_1, \sigma_2) = \frac{1}{P_x P_u} E[\![y(t)x(t-\sigma_1)u(t-\sigma_2)]\!] \qquad (4.139)$$

Note that the cross-kernel is, in general, an asymmetric function of its arguments.

The estimation of h_{2xu} (contrary to h_{2xx} and h_{2uu}) does not theoretically require the use of the response residual $y_0(t) = y(t) - G_0$ in the cross-correlation. However, the use of the response residual in the actual estimation of the cross-kernel will improve the accuracy of the estimate obtained. In general, it is suggested that the highest possible response residual is used in actual evaluations of crosscorrelations, since that improves the accuracy of the kernels estimated by use of finite records.

The Third-Order Term for a Two-Input, One-Output System

The third-order term will have kernels such as $h_{3xxx}(\tau_1, \tau_2, \tau_3)$, $h_{3uuu}(\tau_1, \tau_2, \tau_3)$, $h_{3xuu}(\tau_1, \tau_2, \tau_3)$, $h_{3uxx}(\tau_1, \tau_2, \tau_3)$. It is given by

$$G_3[\{h\}_3; x(t), u(t)]$$

$$= \iiint h_{3xxx}(\tau_1, \tau_2, \tau_3)x(t-\tau_1)x(t-\tau_2)x(t-\tau_3)\,d\tau_1\,d\tau_2\,d\tau_3$$

$$- 3P_x \iint h_{3xxx}(\tau_1, \tau_2, \tau_2)x(t-\tau_1)\,d\tau_1\,d\tau_2$$

$$+ \iiint h_{3uuu}(\tau_1, \tau_2, \tau_3)u(t-\tau_1)u(t-\tau_2)u(t-\tau_3)\,d\tau_1\,d\tau_2\,d\tau_3$$

$$- 3P_u \iint h_{3uuu}(\tau_1, \tau_2, \tau_2)u(t-\tau_1)\,d\tau_1\,d\tau_2$$

$$+ \iiint h_{3xuu}(\tau_1, \tau_2, \tau_3)x(t-\tau_1)u(t-\tau_2)u(t-\tau_3)\,d\tau_1\,d\tau_2\,d\tau_3$$

$$- P_u \iint h_{3xuu}(\tau_1, \tau_2, \tau_2)x(t-\tau_1)\,d\tau_1\,d\tau_2$$

$$+ \iiint h_{3uxx}(\tau_1, \tau_2, \tau_3)u(t-\tau_1)x(t-\tau_2)x(t-\tau_3)\,d\tau_1\,d\tau_2\,d\tau_3$$

$$- P_x \iint h_{3uxx}(\tau_1, \tau_2, \tau_2)u(t-\tau_1)\,d\tau_1\,d\tau_2 \qquad (4.140)$$

and its kernels would be given by

$$h_{3xxx}(\sigma_1, \sigma_2, \sigma_3) = \frac{1}{3!P_x^3}\phi_{y2xxx}(\sigma_1, \sigma_2, \sigma_3) \qquad (4.141)$$

$$h_{3xuu}(\sigma_1, \sigma_2, \sigma_3) = \frac{1}{2P_x P_u^2} \phi_{y2xuu}(\sigma_1, \sigma_2, \sigma_3) \qquad (4.142)$$

etc., where

$$y_2(t) = y(t) - G_0 - G_1[\{h\}_1; x(t), u(t)] - G_2[\{h\}_2; x(t), u(t)] \qquad (4.143)$$

Theoretically, of course, we only need to subtract the response arising from G_1. However, in practice, it is desirable to subtract all lower-order responses because of estimation accuracy considerations.

Three-Input, One-Output System. For a system with three inputs $x(t)$, $u(t)$, $v(t)$, the first-order term will have kernels $h_{1x}(\tau)$, $h_{1u}(\tau)$, $h_{1v}(\tau)$ and the second-order term will have kernels $h_{2xx}(\tau_1, \tau_2)$, $h_{2uu}(\tau_1, \tau_2)$, $h_{2vv}(\tau_1, \tau_2)$, $h_{2xu}(\tau_1, \tau_2)$, $h_{2xv}(\tau_1, \tau_2)$, $h_{2uv}(\tau_1, \tau_2)$. To evaluate these kernels a white-noise experiment needs to be performed where stimuli $x(t)$, $u(t)$, and $v(t)$ are statistically independent Gaussian white-noise signals. From the stimulus–response data of this experiment, the kernels can be evaluated using crosscorrelation. For example,

$$h_{2uu}(\sigma_1, \sigma_2) = \frac{1}{2P_u^2} \phi_{y1uu}(\sigma_1, \sigma_2) \qquad (4.144)$$

and

$$h_{2xv}(\sigma_1, \sigma_2) = \frac{1}{P_x P_v} \phi_{y1xv}(\sigma_1, \sigma_2) \qquad (4.145)$$

where

$$y_1(t) = y(t) - G_0 - G_1[h_{1x}, h_{1u}, h_{1v}; x(t), u(t), v(t)] \qquad (4.146)$$

If the system has more than one output, say m of them, each one is treated separately with a resulting characterization in terms of m separate systems in parallel that share the same inputs. For example, consider a system with two inputs $x(t)$ and $u(t)$ and two outputs $y(t)$ and $w(t)$. This system will have first-order kernels $h_{1x}^y(\tau)$, $h_{1u}^y(\tau)$, $h_{1x}^w(\tau)$, $h_{1u}^w(\tau)$ and second-order kernels $h_{2xx}^y(\tau_1, \tau_2)$, $h_{2uu}^y(\tau_1, \tau_2)$, $h_{2xu}^y(\tau_1, \tau_2)$, $h_{2xx}^w(\tau_1, \tau_2)$, $h_{2uu}^w(\tau_1, \tau_2)$, $h_{2xu}^w(\tau_1, \tau_2)$. These kernels can be again found through appropriate crosscorrelation. For example

$$h_{1u}^y(\sigma) = \frac{1}{P_u} \phi_{yu}(\sigma) \qquad (4.147)$$

and

$$h_{2uu}^w(\sigma_1, \sigma_2) = \frac{1}{2P_u^2} \phi_{w0uu}(\sigma_1, \sigma_2) \qquad (4.148)$$

$$h_{2xu}^w(\sigma_1, \sigma_2) = \frac{1}{P_x P_u} \phi_{w0xu}(\sigma_1, \sigma_2) \qquad (4.149)$$

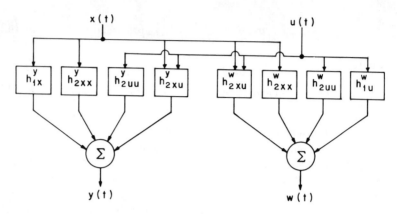

Fig. 4.21. Kernel diagram for two-input–two-output second-order system.

where

$$w_0(t) = w(t) - G_0 \qquad (4.150)$$

(Fig. 4.21). In the frequency domain this system can be conveniently written in matrix form (French and Butz, 1973).

4.5. Other Formulations of the White-Noise Approach

There are several other alternatives to the white-noise approach for testing physiological systems. In this section we briefly mention some of the other formulations only for the sake of completeness, and because they are particularly useful in special cases.

Bose uses an orthogonal class of functions that he calls "gate" functions, which are simply square unit pulses in time in order to partition the function space of the past of the input into nonoverlapping cells (hence orthogonality of the gate functions). This formulation is conceptually simple and it appears that it would be most suitable for systems that have strong saturating elements.

Katzenelson and Gould use the Volterra series and variational calculus techniques, minimizing the mean-square error between system response and model response in order to develop a systematic approach to determining system kernels. This results in a set of simultaneous integral equations, and an iteration procedure is devised for their solution. This approach seems to be computationally taxing, but it may be suitable if optimality in terms of mean-square error is the critical criterion.

In much the same way that Wiener used the family of Laguerre functions to expand the stimulus past, other families of functions can be used for the same purpose. Also, specialized stimuli (such as combinations of one or more impulses) can be used to test the system and from these results to calculate characterizing coefficients or functions.

We propose another alternative approach, which has some common characteristics with some of the above-mentioned approaches. Starting with the basic notion of the functional as the mathematical description of a system and utilizing the white-noise approach, one can devise several schemata for system identification. A very simple one would be the following. A grid is superposed over the past of the input in such a way that it covers the whole memory of the system and the total range of amplitudes of the input (Fig. 4.22). At any time t, the present input and its past are described by a vector of real numbers that gives the ordinates of the grid squares at the fixed times $(t_0, t_1, t_2, \ldots, t_n)$. This vector is put in correspondence with the value, y_0, of the system output at this time, thus forming the input–output vector $(x_0, x_1, \ldots, x_n, y_0)$. As the system is being tested with white noise, new input–output vectors are formed. Eventually, the system will have been exhaustively tested for all combinations of values of the input vectors $x_0, x_1, \ldots, x_n$. All these vectors could be easily stored in some form of auxiliary storage (disk, magnetic tape) of a digital computer and used as the "model" of the system. As an abstraction from this data base one could fit a function $F(x_0, x_1, \ldots, x_n)$ over the whole set of input–output vectors, which would then be the "transfer function" of the system. This function could be used to predict the response of the system to any input.

There are several noteworthy features of this formulation of the white-noise theory. First, it does not require a white-noise input from the statistical point of view since the method simply enumerates input–output correspondences. Instead, a more expedient way would be to put the input under computer control and enumerate all the possible combinations of

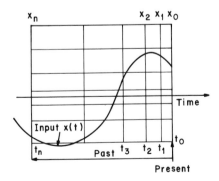

Fig. 4.22. Grid of stimulus past.

vector values $(x_0, x_1, \ldots, x_n)$. This would drastically cut down the testing time required for identifying the system (a white-noise signal is redundant in this sense since it is random and therefore potentially repetitious). Second, the grid square size can be varied depending on its position, thus weighting more heavily the more important regions of the signal. For example, it might be desired to have the squares more densely placed near t_0 than t_n since the immediate past usually affects the present output more than the remote past. Also, the horizontal grid lines could be more densely spaced near the nonlinearity of the system, e.g., where saturation might occur. Third, this formulation is conceptually very simple and it can readily be amended to fit any system peculiarities. Fourth, it can answer many questions about properties of the system under study, provided a suitable computer system exists to manipulate and abstract information from the resulting data base of input–output vectors.

However, this type of approach has also several disadvantages, such as the fact that it would be difficult to recognize, and needlessly complicated to describe, a linear system by it. Also, it would require a rather sophisticated and extensive computing facility to be usefully implemented.

Applicability of the White-Noise Method and the Use of Quasiwhite Test Signals

Introduction

The white-noise method of system identification, i.e., the Wiener formulation of the nonlinear system identification problem in connection with the crosscorrelation technique, appears to be a general, straightforward, and powerful approach to a subject where great mathematical complexity is usually encountered. However, the generality and the elegance of the method is bound to be moderated in actual applications by limitations imposed by reality.

The first reason for this is that the Gaussian white noise (for which the whole method has been designed), since it has an infinite frequency bandwidth and, consequently, infinite power, is not a physically realizable signal. Thus, in actual applications of the method, we have to use an approximate signal that exhibits the properties of the Gaussian white noise within a certain range of interest and up to a determinable degree. This was initially done by using band-limited Gaussian white noise (referred to simply as GWN). GWN has a flat power spectrum up to a characteristic cutoff frequency, which is determined so as to cover the bandwidth of the system being tested. The use of GWN, instead of ideal Gaussian white noise, introduces an estimation error, which varies according to the specific characteristics of each actual case, and which, in general, results in a loss of high frequencies in the kernel estimates.

A second practical restriction, and a source of estimation error in the application of the method, is the finite record length. Experimentation time and data recording time are naturally finite. Therefore, the stimulus and response records with which we compute the crosscorrelations are finite, and, consequently, the averages are calculated within some statistical error. This error, of course, is monotonically decreasing as the record length increases, and, consequently, it can be bounded to a determinable degree.

A third practical restriction is the extent of truncation of the Wiener series, a consequence of the computational capacity required to estimate higher-order kernels. The computation of the crosscorrelation estimates involves a great number of multiplications and additions, and this computational burden rapidly increases as we move to higher-order kernels. Therefore, we usually confine ourselves to the estimation of a few terms of the Wiener series, which ordinarily give a model of acceptable accuracy. This is the reason why the convergence pattern of the functional series is of great practical importance.

A fourth practical restriction is the truncation of the Guassian distribution, since the actual stimulus signal cannot attain infinite values. The error resulting from this restriction is usually insignificant.

Besides all these practical restrictions in the application of the method, there are limitations and errors associated with the numerical operations and the capacity of the digital computer being used to compute the kernel estimates.

Because of these problems in the actual application of the white-noise method we emphasize the compromises that provide the greatest possible advantages with respect to these inherent practical restrictions of the method.

The first approximating signal that comes to mind is the band-limited Gaussian white noise since it is physically realizable while still preserving the basic statistical properties of ideal Gaussian white noise. GWN is a Gaussian random process with a power spectrum flat over a finite range of frequencies, properly chosen to cover the bandwidth of the system under test. The autocorrelation properties of this signal are fairly close to the ones of ideal Gaussian white noise, and that allows its use as an approximating signal in the crosscorrelation technique. (cf. P. Z. Marmarelis, 1972.)

Beyond the problem of physical realizability, an important remaining practical problem is the long computations required for the statistical averages to form with tolerable deviations. Because of this problem, the use of pseudorandom signals based on m sequences (referred to simply as PRS) has been suggested. The PRS (being periodic and deterministic in nature), form the desirable second- and all odd-order autocorrelation functions in much shorter time, because they are constructed so that they eliminate the redundancy of a random signal. However, the higher even-order autocorrelation functions of PRS exhibit inherent anomalies that could cause serious estimation errors in identification of systems with higher-order nonlinearities (Gyftopoulos and Hooper, 1964; Barker and Pradisthayon, 1970).

These two families of approximately white signals have been predominantly used so far in applications of the white-noise method in nonlinear system identification. Note that we consider here only systems with continuous input. If a system has discrete input then a Poisson impulse train can be used as a quasiwhite test signal for its identification (Krausz, 1975.) The choice between GWN and PRS is made in each specific case on the basis of their relative advantages and disadvantages, which are discussed later.

We call these approximating signals "quasiwhite" since they are not really white but are used as such in applications of the white-noise method. Evidently, the construction of a new quasiwhite signal is a matter of creative thinking, and, therefore, their number can be extended. Understandably, the principal concerns of the users of the white-noise method are (a) the reduction of the inevitable estimation error to the minimum possible within the existing practical limitations and (b) the efficiency of the estimation procedure. These are the guidelines on which the choice or the design of a quasiwhite test signal is based. This search remains a challenging subject of the scientific effort in the field of system identification.

In our present study, we include a new family of quasiwhite test signals, which has been shown to possess its own characteristic blend of advantages and disadvantages in applications of the white-noise method (V. Z. Marmarelis, 1977); these are the constant-switching-pace symmetric random signals (CSRS).

In the following we will discuss the basic properties of these three families of quasiwhite signals (GWN, PRS, and CSRS) and the interesting aspects of their use in nonlinear system identification.

5.1. The Band-Limited Gaussian White Noise

The band-limited Gaussian white noise was the first quasiwhite signal to be employed in applications of the white-noise method. GWN is the first approximate signal that comes to mind in an attempt to physically realize ideal Gaussian white noise for which the whole theory had been developed through the remarkable work of a number of investigators (Wiener, 1942, 1958; Bose, 1956; Lee and Schetzen, 1965; Brilliant, 1958; George, 1959; Barrett, 1963). Successful applications of GWN were delayed by several practical limitations and difficulties, and they finally took place mainly in the area of biological systems (P. Z. Marmarelis and Naka, 1972; P. Z. Marmarelis and McCann, 1973; P. Z. Marmarelis and Naka, 1973*a,b,c,d*, 1974*a,b,c,d*; Stark, 1969; McCann, 1974; Lipson, 1975*a,b,c*; Bryant and Segundo, 1976; Moore *et al.,* 1975). The successful application of GWN in biological systems identification established the utility of the Wiener crosscorrelation method, and it signaled its extension into other areas of scientific research (Udwadia and Marmarelis, 1976).

5.1.1. General Description and Generation of GWN

Band-limited Gaussian white noise is a Gaussian random process with a rectangular power spectrum (see Fig. 5.1), the bandwidth B of which is chosen to cover the bandwidth of the system under test. The mean of the GWN is zero and the variance is determined by the dynamic range within which we want to test the operation of the system at hand. In practice we must truncate the tails of the Gaussian distribution beyond a certain number of standard deviations (usually $\pm 3\sigma$). In Fig. 5.1, an actual band-limited distribution-truncated Gaussian white-noise signal is shown, along with the corresponding amplitude distribution.

As discussed later, this quasiwhite signal preserves the basic autocorrelation properties that allow it to be used in nonlinear system identification in connection with the crosscorrelation technique.

The generation of GWN in the laboratory is not a simple task. A variety of methods have been used so far, but there is no universally accepted method of generation. Methods range from filtering of natural sources of approximately white noise to generation within the digital computer.

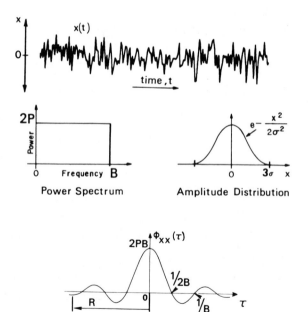

Fig. 5.1 Basic mathematical features of the band-limited distribution-truncated Gaussian white noise.

By "natural" noise sources we mean generators that depend for the *randomness* of their signal on certain probabilistic (random) physical phenomena. Such primary sources of random signals include electronic vacuum tubes, noisy solid state diodes, Zener diodes, and radioactive sources. The primary design requirement for the instrument producing the stimulus is stationarity of the signal.

The main problem with this type of noise generator (which is dependent upon a natural phenomenon) is that the power spectral density drops at low frequencies (about 10 Hz) while physiological systems respond primarily in this low-frequency region. To produce noise with a flat power spectrum starting at dc, demodulation techniques must be used. This has been done (cf. Korn, 1966). An interesting scheme has recently been proposed by French (1974), which depends on the Nyquist sampling theorem. According to it, if a signal is sampled at a frequency $f_s = 1/\Delta t$, then any frequency components of the signal that are greater than $1/2\Delta t$ appear in the spectrum as lower frequencies—in the range of $0-1/2\Delta t$. When we are not interested in very high frequencies (above, say, 100 Hz) we can use this sampling effect to "fold" power from the high frequencies into the low frequencies. There are certain other schemes for generating band-limited white noise with frequency content flat down to dc (cf. Korn, 1966).

A general digital method for generating GWN is based upon a Fourier type of expansion:

$$x(t) = \sum_{n=1}^{N} a_n \sin n\omega_0 t + b_n \cos n\omega_0 t, \qquad 0 \leq t \leq T \qquad (5.1)$$

where a_n and b_n are independent Gaussian random variables with zero mean and variance σ^2 and ω_0 is a fundamental frequency determined by the specified record length T as

$$\omega_0 = 2\pi/T \qquad (5.2)$$

Clearly, this representation is approximate and valid only within the interval $(0, T)$, since it is periodic outside of it. This generation method has the advantage of being analytically well posed and general in the sense that it enables us to generate GWN of any desirable bandwidth. Of course, it has also the disadvantage of possessing a discrete power spectrum instead of a continuous one, and it employs the notion of the Fourier expansion, which is inconsistent with the nature of a random process (aperiodic).

5.1.2. Autocorrelation Properties of GWN and Application in Nonlinear System Identification

Before we study the autocorrelation properties of GWN, we must state concisely what the autocorrelation properties of a signal ought to be in order to be considered quasiwhite and, consequently, usable in connection with the crosscorrelation technique. Also, in order to facilitate discussion of the autocorrelation functions, we must give some basic definitions concerning the argument space of these functions.

Consider the nth-order autocorrelation function of a stationary random signal $x(t)$:

$$\phi_n(\tau_1, \tau_2, \ldots, \tau_n) = E[\![x(t-\tau_1)x(t-\tau_2)\cdots x(t-\tau_n)]\!] \qquad (5.3)$$

Consider the point $(\tau_1, \tau_2, \ldots, \tau_n)$ of the n-dimensional space on which ϕ_n is defined. If at least two of the arguments are identical, the point is called "diagonal." If all the arguments τ_i form exhaustively pairs of identical values the point is called "full diagonal." If all the arguments are different, the point is called "nondiagonal." Clearly, the odd-order autocorrelation functions do not have any full-diagonal points.

The white autocorrelation properties are those for which (a) all the odd-order autocorrelation functions are uniformly zero, and (b) all the even-order autocorrelation functions are zero everywhere except at the full-diagonal points.

A quasiwhite signal must approximately possess these white autocorrelation properties. The approximation is due to the following moderation of requirement (b): The values of the even-order autocorrelation functions of a quasiwhite signal in the close neighborhood of the full-diagonal points ought to be much bigger than their values at the rest of the points of the space.

Clearly, the value of any even-order autocorrelation function of ideal white noise at the full-diagonal points must be infinite, so that its integral over the whole argument space is nonzero. This implies that the even-order statistical moments of the ideal white noise are infinite, which is another manifestation of the infinite power and the physical unrealizability of this signal. In the case of a quasiwhite signal the values of the even-order autocorrelation functions at the full-diagonal points are finite, and their integrals are also finite because of the moderation of requirement (b).

To obtain an insight about the reasons that lead to the above definition of the white autocorrelation properties, we consider the following example. Suppose a nonlinear system is describable by the first- and second-order kernels, i.e.,

$$y(t) = \int_0^\infty k_1(\tau)x(t-\tau)\,d\tau + \int\int^\infty k_2(\tau_1, \tau_2)x(t-\tau_1)x(t-\tau_2)\,d\tau_1\,d\tau_2 \qquad (5.4)$$

According to the crosscorrelation technique, the zero-order Wiener kernel of the system is found by averaging the system response to white noise:

$$h_0 = E[\![y(t)]\!] = P \int_0^\infty k_2(\tau_1, \tau_1)\, d\tau_1 \tag{5.5}$$

since the white autocorrelation properties dictate that

$$E[\![x(t)]\!] = 0 \tag{5.6}$$

$$E[\![x(t-\tau_1)x(t-\tau_2)]\!] = P\delta(\tau_1-\tau_2) \tag{5.7}$$

Proceeding to the evaluation of the first-order Wiener kernel, we have

$$h_1(\sigma_1) = (1/P)E[\![y(t)x(t-\sigma_1)]\!] = k_1(\sigma_1) \tag{5.8}$$

since, again, the white autocorrelation properties dictate that

$$E[\![x(t-\tau_1)x(t-\tau_2)x(t-\sigma_1)]\!] = 0 \tag{5.9}$$

And finally, in the evaluation of the second-order Wiener kernel:

$$h_2(\sigma_1, \sigma_2) = (1/2P^2)E[\![[y(t)-h_0]x(t-\sigma_1)x(t-\sigma_2)]\!]$$
$$= k_2(\sigma_1, \sigma_2) \tag{5.10}$$

since according to the white autocorrelation properties

$$E[\![x(t-\tau_1)x(t-\tau_2)x(t-\sigma_1)x(t-\sigma_2)]\!]$$
$$= P^2[\delta(\tau_1-\tau_2)\delta(\sigma_1-\sigma_2) + \delta(\tau_1-\sigma_1)\delta(\tau_2-\sigma_2)$$
$$+ \delta(\tau_1-\sigma_2)\delta(\tau_2-\sigma_1)] \tag{5.11}$$

Notice that the last expression refers to a white-noise signal with Gaussian amplitude distribution. Similar expressions hold for white noise with any other symmetric amplitude distribution centered at zero. This example illustrates the basic property of white autocorrelation functions, which allows the direct evaluation of Wiener kernels through crosscorrelation.

Once the autocorrelation properties that a quasiwhite signal must possess have been defined, the quasiwhiteness of GWN can be easily manifested. We only need to recall two basic properties of Gaussian random variables: (1) The expected value of the product of an odd number of Gaussian random variables with zero mean is zero; (2) the expected value of the product of an even number of Gaussian random variables is equal to the sum of the products of the expected values of the products of all possible distinct pairs that can be formed. For example, in the case of four Gaussian random variables we have

$$E[\![x_1x_2x_3x_4]\!] = E[\![x_1x_2]\!]E[\![x_3x_4]\!] + E[\![x_1x_3]\!]E[\![x_2x_4]\!] + E[\![x_1x_4]\!]E[\![x_2x_3]\!] \tag{5.12}$$

This is the well-known decomposition property of Gaussian random variables, and it plays a major role in the construction of the Wiener series. Evidently, the number of terms of this sum in the case of $2m$ Gaussian random variables is

$$\frac{2m!}{m!2^m}$$

The usefulness of this decomposition property in the case of the crosscorrelation technique is great. Clearly, the decomposition property enables the higher even-order autocorrelation functions to be expressed in terms of only the second-order autocorrelation function.

On the other hand, the second-order autocorrelation function of GWN is (Fig. 5.1)

$$\phi_2(\tau_1, \tau_2) = 2BP \frac{\sin(2\pi B|\tau_1 - \tau_2|)}{2\pi B|\tau_1 - \tau_2|} \tag{5.13}$$

where B is the bandwidth of GWN and P is its power level. Notice that the variance of the GWN is related to the bandwidth and the power level as

$$\sigma^2 = 2PB \tag{5.14}$$

Clearly, the values of the second-order autocorrelation function are concentrated in a principal lobe around the origin. The width of the principal lobe is $1/B$ and it is double the width of any of the side lobes. The side lobes have clearly much smaller heights than the principal lobe. In fact, the kth side lobe extends from $|\tau_1 - \tau_2| = k/2B$ to $|\tau_1 - \tau_2| = (k+1)/2B$, and for $|\tau_1 - \tau_2| = (k + \frac{1}{2})/2B$ attains a maximum value of $(-1)^k \cdot 2BP/(k + \frac{1}{2})\pi$. Therefore, the ratio of the heights of the principal and the kth side lobe is (absolutely) $(k + \frac{1}{2})\pi$.

In conclusion, the form of the second-order autocorrelation function of GWN in combination with the decomposition property of Gaussian random variables guarantees the fulfillment of the quasiwhite autocorrelation requirements that were previously stated.

The quasiwhiteness of GWN allows its use in nonlinear system identification in connection with the crosscorrelation technique. The kernel estimates obtained, however, only approximate the Wiener kernels of the system. This approximation is usually satisfactory if the bandwidth of the GWN covers the system bandwidth. However, several estimation errors exist, and they are discussed in Chapter 7.

5.2. The Pseudorandom Signals Based on m Sequences

The computational burden accompanying the use of GWN in connection with the crosscorrelation technique has motivated a search for specially structured signals that reduce the natural redundancy of the random quasiwhite processes, while still preserving quasiwhite autocorrelation properties.

This has resulted in the introduction of pseudorandom signals based on m sequences (PRS), which are deterministic periodic signals with autocorrelation properties close to the quasiwhite ones and of very high efficiency (very low redundancy). When we talk about redundancy here, we mean the repetition of identical waveform portions throughout the signal. In addition to their high efficiency, PRS have the advantage of easier generation in the laboratory as compared to GWN. A further important advantage of PRS is the fact that their second-order autocorrelation function is zero in the region outside the neighborhood of origin and within, of course, some limits determined by the period of the signal (since the autocorrelation functions are also periodic). This is an advantage over random quasiwhite signals, which exhibit small nonzero values in this region of their second-order autocorrelation functions that cause some statistical fluctuation error. Nevertheless, PRS exhibit significant imperfections in their higher even-order autocorrelation functions, which offset their superiority in the second-order autocorrelation properties whenever the system possesses higher-order nonlinearities.

Clearly, PRS are most advantageous in identification of linear systems, while the presence of nonlinearities in the system makes the choice between random and pseudorandom quasiwhite test signals a complex one, depending upon the specific characteristics of the case at hand (see Sec. 5.4).

5.2.1. General Description and Generation of PRS

PRS have a special stairlike form (Fig. 5.2). They remain constant within small finite time intervals and switch abruptly at time instants that are integral multiples of a fundamental time interval Δt.

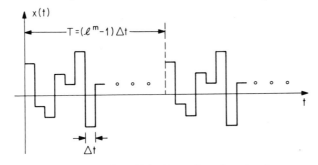

Fig. 5.2. Portion of l-level pseudorandom signal.

The values that they assume are determined by a linear recurrence formula of the form

$$x_i = a_1 \otimes x_{i-1} \oplus a_2 \otimes x_{i-2} \oplus \cdots \oplus a_m \otimes x_{i-m} \qquad (5.15)$$

where all values a_j and x_j correspond to the elements of a specified Galois field with finite population number, and the operations $\{\otimes, \oplus\}$ are defined in the proper way so as to be internal operations for this set of mathematical objects. For example, in the case of a binary pseudorandom signal (BPS) the Galois field has two elements, and, consequently, the operations $\oplus$ and $\otimes$ are defined modulo 2, so that the outcome of the recurrence formula (5.15) is also an element of the same Galois field.

It is evident that a sequence $\{x_i\}$ constructed on the basis of the linear recurrence formula (5.15) is periodic. The size of its period depends on the specific values of the coefficients a_j and the memory extent m of the recurrence formula (for a given Galois field). Among all the sequences $\{x_i\}$ constructed from the members of a certain Galois field and with linear recurrence formulas of memory extent (or order) m, there are some that have the maximum period. Since l^m is the number of all possible distinct arrangements with repetitions of l elements in strings of m, this maximum period is $(l^m - 1)$, where l is the number of elements of the Galois field, and the null string is excluded. Note that l is a prime number.

These maximum period sequences are called m sequences, and they correspond to a special choice of the coefficients $\{a_1, \ldots, a_m\}$. It is known that these special coefficients $\{a_1, \ldots, a_m\}$ coincide with the coefficients of a primitive (or irreducible) polynomial of degree $(m - 1)$ in the respective Galois field (cf. Zierler, 1959). Thus, we can always determine the number of elements l and the order of the recurrence formula m in such a way that we get an m sequence with a desirable period (within the limitations posed by the integral nature of l and m).

The initial string of m values of x_i with which the construction of the m sequence originates is not of importance. Any initial string (except the null one) will give the same m sequence (for a given set of coefficients a_j), merely shifted.

The generation of pseudorandom signals in the laboratory is a relatively simple task. Suppose we have decided upon the number (prime) of values that the signal will attain and the required maximum period [i.e., the order of the linear recurrence formula (5.15)]. Now, we only need to know the coefficients of a primitive polynomial of the specified degree in the respective Galois field. Suppose that such a primitive polynomial is found (tables of such polynomials may be very helpful, cf. Church, 1935). Then we choose an initial string of values and construct the corresponding m sequence with a digital computer using the linear recurrence formula

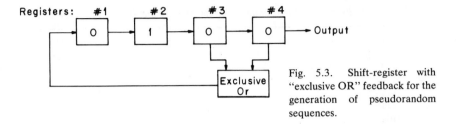

Fig. 5.3. Shift-register with "exclusive OR" feedback for the generation of pseudorandom sequences.

(5.15). The resulting sequence of numbers can subsequently be fed into a digital-to-analog converter to generate the desired pseudorandom signal.

More specialized pieces of hardware can also be used for more efficient generation. For example, a binary m sequence can be generated through a digital shift-register generator.

A digital shift-register consists of a cascade combination of flip-flops. Each flip-flop stores one "bit": 0 or 1. On receipt of a shift (or clock) pulse, the content of each flip-flop is transferred to its neighbor in sequence.

Figure 5.3 shows a pseudorandom number generator. The shift register operates in closed loop with the input to the first stage being fed back from the last two stages. The outputs from the last two stages are fed into an "exclusive OR" gate before being fed into the first stage. This unit produces a 1 output only when its two inputs are different. The truth table describing the operation of an "exclusive OR" unit is given in Table 5.1.

Let us now see how the pseudorandom sequence is generated by the system of Fig. 5.3. Assume that the initial contents of the shift register are

0 1 0 0

Then the output of "exclusive OR" unit is 0. With the next clock pulse, the following pattern results in the register:

0 0 1 0

Now the output of the "exclusive OR" unit is 1. With the next clock pulse the pattern becomes

1 0 0 1

Table 5.1. Truth Table for an "Exclusive OR" Unit

Input A	Input B	Output
0	0	0
0	1	1
1	0	1
1	1	0

Table 5.2. Pseudorandom Sequence Generated by the System of Figure 5.3

Register	Exclusive OR	Register	Exclusive OR
1001	1	0011	0
1100	0	0001	1
0110	1	1000	0
1011	0	0100	0
0101	1	0010	1
1010	1	....	
1101	1	1001	1
1110	1	1100	0
1111	0	:	:
0111	0	:	:

Continuing in a similar manner we obtain the sequence shown in Table 5.2. We note that the fifteenth clock pulse restores the register to the initial state, 1001, and the sequence repeats after that point.

We also note that the system generates the maximum number of all possible four-digit binary numbers except one—0000 never occurs. Notice that if 0000 ever occurred in the sequence the output thereafter would be only zeros.

Therefore, the bit sequence at the output is (with initial state 0100)

$$001001101011110/\text{repeats}$$

If we let 0 correspond to amplitude $-A$ and 1 correspond to $+A$, then the binary signal of Fig. 5.4 results.

Such pseudorandom sequences, produced by shift-registers with feedback, have been studied extensively (cf. W. D. T. Davies, 1970). It can be shown that feedback of the "exclusive OR" output taking inputs from two stage contents will produce maximum length sequences, i.e., of period $2^n - 1$ bits, if the feedback is taken from stages as specified in Table 5.3.

Table 5.3 gives the possible stage numbers in the shift-register from which the output, along with the output from the last stage, could be fed into the "exclusive-OR" gate and fed back into the first stage, in order to obtain a maximum length sequence. Similar results can be obtained if the

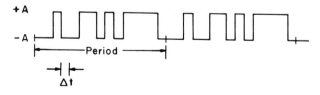

Fig. 5.4. Binary pseudorandom signal.

Table 5.3. Stages That Can Be Combined with the Last Stage of Various Shift-Registers to Generate Maximum-Length Pseudorandom Sequences

Number of stages in shift-register	Stage number giving feedback	Sequence length in bits
5	2	31
6	1	63
7	1 or 3	127
9	4	511
10	3	1023
11	2	2047
15	1, 4, or 7	32767
18	7	262,143
20	3	1,048,575
21	2	2,097,151
22	1	4,194,303
23	5 or 9	8,388,607
25	3 or 7	33,554,431
28	3, 9, or 13	268,435,455
31	3, 6, 7, or 13	2,147,483,647
33	13	8,589,934,591

output of stage $(n - m)$ is taken instead of that of stage m; in this case, we would obtain the delayed reverse of the original sequence (cf. W. D. T. Davies, 1970).

5.2.2. Autocorrelation Properties of PRS and Application in Nonlinear System Identification

The quasiwhiteness of a signal (and consequently its use in connection with the crosscorrelation technique) is manifested through its appropriate autocorrelation properties. Pseudorandom signals based on m sequences exhibit these properties to a reasonable approximation. This is due to the shift-and-add property of the m sequences (cf. Ream, 1970). According to this property the product (of the proper modulo) of any number of sequence elements is another sequence element:

$$x_{k-j_1} \otimes x_{k-j_2} \otimes \cdots \otimes x_{k-j_m} = x_{k-l} \qquad (5.16)$$

where l depends on $j_1, j_2, \ldots, j_m$ but not on k. As a result of this shift-and-add property and the basic structural characteristics of the m sequences (i.e., maximum period and antisymmetry), the odd-order autocorrelation functions are uniformly zero everywhere and the even-order ones approximate quasiwhiteness.

It must be noted that a slight modification must be made in m sequences with even numbers of levels in order to possess the antisymmetric property. This slight modification has been illustrated, for instance, by Simpson (1966) in the case of a binary *m* sequence, and it simply requires the inversion of every other bit of *m* sequence to obtain what he calls the corresponding *n* sequence. This modification results in doubling the period of the sequence, thus alleviating the cause of the problem, namely, the fact that the number of elements in one period of a sequence with even number of levels is odd.

Because of the antisymmetric property, the odd-order autocorrelation functions are perfect (i.e., uniformly zero). Nevertheless, the even-order autocorrelation functions of order higher than the second exhibit some serious imperfections (anomalies), which constitute an important topic of study and source of controversy about the use of PRS in nonlinear system identification. The second-order autocorrelation function is zero everywhere (within a period) except in the neighborhood of the origin, where it is triangularly shaped, as shown in Fig. 5.5. This establishes the PRS as a very effective tool in linear system identification. However, the higher even-order autocorrelation functions exhibit some anomalies distributed all around their argument space, and, therefore, the effectiveness of PRS in nonlinear system identification is significantly reduced. These anomalies, first observed by Gyftopoulos and Hooper (1964, 1967), have been studied by Barker and Pradisthayon (1970) and Barker *et al.* (1972). They showed that these anomalies are due to existing linear relationships among the elements of the sequence and that their exact position and magnitude can be determined through a laborious algorithm related to polynomial division. In any case, these anomalies are proved to be inherent and inevitable characteristics of the *m* sequences, directly and tightly related to their deterministic nature and their mathematical structure.

These anomalies cause estimation errors whenever nonlinearities are present. The magnitude of these estimation errors, as well as their relative

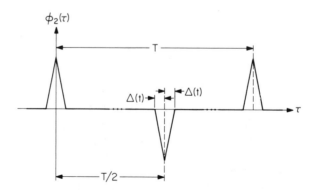

Fig. 5.5. Second-order autocorrelation function of antisymmetric pseudorandom signals.

severity (as compared to GWN), is still a subject under study. It is evident, however, that this depends on the specific system under study, as well as on the specific PRS or GWN that happens to be used. Barker *et al.* (1972) studied several PRS (binary, ternary, and quinary) trying to compare their relative virtues, and determined some optimum PRS, according to a criterion of performance that weighted the degree of exhibited anomalies.

Despite the presence of anomalies, the PRS have been proven useful and efficient quasiwhite signals, providing satisfactory results in several applications (Balcomb *et al.*, 1961; Briggs *et al.*, 1967; O'Leary *et al.*, 1975). Whether or not they should be preferable to other quasiwhite signals depends on considerations of the specific case at hand.

A very important point, which ought to be emphasized, is that the functional series, which are orthogonal with respect to a specific PRS, must be slightly modified from the original Wiener series, in order to accomodate the moments of the PRS, which are different, in general, from the moments of GWN. Consequently, the kernels estimated by the use of a PRS are different from the Wiener or Volterra kernels of the system and are characteristic of the specific PRS and the corresponding functional series.

This is easily seen from the relations between the estimated kernels using a PRS and the Volterra kernels of the system. To illustrate this, let us consider the estimation of the zero-order kernel h_0 of the zero-memory system:

$$y = e^x \tag{5.17}$$

Using a PRS we obtain

$$\hat{h}_0 = E[\![e^x]\!]$$

$$= \sum_{n=0}^{\infty} \frac{E[\![x^n]\!]}{n!} = \sum_{k=0}^{\infty} \frac{m_{2k}}{2k!} \tag{5.18}$$

where m_{2k} is the $2k$th moment of the PRS.

Similar expressions hold for all orders of kernels and for finite-memory systems. They clearly demonstrate the dependence of the estimated kernels upon the moments of the PRS used. Further, if we attempt to orthogonalize the functional series with respect to a certain PRS, in the same way that Wiener orthogonalized the functional series with respect to Gaussian white noise, we realize that the resulting orthogonal functionals depend upon the even-order moments of the respective PRS. Thus, both the kernels and the functionals depend upon the moments of the respective PRS.

5.3. The Constant-Switching-Pace Symmetric Random Signals

In previous sections we discussed the properties of two families of quasiwhite signals that have been used in applications of the white-noise method. In this section, we introduce a new family of quasiwhite random signals that can be used in connection with the crosscorrelation technique for the identification of nonlinear systems. These new test signals combine the stairlike form of the PRS with the random character of GWN, and, consequently, they exhibit a new blend of advantages and disadvantages. (See V. Z. Marmarelis, 1975).

5.3.1. General Description and Generation of CSRS

There are two basic defining characteristics of each member of the CSRS family: (1) The value of the signal switches randomly and independently at all time instants that are integral multiples of an elementary finite time interval Δt, attaining values according to a symmetric probability density function; and (2) the value of the signal remains constant between two successive switching times (Fig. 5.6).

The fundamental time interval Δt is called the "step" of the CSRS, and it directly determines the bandwidth of the signal. Evidently, as the step Δt decreases, the bandwidth of the signal increases and asymptotically approximates ideal white noise. The symmetric probability density function $p(x)$ with which a CSRS $x(t)$ is generated has zero mean, and, consequently, all its odd-order moments are zero. Additionally, the even-order moments of $p(x)$ ought to exist. This is a condition that is always satisfied in practice, since we must have a finite domain for the probability density function when we generate the signal in the laboratory. Similarly, the probability density function becomes, in practice, always discrete when a digital computer is used to generate the signal. The limits of this discretization are posed by the word length of the computer. In theory,

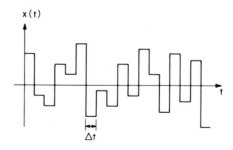

Fig. 5.6. Portion of CSRS.

however, the mathematical definition of a CSRS allows the probability density $p(x)$ to be continuous and of infinite domain, as long as the even-order moments exist.

The stairlike form of a CSRS is a feature compatible with the use of digital computers in data processing. The handling of continuous signals with digital computers requires their discretization through a constant-rate sampling procedure, while the complete recovery of the original signal is not (in general) possible, unless the signal has a special form (stairlike, piecewise linear, etc.). Thus, the inevitable discretization of a continuous signal within the digital computer leads naturally to the conception of a stairlike constant-switching-pace signal. When used intentionally this eliminates errors resulting from the discretization and assures the complete recovery of the original signal.

Clearly, the defining prescriptions of the CSRS family are fairly general and simple, providing the user with great flexibility in choosing the test signal that best fits the special considerations of a specific problem. In the following section, it will be shown that merely the statistical independence of any two steps of a CSRS, along with the fact that all the odd-order moments of $p(x)$ are zero and the even-order ones exist, is sufficient to guarantee the quasiwhiteness of $x(t)$ within the frequency range posed by the specified step length Δt.

5.3.2. Autocorrelation Properties of CSRS and Application in Nonlinear System Identification

At first, we note that every member of the CSRS family is by construction a stationary and ergodic process. For a given step length Δt and a proper probability distribution $p(x)$, an ensemble of random processes $x(t)$ is defined within the CSRS family. The ergodicity of $x(t)$ allows us to define the autocorrelation functions in both the temporal and the probabilistic sense. Thus, the nth-order autocorrelation function of $x(t)$ is

$$\phi_n(\tau_1, \tau_2, \ldots, \tau_n) = E[\![x(t-\tau_1)x(t-\tau_2)\cdots x(t-\tau_n)]\!]$$

$$= \lim_{T \to \infty} \frac{1}{2T} \int_{-T}^{T} x(t-\tau_1)x(t-\tau_2)\cdots x(t-\tau_n)\, dt \qquad (5.19)$$

It has been shown (V. Z. Marmarelis, 1975) that the autocorrelation functions of a CSRS as defined by Eq. (5.19) are those of a quasiwhite signal, namely, that the odd-order autocorrelation functions are uniformly zero, while the even-order ones are zero everywhere except at the diagonal strips. Note that the diagonal strips are areas within Δt (the step length of a CSRS) around every full diagonal of the argument space (i.e., where the arguments form exhaustively pairs of identical values).

In practice, we always have finite-length sample signals and none of the expressions in Eq. (5.19) can actually be evaluated. Hence, we are practically restricted to obtaining only an estimate of the autocorrelation function, usually by time averaging, as

$$\hat{\phi}_n(\tau_1, \tau_2, \ldots, \tau_n) = \frac{1}{T - T_m} \int_{T_m}^{T} x(t - \tau_1)x(t - \tau_2) \cdots x(t - \tau_n)\, dt$$

$$(5.20)$$

where T is the temporal length of the sample signal $x(t)$ and

$$T_m = \max\{\tau_1, \tau_2, \ldots, \tau_n\}$$

The estimate $\hat{\phi}_n(\tau_1, \ldots, \tau_n)$ is a random variable itself and its statistical properties must be studied in order to achieve an understanding of the kernel estimates obtained by the crosscorrelation technique.

It is found that the expected value of $\hat{\phi}_n(\tau_1, \ldots, \tau_n)$ is $\phi_n(\tau_1, \ldots, \tau_n)$, which makes it an unbiased estimate. Also, the probability limit of $\phi_n(\tau_1, \ldots, \tau_n)$ is $\phi_n(\tau_1, \ldots, \tau_n)$, which makes it a consistent estimate. Note also that the variance of $\hat{\phi}_n(\tau_1, \ldots, \tau_n)$ at all points tends to zero asymptotically with increasing record length, and the values of $\phi_n(\tau_1, \ldots, \tau_n)$ tend to those described above.

The surface $\hat{\phi}_n(\tau_1, \ldots, \tau_n)$ appears to have apexes corresponding to the nodal points (i.e., the points with ordinates that are integral multiples of Δt) of the n-dimensional space. These apexes are connected with $(n + 1)$-dimensional surface segments which are of first degree with respect to each argument τ_i. The direct implication of this morphology is that the "extrema" of the surface $\hat{\phi}_n(\tau_1, \ldots, \tau_n)$ must be sought among its apexes (i.e., among the nodal points).

To illustrate this, we consider the second-order autocorrelation function of a CSRS (Fig. 5.7):

$$\phi_2(\tau_1, \tau_2) = \begin{cases} m_2(1 - |\tau_1 - \tau_2|/\Delta t) & \text{for } |\tau_1 - \tau_2| \leq \Delta t \\ 0 & \text{for } |\tau_1 - \tau_2| > \Delta t \end{cases} \qquad (5.21)$$

We established above the quasiwhiteness of the CSRS family, which justifies their use in nonlinear system identification through the crosscorrelation technique. The kernel estimates that are obtained through the use

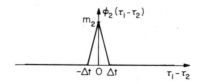

Fig. 5.7. Second-order autocorrelation function of CSRS.

of CSRS correspond to a functional series that is different in structure from the Wiener series. This structural difference is due to the statistical properties of the CSRS, as expressed by the moments of the amplitude probability distribution, which are different in general from the ones of GWN.

More specifically, the Gaussian amplitude distribution possesses the important property of being describable by only its first two moments. This, along with the decomposition property of products of Gaussian random variables, results in great simplification of the expressions describing the orthogonal Wiener functionals. In the general case of a CSRS, however, the complete description of the amplitude probability distribution requires all of its moments. This results in a certain complexity of the form of the CSRS orthogonal functionals. Nevertheless, the construction of the CSRS functionals is made routinely on the basis of an orthogonalization procedure similar to the one that was used in the construction of the Wiener series. It must also be noted that the orthogonality of the CSRS functionals is only approximate and based on the assumption that the bandwidth of the respective CSRS is broad enough with respect to the system bandwidth so that the deconvolution takes place with acceptable accuracy.

Clearly, the structural form of the CSRS functional series depends on the even-order moments and the step length of the associated CSRS. In the special case where a Gaussian amplitude distribution is chosen for the CSRS, the CSRS functional series takes the exact form of the Wiener series, where the power level of the GWN is equal to the product of the second moment and the step length of the CSRS. Thus, it becomes clear that the CSRS functional series is a more general orthogonal functional expansion than the Wiener series, extending the basic idea of orthogonal expansion using Volterra-type functionals throughout the space of symmetric probability distributions.

This generality is achieved at the expense of more complexity in the functional expressions. The advantages that such a generalization of the orthogonal functional series provides are those of any optimization problem where the parameter space is augmented. The augmentation of the parameter space provides greater flexibility and allows the search (and usually the achievement) of new global maxima of a certain "utility function."

The orthogonal functionals that correspond to a CSRS have the form

$$G_0^*[g_0; x(t'), t' \leq t] = g_0 \tag{5.22}$$

$$G_1^*[g_1(\tau_1); x(t'), t' \leq t] = \int_0^\infty g_1(\tau_1)x(t - \tau_1)\, d\tau_1 \tag{5.23}$$

$$G_2^*[g_2(\tau_1, \tau_2); x(t'), t' \le t] = \int_0^\infty \int_0^\infty g_2(\tau_1, \tau_2)x(t - \tau_1)x(t - \tau_2)\, d\tau_1\, d\tau_2$$

$$- (m_2\Delta t) \int_0^\infty g_2(\tau_1, \tau_1)\, d\tau_1 \qquad (5.24)$$

$$G_3^*[g_3(\tau_1, \tau_2, \tau_3); x(t'), t' \le t]$$

$$= \int_0^\infty \int_0^\infty \int_0^\infty g_3(\tau_1, \tau_2, \tau_3)x(t - \tau_1)x(t - \tau_2)x(t - \tau_3)\, d\tau_1\, d\tau_2\, d\tau_3$$

$$- 3(m_2\Delta t) \int_0^\infty \int_0^\infty g_3(\tau_1, \tau_2, \tau_2)x(t - \tau_1)\, d\tau_1\, d\tau_2$$

$$- [(m_4/m_2 - 3m_2)\Delta t^2] \int_0^\infty g_3(\tau_1, \tau_1, \tau_1)x(t - \tau_1)\, d\tau_1 \qquad (5.25)$$

etc., where $x(t)$ is a CSRS, Δt is its step length, and m_2, m_4, etc. are the second, fourth, etc. moments of its amplitude probability density function $p(x)$.

The expressions for higher-order functionals become quite involved, but their derivation can be done routinely on the basis of a Gram–Schmidt type of orthogonalization procedure.

It must be pointed out that the integral terms of the G^* functionals that contain higher even-order moments (> 2) contain also a higher power of Δt as a factor. This makes them significantly smaller than the terms containing only the second moment, since Δt usually attains small values. Therefore, for very small values of Δt (which is often the case in practice) the G^* functionals become (for all practical purposes) the same as the G functionals. This implies in turn that, whenever Δt is very small, the CSRS kernels are approximately the same as the Wiener kernels except possibly at the diagonal points. Note that in this case the corresponding GWN power level is equal to $(m_2\Delta t)$.

The power spectrum of CSRS with step length Δt and second moment m_2 is shown in Fig. 5.8. Clearly, the bandwidth of the signal is inversely proportional to Δt, and it approaches ideal white noise as Δt approaches zero (provided that the power level $P = m_2\Delta t$ remains finite). Clearly the degree of orthogonality of the G^* functionals monotonically increases as Δt is decreased, since the G^* functionals are constructed orthogonal under the assumption of infinite stimulus bandwidth. However, for all practical purposes, it usually suffices that the bandwidth of the CSRS covers the bandwidth of the system under study.

Notice that the basic structural form of the G^* functionals is the same as the Wiener G functionals, i.e., the odd- (even-) order functionals consist solely of all odd- (even-) order integral terms of equal and lower order.

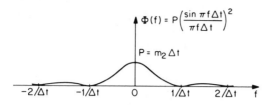

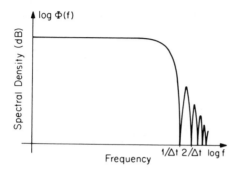

Fig. 5.8. The power spectrum of CSRS.

Notice also that if a Gaussian probability density function is chosen for a CSRS, then $m_4 = 3m_2^2$ and, consequently, G_3^* becomes exactly like the G_3 Wiener functional, with power level $P = m_2\Delta t$.

The actual procedure of crosscorrelation is basically the same as in the GWN case. That is, in order to estimate the nth-order kernel, we cross-correlate the nth-order response residual with n time-shifted versions of the stimulus and normalize the outcome:

$$\hat{g}_n(\sigma_1, \ldots, \sigma_n) = C_n E[\![y^{(n)}(t) x(t - \sigma_1) \cdots x(t - \sigma_n)]\!] \qquad (5.26)$$

where

$$y^{(n)}(t) = y(t) - \sum_{i=0}^{n-1} G_i^*[g_i(\tau_1, \ldots, \tau_i); x(t'), t' \le t] \qquad (5.27)$$

and C_n is the proper normalizing factor.

In the case of GWN, the normalizing factor C_n is $1/n!P^n$, where P is the power level of the GWN. In the case of CSRS, the normalizing factors differ for the diagonal and nondiagonal points. For the nondiagonal points, the normalizing factor is that of the GWN case:

$$C_n = 1/n!P^n \qquad (5.28)$$

where $P = m_2\Delta t$.

However, the determination of the appropriate normalizing factors for the diagonal points requires the evaluation of the volume under the corresponding autocorrelation function surface.

This is not a problem in practice, because we always confine ourselves to estimating the first few kernels (usually up to the second order) and thus only need the normalizing factors for these limited cases. For example, in the second-order case the normalizing factor can be easily evaluated on the basis of our knowledge about the form and structure of the autocorrelation functions of the CSRS. Namely, the second-order crosscorrelation gives:

$$\psi_2(\sigma_1, \sigma_2) = E[\![y(t)x(t-\sigma_1)x(t-\sigma_2)]\!]$$

$$= E[\![G_2^*(t)x(t-\sigma_1)x(t-\sigma_2)]\!]$$

$$= \int\int_0^\infty g_2(\tau_1, \tau_2)E[\![x(t-\tau_1)x(t-\tau_2)x(t-\sigma_1)x(t-\sigma_2)]\!]\, d\tau_1\, d\tau_2$$

$$- (m_2\Delta t)\int g_2(\tau, \tau)\, d\tau E[\![x(t-\sigma_1)x(t-\sigma_2)]\!]$$

$$= \begin{cases} 2(m_2\Delta t)^2 g_2(\sigma_1, \sigma_2) & \text{for the nondiagonal points} \\ (m_4 - m_2^2)\Delta t^2 g_2(\sigma, \sigma) & \text{for the diagonal points} \end{cases} \tag{5.29}$$

Therefore the normalizing factors for the second-order kernel are

$$C_2 = \begin{cases} 1/2(m_2\Delta t)^2 & \text{for the nondiagonal points} \\ 1/(m_4 - m_2^2)\Delta t^2 & \text{for the diagonal points} \end{cases} \tag{5.30}$$

We will now study the relation between the Volterra and the CSRS kernels of a system. Our objective is also to demonstrate the dependence of the CSRS kernels upon the moments and the step length of the specific CSRS that is used to estimate the kernels.

For simplicity of expression, we confine ourselves to the nondiagonal points of the CSRS kernels. The resulting expressions for the CSRS kernels in terms of the Volterra kernels are

$$g_{2n}(\sigma_1, \ldots, \sigma_{2n}) = \sum_{m=n}^{\infty} C_{m,n}(P_1)$$

$$\times \int_0^\infty \cdots \int_0^\infty k_{2m}(\tau_1, \ldots, \tau_{2m-2n}, \sigma_1, \ldots, \sigma_{2n})\, d\tau_1 \cdots d\tau_{2m-2n}$$

$$+ \sum_{l=1}^{m-n} \Delta t^l \int_0^\infty \cdots \int_0^\infty D_{l,m,n}(P_1, \ldots, P_{l+1})$$

$$\times k_{2m}(\tau_1, \ldots, \tau_{2m-2n-2l}, \sigma_1, \ldots, \sigma_{2n})\, d\tau_1 \cdots d\tau_{2(m-n-l)} \tag{5.31}$$

where P_k is a "generalized power level of kth order" defined as

$$P_k = m_{2k}\Delta t^k \tag{5.32}$$

$C_{m,n}$ and $D_{l,m,n}$ are rational expressions of these generalized power levels, and $k_i(\tau_1, \ldots, \tau_i)$ are the Volterra kernels of the system. Similar expressions hold for the odd-order CSRS kernels. Note that the coefficients $C_{m,n}$ and $D_{l,m,n}$ attain values of the same order of magnitude. Consequently, the terms of the second summation in the expression above are usually negligible in comparison with the terms of the first summation, since Δt is usually very small. Hence, the CSRS kernels at the nondiagonal points of the argument space are approximately the same as the Wiener kernels (as long as they have the same power level $P = m_2\Delta t$), since the coefficient $C_{m,n}(P_1)$ is the same as the coefficient found in the relation between the Wiener and the Volterra kernels [cf. Eq. (4.50)]. The only difference between the CSRS and the Wiener kernels of a system (at the nondiagonal points) is contained in the second summation terms, which are usually negligible for very small Δt.

5.3.3. An Analytical Example

As an analytical example of the parametric dependence of the CSRS functional series, consider a third-order Volterra system (i.e., a system for which $k_n(\tau_1, \tau_2, \ldots, \tau_n) \equiv 0$ for $n > 3$). If $k_0 = 0$, the system response to a CSRS $x(t)$ is

$$y(t) = \int_0^\infty k_1(\tau_1)x(t-\tau_1)\,d\tau_1 + \int\int_0^\infty k_2(\tau_1, \tau_2)x(t-\tau_1)x(t-\tau_2)\,d\tau_1\,d\tau_2$$

$$+ \int\int\int_0^\infty k_3(\tau_1, \tau_2, \tau_3)x(t-\tau_1)x(t-\tau_2)x(t-\tau_3)\,d\tau_1\,d\tau_2\,d\tau_3 \quad (5.33)$$

and the CSRS kernels of the system are (for the nondiagonal points)

$$g_0 = (m_2\Delta t)\int_0^\infty k_2(\tau_1, \tau_1)\,d\tau_1 \quad (5.34)$$

$$g_1(\sigma_1) = k_1(\sigma_1) + 3(m_2\Delta t)\int_0^\infty k_3(\sigma_1, \tau_1, \tau_1)\,d\tau_1$$

$$+ \left[\left(\frac{m_4}{m_2} - 3m_2\right)\Delta t^2\right]k_3(\sigma_1, \sigma_1, \sigma_1) \quad (5.35)$$

$$g_2(\sigma_1, \sigma_2) = k_2(\sigma_1, \sigma_2) \quad (5.36)$$

$$g_3(\sigma_1, \sigma_2, \sigma_3) = k_3(\sigma_1, \sigma_2, \sigma_3) \quad (5.37)$$

It is interesting to note that the Wiener kernels of this system are

$$h_0 = P\int_0^\infty k_2(\tau_1, \tau_1)\,d\tau_1 \quad (5.38)$$

$$h_1(\sigma_1) = k_1(\sigma_1) + 3P \int_0^\infty k_3(\sigma_1, \tau_1, \tau_1) \, d\tau_1 \qquad (5.39)$$

$$h_2(\sigma_1, \sigma_2) = k_2(\sigma_1, \sigma_2) \qquad (5.40)$$

$$h_3(\sigma_1, \sigma_2, \sigma_3) = k_3(\sigma_1, \sigma_2, \sigma_3) \qquad (5.41)$$

where P is the power level of GWN. In other words, the Wiener kernels are a special case of CSRS kernels, where $m_4 = 3m_2^2$ (i.e., when the amplitude probability distribution is Gaussian).

We can also observe the difference in the order of magnitude between the second and the third terms of $g_1(\sigma_1)$, for small Δt.

Clearly, the second- and third-order CSRS kernels are identical to the Volterra kernels because of the absence of nonlinearities of order higher than third. The zero-order CSRS kernel depends upon the second-order Volterra kernel, and the first-order CSRS kernel depends upon the first- and third-order Volterra kernels in accordance with Eq. (5.31).

The difference between the Volterra and the CSRS kernels of zero and first order reflects the fact that a CSRS functional of any order depends upon the higher-order Volterra functionals, thus providing a different span of the function space of the system response. This different span is expected to be more efficient for expanding the system response to a CSRS stimulus, because of the orthogonality of the CSRS functionals.

Recalling that the Volterra kernels constitute a nonparametric description of the system (i.e., they depend only upon the functional derivatives of the system operator and not upon any stimulus characteristics, like the power level, etc.) the expressions above state very eloquently the dependence of the CSRS kernels upon the even moments and the step length of the associated CSRS.

What is of importance in system modeling is the accuracy (in the mean-square sense) of the model-predicted response to a given stimulus. We will study now the improvement of this accuracy when we use a CSRS model, as opposed to a Volterra model of the same order. To study this, we will simply consider the zero-order model of the system above. The MSE of the zero-order Volterra model response is

$$e_0^2 = E[y^2(t)] \qquad (5.42)$$

The MSE of the zero-order CSRS model response is

$$\varepsilon_0^2 = E[[y(t) - g_0]^2]$$

$$= E[y^2(t)] + g_0^2 - 2g_0 E[y(t)] \qquad (5.43)$$

Therefore, the improvement in accuracy of the zero-order model-predicted response, using a CSRS model instead of a Volterra model, is

$$i_0 = e_0^2 - \varepsilon_0^2$$

$$= 2g_0 E[y(t)] - g_0^2 \qquad (5.44)$$

If $x(t)$ is the CSRS stimulus with which the model was estimated, then

$$i_0 = g_0^2$$

$$= \left[P_1 \int_0^\infty k_2(\tau_1, \tau_1) \, d\tau_1 \right]^2 \geq 0 \qquad (5.45)$$

Therefore, we always have a positive (or zero) improvement in accuracy with the zero-order CSRS model in predicting the system response to the CSRS stimulus. This improvement clearly depends on the first-order power level of the CSRS stimulus.

Let us now study this measure of improvement (or deterioration) in the accuracy of the model-predicted response to several other stimuli, when we are using the previous CSRS zero-order model instead of the Volterra model of the same order.

If $x(t)$ is another CSRS with first-order power level P_1^*, then

$$i_0 = P_1(2P_1^* - P_1) \left[\int_0^\infty k_2(\tau_1, \tau_1) \, d\tau_1 \right]^2 \qquad (5.46)$$

Thus, we can have improvement or deterioration in the accuracy of the model response depending on the relative size of the power levels. A similar expression holds in the case of GWN, PRS, or any other quasiwhite signal.

If $x(t)$ is an arbitrary signal, then

$$i_0 = P_1 \int_0^\infty k_2(\tau_1 \tau_1) \, d\tau_1 \left\{ 2 \int_0^\infty k_1(\tau_1)\phi_1(\tau_1) \, d\tau_1 \right.$$

$$+ 2 \iiint_0^\infty k_3(\tau_1, \tau_2, \tau_3)\phi_3(\tau_1, \tau_2, \tau_3) \, d\tau_1 \, d\tau_2 \, d\tau_3$$

$$\left. + \iint_0^\infty k_2(\tau_1, \tau_2)[2\phi_2(\tau_1, \tau_2) - P_1\delta(\tau_1 - \tau_2)] \, d\tau_1 \, d\tau_2 \right\} \qquad (5.47)$$

where

$$\phi_i(\tau_1, \ldots, \tau_i) = \frac{1}{T} \int_0^T x(t - \tau_1) \cdots x(t - \tau_i) \, dt, \qquad i = 1, 2, 3 \qquad (5.48)$$

Equation (5.47) clearly demonstrates the fact that the improvement (or deterioration) in this case depends upon the autocorrelation functions ϕ_i of the stimulus. This fact leads us to a basic conclusion with respect to the system models that are obtained using quasiwhite signals: The performance of the model (in the MSE sense) depends crucially on the relation of the autocorrelation functions of the stimulus with the ones of the associated quasiwhite signal.

Another important observation is that the improvement in accuracy of the zero-order model in the example considered becomes maximum if and only if

$$E[y(t)] = g_0 \tag{5.49}$$

as is evident from the derivatives:

$$\frac{\partial i_0}{\partial P_1} = 2 \int_0^\infty k_2(\tau_1, \tau_1) \, d\tau_1 [E[y(t)] - g_0] \tag{5.50}$$

$$\frac{\partial^2 i_0}{\partial P_1^2} = -2 \left[\int_0^\infty k_2(\tau_1, \tau_1) \, d\tau_1 \right]^2 \tag{5.51}$$

Thus, the improvement is maximized in the case of the CSRS stimulus with which the model was estimated (as was expected), but this may also be true for other stimuli for which Eq. (5.49) holds. Thus, for a given arbitrary stimulus there is always, in this case, a CSRS that gives the optimum zero-order model. This CSRS is specified by its first-order power level:

$$P_1 = E[y(t)] \bigg/ \int_0^\infty k_2(\tau_1, \tau_1) \, d\tau_1 \tag{5.52}$$

Of course, as the order of the system nonlinearity and of the model increases, the analytical expressions describing the dependence of the model accuracy upon the power levels of the CSRS become complicated very rapidly. However, the basic remark can be generalized to state that for a given system and a given stimulus there are CSRS, specified by some values of generalized power levels, that give the model of a certain order with the highest accuracy in predicting the system response to the given stimulus.

It must be emphasized that these optimal CSRS are specified strictly by their generalized power levels as long as the stimulus bandwidth remains broad enough so that the CSRS functional series can be considered approximately orthogonal. However, if Δt is very small, then the determining factor for the optimality of the stimulus becomes simply the first-order power level $(m_2 \Delta t)$, which corresponds to the power level of the GWN.

5.4. Comparative Study of the Use of GWN, PRS, and CSRS in System Identification

The quasiwhite signals that have been used so far in system identification through crosscorrelation are GWN, PRS, and CSRS. In the process of deciding which one of these signals is preferable in a specific application, one is faced with a complicated problem, because each one of these signals exhibits its own characteristic set of advantages and disadvantages.

An appreciation of these relative advantages and disadvantages is a complex task and often highly circumstantial. Of course, there are some universal criteria that can be used in this relative appreciation; nevertheless, the special characteristics of a specific application can introduce a variety of influential factors.

Of course, the determinants of the decision are usually not simply and clearly outlined. The decision-making process is complicated and not always free of errors or even psychological bias.

Below we discuss the most basic considerations that the investigator ought to have in mind in attempting to choose the test signal that (according to a limited number of basic criteria) best suits his or her specific application.

5.4.1. Discussion on Relative Advantages and Disadvantages of GWN, PRS, and CSRS

In review, the principal advantages and disadvantages of each one of these families of quasiwhite signals are as follows:

(*I*) *For the GWN.* The main advantages of GWN derive from its Gaussian nature and the fact that it has traditionally established a solid reputation among the users of the Wiener approach and the crosscorrelation technique, so that more relevant literature can be found if wanted. Its Gaussian nature secures the simplest and most elegant expressions for the orthogonal functional series (in this case the original Wiener series) and related matters (like relations between estimated kernels and Volterra kernels, the normalizing factors of the crosscorrelation estimates, etc.), simply because of the decomposition property of Gaussian random variables (which allows all the high even autocorrelation functions to be expressed in terms of the second one). Additionally, GWN is a signal with rich information content, and it can be expected to provide a good model for a great variety of inputs.

The main disadvantages of GWN are as follows: First, the actual generation of GWN in the laboratory is a relatively complex task in comparison to the straightforward procedure of generating PRS or CSRS.

Second, there are some imperfections in the autocorrelation functions due to side lobes and the truncation of the Gaussian distribution. Third, the computational burden of reducing statistical errors to an acceptable degree can become heavy. Fourth, the error analysis is complicated by the perplexing analytical form that the autocorrelation functions attain for each actual method of GWN generation.

(*II*) *For the PRS.* The main advantages of PRS are the following: First, they are generated in a relatively simple way in the laboratory. Second, they require relatively short records in order to form the desirable autocorrelation functions and consequently, they reduce significantly the computational burden. This reduction becomes even more dramatic when a binary or a ternary PRS is used, and when the special form of these signals is exploited using proper pieces of software and/or hardware.

The main disadvantages of PRS are as follows: First, they exhibit anomalies in the higher (>2) even-order autocorrelation functions, which may induce considerable estimation errors if the system contains significant nonlinearities. Second, the analytical expressions concerning the corresponding functional series and related matters (i.e., relation of PRS kernels to Volterra kernels, normalizing factors of the crosscorrelation estimates, etc.) are fairly complicated. Third, the error analysis is quite difficult, because of the complex method by which the anomalies in position and magnitude are determined.

(*III*) *For the CSRS.* The main advantages of the CSRS are the following: First, they are generated in a simple way, easily implemented in the laboratory. Second, their autocorrelation functions do not exhibit any deterministic kind of imperfections, within the frequency limits posed by the signal bandwidth (which must cover the system bandwidth). Third, the error analysis is greatly facilitated by the convenient form that the autocorrelation functions attain and the simple structure of CSRS. The thorough analysis of the estimation errors allows, in turn, the design of an optimum test. Fourth, they provide the user with variety and flexibility in choosing the signal with the number of levels and probability distribution that fits best the specific case at hand and provides the model with the highest potential accuracy.

The main disadvantages of CSRS are as follows: First, they require fairly long records in order to reduce the statistical fluctuation error to acceptable limits. This results in a heavy computational burden as in the case of GWN. However, the computational burden can be considerably reduced with binary or ternary CSRS, exploiting the special form of these signals by employing proper pieces of hardware and/or software. Second, the analytical expressions concerning the corresponding functional series and related matters (i.e., relation of CSRS kernels with Volterra kernels, normalizing factors of the crosscorrelation estimates, etc.) are fairly complicated. Nevertheless, they are a little simpler than in the case of PRS, since it is easier to evaluate the even-order autocorrelation functions of CSRS than the ones of PRS.

Besides these advantages and disadvantages of GWN, PRS, and CSRS, there may be other factors that become important in a specific situation because of special experimental or computational considerations. Therefore, the choice of the proper quasiwhite test signal in a specific case is still considerably a case-to-case matter relying on subjective appreciation and relative weighing of a variety of effectual factors.

In any case, we consider it essential for the prospective user of the crosscorrelation method to know and consider seriously the principal advantages and disadvantages of the available quasiwhite signals, in order to retain a scientific approach to a task that still has some artistic flavor.

5.4.2. Computer-Simulated Applications of GWN, PRS, and CSRS

The systems we consider in these computer-simulated applications are the ones shown in Figs. 5.9–5.11, since they include some of the most interesting cases of system nonlinearities.

More specifically, the system of Fig. 5.9 has up to second-order nonlinearities; therefore, a complete model of it can be actually estimated.

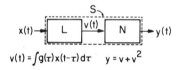

$$v(t) = \int g(\tau)x(t-\tau)d\tau \qquad y = v + v^2$$

Fig. 5.9. Cascade nonlinear system of second order.

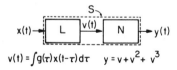

$$v(t) = \int g(\tau)x(t-\tau)d\tau \qquad y = v + v^2 + v^3$$

Fig. 5.10. Cascade nonlinear system of third order.

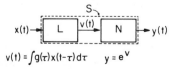

$$v(t) = \int g(\tau)x(t-\tau)d\tau \qquad y = e^v$$

Fig. 5.11. Cascade nonlinear system of infinite order.

The system of Fig. 5.10 has up to third-order nonlinearities with the third-order term being of size comparable to the first- and second-order terms; thus, the incomplete second-order model that is estimated in practice will contain only part of the quantity corresponding to the third-degree polynomial term (see example in Sec. 5.3), and the effectiveness of this probing into the third-degree term depends upon the fourth-order autocorrelation function (recall that the fourth-order autocorrelation function is the first one where the pseudorandom signals exhibit anomalies).

Finally, the system of Fig. 5.11 has nonlinearities of all orders, while the size of the higher-order terms is rapidly decreasing; thus, the incomplete second-order model that is estimated will contain parts of the quantities corresponding to terms of all orders, with the relative contribution decreasing as the order of the term increases.

The test signals that are used in these applications have characteristics that make them comparable from the system identification point of view.

More specifically, they all have the same record length $T = 1968$ sec and sampling interval $DT = 0.15$ sec. The record length corresponds to one period of a ternary pseudorandom signal being generated by an eighth-order linear recurrence formula ($3^8 - 1 = 6560$ steps) and having a step length $\Delta t = 0.3$ sec ($6560 \times 0.3 = 1968$ sec).

The CSRS family is represented in these applications by a ternary equirandom signal of the same record length and step size as the pseudorandom ternary signal. The operational range for both the PRS and the CSRS is $A = 1$ stimulus unit.

Owing to the fact that the amplitude histogram of one period of the pseudorandom ternary signal has approximately uniform profile (i.e., 2187 step values are $+1$'s, 2187 step values are -1's, and 2186 step values are 0's), the pseudorandom and the equirandom ternary test signals have approximately the same power level $P = 0.2$. That makes them comparable from the system identification point of view.

Making the GWN comparable to the PRS and the CSRS is more complicated, since there is no exact correspondence defining its frequency bandwidth. The power spectrum of the PRS and the CSRS is shown in Fig. 5.8, and the frequency where it first vanishes in this application is 3.33 Hz. Thus, it is reasonable to take a bandwidth of approximately 1.7 Hz for the GWN test signal. For another thing, owing to the different statistical moments of a Gaussian and an equirandom ternary amplitude probability distribution, the requirement of having the same power level in all cases will force us to have an operational range for the GWN that is different from the one of PRS and CSRS. Thus, the appropriate operational range for the GWN is determined from the specified GWN bandwidth $B = 1.7$ Hz and power level $P = 0.2$ [cf. Eq. (5.14)].

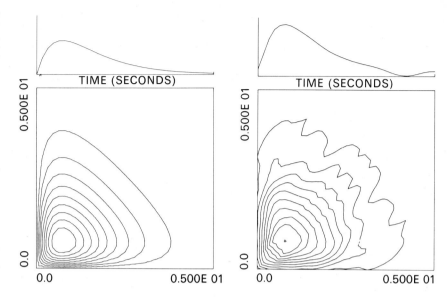

Fig. 5.12. First- and second-order Volterra kernels of the system in Fig. 5.9.

Fig. 5.13. First- and second-order GWN kernel estimates of the system in Fig. 5.10.

Thus, the criteria we use to determine the GWN, PRS, and CSRS test signals, so that they are comparable from the system identification point of view are (1) the same temporal record length; (2) the same number of sample points; (3) the same power level (of first order); and (4) approximately the same frequency bandwidth.

Clearly, criteria (3) and (4) allow a certain degree of arbitrariness, which is consistent with the approximate nature of this study.

For the system of Fig. 5.9 (Second-Order Nonlinearity). The first- and second-order Volterra kernels of the system are shown in Fig. 5.12. The percentage MSEs of the first-order kernel estimates are

GWN: 0.71%,   PRS: 0.37%,   CSRS: 0.66%

The percentage MSEs of the second-order kernel estimates are

GWN: 3.12%,   PRS: 5.49%,   CSRS: 3.28%

First- and second-order kernel estimates of the third-order system are shown in Figs. 5.13–5.15. The first-order kernels illustrate Eq. (5.35).

The percentage MSEs of the second-order model-predicted responses are

GWN: 1.22%,   PRS: 1.88%,   CSRS: 1.03%

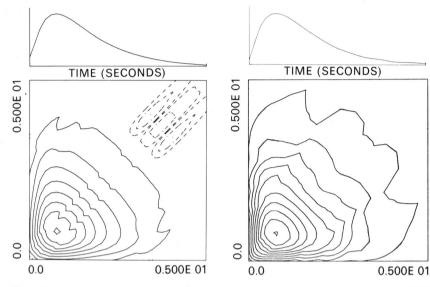

Fig. 5.14. First- and second-order PRS kernel estimates of the system in Fig. 5.10.

Fig. 5.15. First- and second-order CSRS kernel estimates of the system in Fig. 5.10.

The percentage MSEs of the second-order model-predicted responses to (1) a pulse stimulus of height 0.5 and duration 10 sec, (2) a sinusoidal stimulus of frequency 0.2 Hz and amplitude 1, and (3) an arbitrary stimulus of 25 sec long are given in Table 5.4. The model-predicted responses to the arbitrary stimulus and the actual system response are shown in Fig. 5.16.

The results above demonstrate the deterioration of the PRS autocorrelation properties in the higher even-order autocorrelation functions (since the PRS kernel estimate of first order is the best, while the second order is the worst in the group). The demonstrated difference between GWN and CSRS may be due to statistical variation relating to the specific sample signals that have been used.

Table 5.4. Percentage MSEs of Second-Order Model Responses to Various Stimuli for the System Shown in Figure 5.9

Quasiwhite test signal	Stimulus		
	pulse (%)	sinusoidal (%)	arbitrary (%)
GWN	0.46	0.91	0.26
PRS	0.69	1.13	1.49
CSRS	0.34	0.77	0.12

Table 5.5. *Percentage MSEs of Second-Order Model Responses to Various Stimuli for the System Shown in Figure 5.10*

Quasiwhite test signal	Stimulus	
	pulse (%)	arbitrary (%)
GWN	1.99	13.23
PRS	3.80	14.92
CSRS	2.10	13.45

For the System of Fig. 5.10 (Third-Order Nonlinearity). The percentage MSEs of the second-order model-predicted responses are

GWN: 27.32%,   PRS: 30.08%,   CSRS: 25.86%

The percentage MSEs of the second-order model-predicted responses to a pulse stimulus of height 0.5 and duration 10 sec, and an arbitrary stimulus of 25 sec long, are given in Table 5.5.

For the system of Fig. 5.11 (Exponential Nonlinearity). The percentage MSEs of the first-order model-predicted responses are

GWN: 34.42%,   PRS: 33.31%,   CSRS: 31.22%

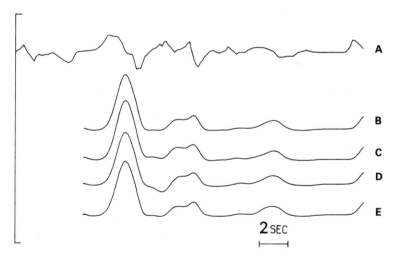

2 SEC

Fig. 5.16. (A) Arbitrary stimulus, (B) system response to arbitrary stimulus, (C) GWN model-predicted response, (D) PRS model-predicted response, (E) CSRS model-predicted response.

Table 5.6. Percentage MSEs of Second-Order Model Responses to Various Stimuli for the System Shown in Figure 5.11

Quasiwhite test signal	Stimulus	
	pulse (%)	arbitrary (%)
GWN	0.90	4.58
PRS	0.83	4.73
CSRS	0.77	4.07

The percentage MSEs of the second-order model-predicted responses are

$$\text{GWN: } 10.12\%, \quad \text{PRS: } 11.83\%, \quad \text{CSRS: } 9.02\%$$

The percentage MSEs of the second-order model-predicted responses to the previous pulse and arbitrary stimuli are given in Table 5.6.

The results obtained demonstrate beyond any statistical or circumstantial deviation the comparable efficacy of the GWN, PRS, and CSRS quasiwhite test signals in nonlinear system identification. This conclusion is not limited to the specific systems that were studied in this example. It applies to the general case, except possibly in a few singular situations.

5.5. Validation of Generated Quasiwhite Test Signals

In the previous sections we discussed generation methods and the basic statistical properties of some quasiwhite test signals that can be used in system identification with the crosscorrelation technique. Of course, a necessary step in the actual application of the method is the validation of the test signals, to determine whether they possess the required statistical properties.

As discussed in Sec. 5.1, the most important and necessary property of these signals is the quasiwhiteness of their autocorrelation functions of all orders. An exhaustive validation test for all autocorrelation functions is an infeasible task. Therefore, we confine ourselves in practice to validating the first few autocorrelation functions (usually only the mean of the signal and the second-order autocorrelation function), as well as some other important statistical characteristics like stationarity, amplitude probability distribution, and spectral density.

5.5.1. Check on Autocorrelation Functions

Under the usual circumstances we test the first two autocorrelation functions. The first one (the mean of the signal) ought to be zero, and the second one ought to be zero everywhere but in the neighborhood of the origin. In the case of random signals an estimate of the autocorrelation function is obtained that must be subsequently tested for its expected value with a statistical test. For instance, if the mean of the signal is to be checked, the estimate is

$$\hat{m} = \frac{1}{N} \sum_{k=1}^{N} x_k \qquad (5.53)$$

Let us assume that the sampling interval is such that the samples x_k are statistically independent. Then, if σ^2 is the variance of the process (assumed stationary), $\hat{m}$ has a Gaussian distribution with zero mean and variance equal to σ^2/N. On the basis of this fact, a statistical test may be performed to check the hypothesis of zero as expected value of $\hat{m}$ at some level of significance.

5.5.2. Check on Stationarity

Checking the stationarity of a random signal requires the testing of the time invariance of several statistical measures of the signal. To make a complete statement on the stationarity of a random signal, an exhaustive testing of all possible independent statistical measures (statistics) of the signal is required. The most popular, simple, and complete set of statistics consists of the time moments of the signal. The nth-order time moment is estimated from a portion of the signal, which is represented as a discrete data set of samples and is evaluated by averaging the nth powers of these samples:

$$\hat{m}_n = \frac{1}{N} \sum_{k=1}^{N} x_k^n \qquad (5.54)$$

A stationarity test for all these time moments appears to be an impossible task. Thus we arrive at the notion of *weak* stationarity, according to which only the first two moments ought to be checked. It is evident that in the case of a Gaussian process the weak stationarity implies strong stationarity, since a Gaussian distribution is completely determined by its first two moments. Other probability distributions may have a different number of independent determining parameters (for example, the Poisson distribution has one). Thus, if we know the underlying amplitude probability distribution of the signal analytically, then we only have a finite number of independent moments to check. If the probability distribution is not known, then some reasonable assumption is made and the resulting independent moments are checked.

The check of the time invariance of a certain statistic can be done through the so-called "run test" (cf. Bendat and Piersol, 1971).

The "run test" is a special-purpose statistical test, which applies in cases of stationarity testing where we cannot assume any kind of underlying probability distribtuion for our data. According to the "run test," given a random time series $\{x_1, x_2, \ldots, x_N\}$ we form k groups of M successive values each, so that $N = kM$. Then we compute a statistic d_i (like the sample mean or the sample variance, etc.) from each one of the k groups using its M samples.

In this way, we obtain the sequence of the statistics $\{d_1, d_2, \ldots, d_k\}$. We compute the median d_m of the population $\{d_1, \ldots, d_k\}$, and the differences:

$$f_i = d_i - d_m, \qquad i = 1, 2, \ldots, k \tag{5.55}$$

Finally, we form the sequence of the signs (positive or negative) of these differences and count the number of times the sign changes in the difference sequence. This number plus one is the number of runs in the sequence. Then, we compare this number to the bounds given in Table 5.7, which are the bounds of a confidence interval that the hypothesis of stationarity of the time series, with respect to the statistic d_i, is not rejected (at some significance level α). Notice that the bound numbers of the table have been computed as confidence-interval bounds of a Gaussian random variable (the number of runs) with mean and variance given by

$$(\text{mean}) = \frac{k}{2} + 1 \tag{5.56}$$

$$(\text{variance}) = \frac{k(k-2)}{4(k-1)} \tag{5.57}$$

where k is the number of statistics in the sequence. Of course it is still possible that the hypothesis of stationarity is not rejected while the process is actually nonstationary. This risk is related to the significance level α. Besides this risk, the "run test" is unable to detect periodic nonstationarities that have a period comparable to the temporal length of each one of the k groups from which the statistics are computed. However, periodic nonstationarities are usually detected as spikes in the power spectrum of the signal (cf. Bendat and Piersol, 1971).

Another way to test linear trend of a time sequence of statistics is to compute the correlation coefficient r between the statistics d_i and the order i of each one of them and then use the new statistic

$$w = \tfrac{1}{2} \ln \left(\frac{1+r}{1-r} \right) \tag{5.58}$$

Table 5.7. Confidence Bounds in "Run Test"[a]

Total number of statistics d_i	Significance level α					
	0.01		0.025		0.05	
	lower bound	upper bound	lower bound	upper bound	lower bound	upper bound
10	2	9	2	9	3	8
12	2	11	3	10	3	10
14	3	12	3	12	4	11
16	4	13	4	13	5	12
18	4	15	5	14	6	13
20	5	16	6	15	6	15
22	6	17	7	16	7	16
24	7	18	7	18	8	17
26	7	20	8	19	9	18
28	8	21	9	20	10	19
30	9	22	10	21	11	20
32	10	23	11	22	11	22
36	11	26	12	25	13	24
40	13	28	14	27	15	26
50	17	34	18	33	19	32
60	21	40	22	39	24	37
70	25	46	27	44	28	43
80	30	51	31	50	33	48
90	34	57	36	55	37	54
100	38	63	40	61	42	59
110	43	68	45	66	46	65
120	47	74	49	72	51	70
130	52	79	54	77	56	75
140	56	85	58	83	60	81
150	61	90	63	88	65	86
160	65	96	68	93	70	91
170	70	101	72	99	74	97
180	74	107	77	104	79	102
190	79	112	82	109	84	107
200	84	117	86	115	88	113

[a] Source: Bendat, J. S., and Piersol, A. G. (1971). *Random Data: Analysis and Measurement Procedures*, Wiley-Interscience, New York.

to perform a statistical test against the hypothesis that w is normally distributed with mean and variance

$$\mu_w = \tfrac{1}{2} \ln \left(\frac{1+\rho}{1-\rho} \right) \tag{5.59}$$

$$\sigma_w^2 = \frac{1}{k-3} \tag{5.60}$$

where ρ is the hypothetical correlation coefficient. It is evident that in the case in which we simply want to check stationarity, ρ is set equal to zero.

In cases where the assumption of an underlying Gaussian distribution can be made for our data, a t-statistic test can be used for a sequence of sample means or a χ^2-statistic test for a sequence of sample variances.

5.5.3. Check on Amplitude Distribution

There are two main ways to test the amplitude probability distribution of a signal. One is to test several parameters of the assumed distribution versus the sample estimates obtained from the record data, provided that the distribution of those estimators is known. The other is to test the amplitude histogram of the sample signal versus the assumed (hypothesized) distribution using a chi-square test.

5.5.4. Check on Power Spectrum

In order to check the suitability of the power spectrum of a generated quasiwhite test signal, we need to employ the proper statistical test. This will be illustrated in the following for the case of band-limited Gaussian white noise (GWN).

In this case we need to check whether the expected value of the power spectrum of the generated signal is flat over the specified range of frequencies. We must note that the computed power spectrum of a sample signal will exhibit some statistical deviations due to the finite record length. The statistical test aims at checking the significance of these observed deviations for the purpose of qualifying them (or not) as random discrepancies from the hypothesized situation (flat spectrum).

To be able to run such a statistical test, we need to know the statistical characteristics of the power spectrum of GWN. To facilitate the study of these statistical characteristics, let us assume that a Gaussian stationary random process $x(t)$ with zero time-average can be represented within a finite time interval T by a Fourier series expansion:

$$x(t) = \sum_{n=1}^{\infty} (a_n \cos n\omega_0 t + b_n \sin n\omega_0 t); \qquad 0 \le t \le T, \quad \omega_0 = \frac{2\pi}{T} \qquad (5.61)$$

where a_n and b_n are uncorrelated Gaussian random variables with zero mean. Note that the Fourier expansion of a random process is strictly valid only in the limit (i.e., when T goes to infinity); however, the expansion over a finite interval T allows us to obtain an approximate but useful insight into the statistical character of the process.

The defining relations for the coefficients are:

$$a_n = \frac{2}{T} \int_0^T x(t) \cos n\omega_0 t \, dt \tag{5.62}$$

$$b_n = \frac{2}{T} \int_0^T x(t) \sin n\omega_0 t \, dt \tag{5.63}$$

The variance of these Fourier coefficients is given by

$$\text{Var} \llbracket a_n \rrbracket = \frac{4}{T^2} \int_0^T \int_0^T E\llbracket x(t)x(t') \rrbracket \cos n\omega_0 t \cos n\omega_0 t' \, dt \, dt'$$

$$= \frac{2}{T} \int_0^T \phi_{xx}(\tau) \cos n\omega_0 \tau \, d\tau$$

$$= \text{Var} \llbracket b_n \rrbracket \tag{5.64}$$

where $\phi_{xx}(\tau)$ is the second-order autocorrelation function of $x(t)$.

Recall that the power spectrum is the Fourier transform of the second-order autocorrelation function. Consequently, the spectral density at each frequency ($n\omega_0$) is the sum of the variances of a_n and b_n.

Note now that in the case of band-limited Gaussian white noise the spectral density is constant up to the cutoff frequency B and zero beyond that frequency. Therefore, in this case

$$\text{Var} \llbracket a_n \rrbracket = \text{Var} \llbracket b_n \rrbracket = P \tag{5.65}$$

for $n = 1, 2, \ldots, N$, where $N = BT$ and P is the power level of the GWN.

In other words, the spectral density function can be written as

$$S(\omega) = \sum_{n=1}^{N} (a_n^2 + b_n^2)\delta(\omega - n\omega_0) \tag{5.66}$$

This implies directly that the spectral density at a certain frequency ($n\omega_0$), after being normalized by P, follows a chi-square distribution with two degrees of freedom. To test the statistical properties of the spectral density of GWN, we calculate a chi-square statistic. The signal spectral density computed at some frequency ($2\pi n/T$) is divided by the hypothesized power level P, and the resulting value $\chi^2_{(n)}$ is checked against the confidence bounds of a chi-square distribution with two degrees of freedom for some significance level α. If

$$\chi^2_{2;\alpha/2} \leq \chi^2_{(n)} \leq \chi^2_{2;(1-\alpha/2)} \tag{5.67}$$

the hypothesis is not rejected. Sometimes in practice, because of the big variance of the spectral density estimate, a smoothing procedure precedes the statistical test. Notice that a smoothing procedure, either as an ensemble averaging of independent records, or as an interval averaging of spectral density values at contiguous frequencies within the interval, will result in an increase in the degrees of freedom. Specifically, if Δf is the frequency interval where contiguous values of spectral density are averaged, then the degrees of freedom of the resulting chi-square statistic become

$$n = 2\Delta f T \tag{5.68}$$

In the case where averaging does not take place, $\Delta f = 1/T$ and therefore $n = 2$.

5.5.5. Check on Independence of Multiple Stimuli

In the application of the white-noise method to multi-input systems the need arises for statistically independent stimuli. This independence should be validated in the laboratory. This validation is performed by computation of the crosscorrelation of any two of the stimuli. The expected value of this crosscorrelation at any time is zero if the stimuli are independent.

The statistical test is illustrated below for the case of two GWN stimuli $x(t)$ and $u(t)$ and for zero argument (time shift) of their crosscorrelation function.

The procedure to be followed in practice is as follows:

(1) Compute the correlation coefficient ρ_{xu} of the sample records $\{x_i\}$ and $\{u_i\}$:

$$\rho_{xu} = \sigma_{xu}/\sigma_x\sigma_u \tag{5.69}$$

where σ_x, σ_u, and σ_{xu} are given by

$$\sigma_x^2 = \frac{1}{N} \sum_{i=1}^{N} x_i^2 \tag{5.70}$$

$$\sigma_u^2 = \frac{1}{N} \sum_{i=1}^{N} u_i^2 \tag{5.71}$$

$$\sigma_{xu} = \frac{1}{N} \sum_{i=1}^{N} x_i u_i \tag{5.72}$$

(2) Compute the statistic:

$$w = \frac{1}{2} \ln \left(\frac{1 + \rho_{xu}}{1 - \rho_{xu}} \right) \tag{5.73}$$

(3) For uncorrelated signals w has a Gaussian distribution with zero mean and variance:

$$\sigma^2 = 1/(N - 3) \tag{5.74}$$

If

$$|w| \le Z_{\alpha/2}/(N-3)^{1/2} \tag{5.75}$$

(where $Z_{\alpha/2}$ is determined from a standard Gaussian distribution for a significance level α), then the hypothesis of statistical independence between $x(t)$ and $u(t)$ is accepted at the significance level α.

 Example. Suppose we want to test the statistical independence of two sample records $\{x_i\}$ and $\{u_i\}$ at the 5% significance level. Then

$$Z_{\alpha/2} = 1.96$$

(from a table of the standard Gaussian distribution). Let the number of samples in each record be $N = 900$. Now, compute the statistic w as given by Eq. (5.73) for every value of the argument of their crosscorrelation function. If

$$|w| \le 0.065$$

for every value of their crosscorrelation function, then the hypothesis of statistical independence between $\{x_i\}$ and $\{u_i\}$ is accepted at 5% significance level; otherwise, it is rejected.

Methods of Computation of System Kernels

Introduction

The objective of functional identification is the determination of system kernels that furnish a complete description of the stimulus–response functional relation.

Since the formulation of the method by Wiener and his colleagues (Wiener, 1942, 1958; Bose, 1956; Brilliant, 1958; George, 1959; Katzenelson and Gould, 1962, 1964; Lee and Schetzen, 1965; Schetzen, 1965a,b, 1974), one principal difficulty has hampered attempts to apply the method practically: the long computations required in estimating the system kernels. However, recent developments in computer hardware, numerical techniques (such as the introduction of the fast Fourier algorithm), as well as new approaches to the problem (such as the use of binary and ternary stimuli or the optimal choice of test parameters) have greatly alleviated this difficulty and have made the practical estimation of system kernels a manageable task.

In this chapter we examine some of the computational considerations and present techniques that can be employed in estimating kernels. In this whole discussion, the crosscorrelation approach to kernel estimation is used, for reasons concerning the theoretical advantages of this approach (cf. Sec. 4.3), as well as advantages with regard to application to physiological systems (cf. Chapter 10).

6.1. Computational Considerations for Kernel Measurement

The main difficulty in the computation of kernels is the calculation of the necessary higher-order correlation functions, since estimation of the nth-order kernel necessitates estimation of the nth-order crosscorrelation (cf. Sec. 4.3),

$$\phi_{yxx\cdots x}(\tau_1, \ldots, \tau_n) = \frac{1}{T} \int_0^T \int \cdots \int y(t) x(t-\tau_1) \cdots x(t-\tau_n) \, dt \quad (6.1)$$

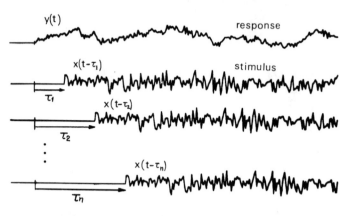

Fig. 6.1. Computation of nth-order crosscorrelation.

where T is the length of the data record, $y(t)$ is the response signal, and $x(t)$ is the white-noise stimulus signal. Signals $x(t - \tau_i)$ and $y(t)$ exist over the time interval $[0, T]$ and are assumed to be zero for all other times. We may visualize the nth-order crosscorrelation of response $y(t)$ and stimulus $x(t)$ as in Fig. 6.1. Shifting of the stimulus $x(t)$, multiplying, and averaging are involved.

A simple trapezoidal rule is used to estimate the integral of Eq. (6.1). More accurate integration schemes may, of course, be used, but the resulting improvement, in practice, is much smaller than other sources of error such as statistical variance of the estimates, physiological noise, experimental measurement errors, etc., while their sophistication will cloud the present analysis without increasing the generality of the basic results. We have, therefore,

$$\phi_{yxx\cdots x}(\tau_1, \tau_2, \ldots, \tau_n) = \frac{1}{N}\left\{ \sum_{i=1}^{N} y(t_i)x(t_i - \tau_1) \cdots x(t_i - \tau_n) \right.$$
$$-\tfrac{1}{2}[y(t_1)x(t_1 - \tau_1) \cdots x(t_1 - \tau_n)$$
$$\left. + y(t_N)x(t_N - \tau_1) \cdots x(t_N - \tau_n)] \right\} \qquad (6.2)$$

when records $y(t)$ and $x(t)$ are sampled every Δt:

$$y(t_1), y(t_2), \ldots, y(t_N)$$
$$x(t_1), x(t_2), \ldots, x(t_N)$$
$$t_k = k\Delta t, \qquad k = 1, 2, \ldots, N$$
$$N = T/\Delta t \text{ (number of record samples)}$$

Since N is usually fairly large (at least about 2,000 in practice), we may approximate Eq. (6.2) for the purposes of this discussion by

$$\phi_{yxx\cdots x}(\tau_1, \tau_2, \ldots, \tau_n) = \frac{1}{N} \sum_{i=1}^{N} y(t_i)x(t_i - \tau_1) \cdots x(t_i - \tau_n) \qquad (6.3)$$

i.e., by a rectangular rule of integration. The extent to which the crosscorrelation should be estimated (i.e., how big $\tau_1, \tau_2, \ldots, \tau_n$ can be before $\phi_{yx\cdots x}$ becomes nearly zero) depends on the system memory μ_n, which may depend on the kernel order. Here we assume that it is constant for all kernels; for example, we choose it to be the largest of the μ_n. Therefore each τ_k must take m values, where

$$m = \mu/\Delta t + 1 \qquad (6.4)$$

and each $\phi_{yxx\cdots x}(\ )$ must be computed for all of these values of its arguments $\tau_1, \tau_2, \ldots, \tau_n$ (Fig. 6.2). However, a considerable saving results from the fact that the crosscorrelation is symmetric with respect to its arguments, and therefore all permutations of a given combination of arguments are redundant. This results in a reduction of the kernel values that need to be computed by a factor equal to the order of the kernel factorial. Equation (6.3) can be written as

$$\phi_{yxx\cdots x}(k_1, k_2, \ldots, k_n) = \frac{1}{N} \sum_{i=1}^{N} y(i)x(i - k_1) \cdots x(i - k_n) \qquad (6.5)$$

where $\tau_i = k_i \Delta t$, and

$$k_1 = 0, 1, 2, \ldots, k_2$$
$$k_2 = 0, 1, 2, \ldots, k_3$$
$$\vdots$$
$$k_n = 0, 1, 2, \ldots, m - 1$$

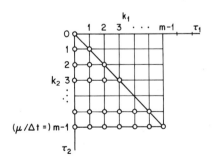

Fig. 6.2. Points of the $h_2(k_1, k_2)$ matrix to be computed.

For example, the first-order correlation is

$$\phi_{yx}(k) = \frac{1}{N} \sum_{i=1}^{N} y(i)x(i-k) \qquad (6.6)$$

It should be noted that since the crosscorrelation is an average, if the signals $x(t)$, $y(t)$ are zero outside the $[0, T]$ interval, an unbiased estimator of this average must be

$$\hat{\phi}_{yx}(k) = \frac{1}{N-k} \sum_{i=1}^{N} y(i)x(i-k) \qquad (6.7)$$

rather than Eq. (6.6). However, it can be shown (cf. Parzen, 1962) that the statistical variance of $\hat{\phi}_{yx}$ is greater than that of ϕ_{yx}, even though ϕ_{yx} is a biased estimator. For this reason, and since for our purposes in practice the maximum value of k [i.e., $(m-1)$] is of the order of $1/10$ or less of N, we will employ the estimator of Eq. (6.6).

The amount of computation increases with the order of the computed correlation, the length of the record, and the extent to which each correlation (kernel) is computed. Considering that the correlations (kernels) are symmetric functions of their arguments, it can be shown that the number of points of the nth-order kernel that we have to calculate (for $n < m$) is given by

$$\binom{n+m-1}{n} = \frac{(m+n-1)(m+n-2) \cdots m}{n!}$$

For example, the second-order kernel $(n = 2)$ needs to be computed only at

$$\frac{(m+1)m}{2} \quad \text{points}$$

Figure 6.2 shows these points. Indeed, it can be shown by simple induction that

$$1+2+3+\cdots+m = \frac{(m+1)m}{2}$$

Of more interest, however, is the number of multiplications required for the computation of each kernel correlation, since multiplication is a time-consuming operation for a digital computer. In order to compute one point of the correlation for some fixed $(k_1, k_2, \ldots, k_n)$, and if $x(t)$, $y(t)$ are zero outside the interval $[0, T]$, we require [from Eq. (6.5)]

$$n(N - \max\{k_1, k_2, \ldots, k_n\}) \quad \text{multiplications}$$

To simplify matters, we can approximate the expression above (on the average) by

$$n(N - m/2)$$

Thus, the number of multiplications required for the calculation of the nth-order kernel is given by

$$(\text{number of multiplications}) = n\left(N - \frac{m}{2}\right)\left[\frac{(m+n-1)(m+n-2)\cdots m)}{n!}\right]$$

$$(6.8)$$

In practice there is, of course, the usual tradeoff between computation time and available storage space. Computing time (i.e., number of multiplications) can be reduced by storing intermediate results. As the storage requirements increase with the order of the computed kernel there will be a sharp increase in computing when we are forced to use auxiliary storage (disk, tapes) to hold the intermediate results or even to store the final result.

Let α_n be a constant (dependent on the order n) that accounts for time spent in addressing, storing, etc. Then the total computation time is approximately

$$T_n = \alpha_n\left(N - \frac{m}{2}\right)n\left[\frac{(m+n-1)(m+n-2)\cdots m}{n!}\right] \qquad (6.9)$$

where N is the total number of sample points in the record and m is given by Eq. (6.4). From Eq. (6.9) we have for the first four kernels

$$T_1 = \alpha_1\left(N - \frac{m}{2}\right)m \qquad (6.10)$$

$$T_2 = \alpha_2\left(N - \frac{m}{2}\right)(m^2 + m) \qquad (6.11)$$

$$T_3 = \alpha_3\left(N - \frac{m}{2}\right)\left(\frac{m^3 + 3m^2 + 2m}{2}\right) \qquad (6.12)$$

$$T_4 = \alpha_4\left(N - \frac{m}{2}\right)\left(\frac{m^4 + 6m^3 + 11m^2 + 6m}{6}\right) \qquad (6.13)$$

The values of factors $\alpha_1, \alpha_2, \ldots, \alpha_n$ depend much on the particular digital machine used and the size of core memory. The latter in fact is the more significant factor since it determines whether all data (N samples) fit in core or whether auxiliary storage (disk, tape, etc.) must be used, with the correlations being computed from segments of the data. In this respect, also, the memory extent m and order n of the computed kernel come into play. To simplify matters and get some idea of the length of computing times, we assume that $\alpha_1 = \alpha_2 = \cdots = \alpha_n = 10\ \mu\text{sec/multiplication}$, which is the order of multiplication time for a common digital computer. Then, computing times for the first three kernels would be as given in Table 6.1.

Table 6.1. Typical Computing Times for the Estimation of the First Three Kernels[a]

N	m = 50			m = 100		
	T_1	T_2	T_3	T_1	T_2	T_3
1000	$\frac{1}{2}$ sec	25 sec	11 min	1 sec	1.5 min	1.3 hr
2000	1 sec	50 sec	22 min	2 sec	3 min	2.6 hr
5000	2.5 sec	2 min	1 hr	5 sec	7.5 min	6.5 hr

[a]N = number of data points of input (output), m = number of data points of kernel.

It can be seen that computing time increases quickly with the order of the kernel, a severe limitation on the order of the kernel that can be computed by the straightforward means discussed in this section. Fortunately, for those physiological systems that have been studied, the contribution of the kernels decreases very rapidly with their order, making it sufficient to compute just the first two or three in order to describe the system quite accurately. This represents a vast improvement over the usual approach of using linear techniques, which *at best* amount to measuring only the first-order kernel $h_1(\tau)$. Moreover, we note that, for a sine-wave stimulus of frequency f, the nth-order kernel gives rise to the nth harmonic (of frequency nf). However, the harmonic content of periodic waveforms, such as those encountered in physiological signals, usually decreases quite fast. Therefore the contributions to the response by the higher-order kernels should decrease just as fast.

In the next few sections we discuss techniques for obtaining the crosscorrelation functions with much shorter computing times. These in part alleviate the problem of computing the higher-order kernels. It should be noted that it is quite common, in practice, for the higher-order kernels to have shorter memory than the lower-order ones. This will provide for additional computational time-savings.

6.2. Time-Domain Approaches to Kernel Computation

There are several computational shortcuts that can be employed in increasing the efficiency of estimating the system kernels in the time domain. Most of these are easily implementable and suitable for the small computer existing in most physiology laboratories. Because of the limited size of immediate storage in these computers we are also faced with a problem in dealing with the long arrays of the stimulus–response data. Methods to circumvent this problem are also discussed in this section.

6.2.1. Utilization of Intermediate Products

It is noted that if the summation in Eq. (6.5) is expanded and written explicitly, many of the terms have many common factors. They can be factored out, resulting in great savings in the total number of multiplications needed for the estimation of the crosscorrelation function.

The computation time for the first-order kernel is not affected by this method, but this time is short anyway and it does not present a problem. For example, consider the computation of the second-order kernel (correlation):

$$\phi_{yxx}(k_1, k_2) = \frac{1}{N} \sum_{i=1}^{N} y(i)x(i-k_1)x(i-k_2) \qquad (6.14)$$

where

$$k_1 = 0, \ldots, k_2$$
$$k_2 = 0, \ldots, m-1$$
$$m = \mu/\Delta t + 1$$

and μ is the memory of the system. As an illustration, $N = 10$ and $m = 4$. Then, the diagonal points are estimated as

$$N\phi_{yxx}(0, 0) = y_1 x_1 x_1 + y_2 x_2 x_2 + \cdots + y_{10} x_{10} x_{10}$$
$$N\phi_{yxx}(1, 1) = y_2 x_1 x_1 + y_3 x_2 x_2 + \cdots + y_{10} x_9 x_9$$
$$N\phi_{yxx}(2, 2) = y_3 x_1 x_1 + y_4 x_2 x_2 + \cdots + y_{10} x_8 x_8$$
$$N\phi_{yxx}(3, 3) = y_4 x_1 x_1 + y_5 x_2 x_2 + \cdots + y_{10} x_7 x_7$$

Notice that the products $x_1 x_1, x_2 x_2, \ldots, x_9 x_9$ appear as common factors. Therefore, if these products are computed once and then saved for the kernel computation along the diagonal we would need only

$$(10) + (10 + 9 + 8 + 7) = 44 \text{ multiplications}$$

instead of

$$(10 + 9 + 8 + 7) + (10 + 9 + 8 + 7) = 68 \text{ multiplications}$$

a considerable savings for the computation of the diagonal kernel values. Similarly,

$$N\phi_{yxx}(0, 1) = y_2 x_2 x_1 + y_3 x_3 x_2 + \cdots + y_{10} x_{10} x_9$$
$$N\phi_{yxx}(1, 2) = y_3 x_2 x_1 + y_4 x_3 x_2 + \cdots + y_{10} x_9 x_8$$
$$N\phi_{yxx}(2, 3) = y_4 x_2 x_1 + y_5 x_3 x_2 + \cdots + y_{10} x_8 x_7$$

Therefore, if the common product terms $x_2x_1, x_3x_2, \ldots, x_9x_8$ are computed only once and then saved, we would need only

$$(9)+(9+8+7)=33 \text{ multiplications}$$

instead of

$$(9+8+7)+(9+8+7)=48 \text{ multiplications}$$

Thus, in this scheme, the kernel values are computed along the diagonal first and then along the lines parallel to it. It should be noted that the only requirement in this scheme of kernel computation is an increase of storage by N locations to hold the intermediate (common factor) products. If this is a small number (less than 1000) this requirement is by no means severe.

In general, the number of multiplications for estimation of the second-order kernel along the diagonal, is, according to this scheme,

$$N+[N+(N-1)+\cdots+(N-m+1)]$$

Along the first parallel to the diagonal it is

$$(N-1)+[(N-1)+\cdots+(N-m+1)]$$

and continuing along the rest of the parallel lines to the diagonal (Fig. 6.3)

$$(N-2)+[(N-2)+\cdots+(N-m+1)]$$
$$\vdots$$
$$(N-m+1)+[N-m+1]$$

Adding all these together (to get the total number of multiplications) we obtain

$$2N+3(N-1)+4(N-2)+\cdots+(m+1)(N-m+1)$$
$$=N(2+3+\cdots+m+1)-[1\cdot3+2\cdot4+3\cdot5+\cdots+(m-1)(m+1)]$$
$$=N(1+2+3+\cdots+m)$$
$$\quad-[(2-1)(2+1)+(3-1)(3+1)+\cdots+(m-1)(m+1)]$$
$$=N(1+2+\cdots+m)-[2^2-1^2+3^2-1^2+\cdots+m^2-1^2]$$

Recalling that

$$1+2+3+\cdots+m=\frac{m(m+1)}{2}$$

$$1^2+2^2+3^2+\cdots+m^2=\frac{m(m+1)(2m+1)}{6}$$

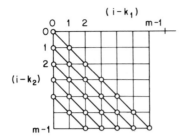

Fig. 6.3. Lines of computational order in case of intermediate products storage.

we finally have for the total number of multiplications

$$M'_2 = N\left[\frac{m(m+1)}{2}\right] - \frac{m(m+1)(2m+1)}{6} + m \qquad (6.15)$$

as compared to

$$M_2 = \left(N - \frac{m}{2}\right)(m^2 + m) \qquad (6.16)$$

for the straightforward method of the previous section. Since $N > 10m$ and m is 50–100, we can approximate

$$M'_2 = N\frac{m(m+1)}{2} \qquad (6.17)$$

$$M_2 = N(m^2 + m) \qquad (6.18)$$

So the ratio of numbers of multiplications in those two cases is

$$M_2/M'_2 \approx 2 \qquad (6.19)$$

This method, therefore, would result in savings of a factor of 2 for the second-order kernel. This factor increases considerably for the third-order kernel provided there is enough space to save the intermediate products $x_i x_j x_k$; otherwise it remains of the order of 2, if only $x_i x_j$ products are saved. For the typical computer of 10-μsec multiply time we have the values given in Table 6.2.

6.2.2. Treatment of Long Stimulus–Response Records

The typical physiology laboratory is equipped with a small or medium-size computer. Therefore, the stimulus–response data will normally not fit in core memory and instead are stored in auxiliary storage (disk, tape). They are later brought into core piece by piece. The kernel (correlation) functions can still be computed by the following procedure. Let us take the

Table 6.2. Typical Computing Times for Second-Order
Kernel Estimation Using the Straightforward Method (T_2)
or by Storing Intermediate Products (T_2')[a]

	$m = 50$		$m = 100$	
N	T_2	T_2'	T_2	T_2'
1000	25 sec	12 sec	1.5 min	40 sec
2000	50 sec	24 sec	3 min	1.4 min
5000	2 min	1 min	7.5 min	3.6 min

[a]N and m are as defined in the footnote to Table 6.1.

case of the second-order kernel (the first-order kernel being certainly much easier to compute following a similar procedure). We need to compute

$$\phi_{yxx}(k_1, k_2) = \frac{1}{N} \sum_{i=1}^{N} y(i)x(i-k_1)x(i-k_2) \qquad \begin{cases} k_1 = 0, \ldots, m-1 \\ k_2 = 0, \ldots, k_1 \end{cases}$$

$$(6.20)$$

This method is based on the observation that the maximum difference in subscripts between $y(i)$, $x(i-k_1)$ and $x(i-k_2)$ is m. Therefore, we only need to multiply data samples that are at most $m\Delta t$ apart, and consequently only these have to be in core at that time. There are, at this point, two possibilities: Either there is enough space to hold all the $m^2/2 + m/2$ values of ϕ_{yxx}, or there is not. Let us consider first the former possibility.

We bring into core the first $2m$ data points,

$$y_1, y_2, \ldots, y_m, y_{m+1}, \ldots, y_{2m}$$

$$x_1, x_2, \ldots, x_m, x_{m+1}, \ldots, x_{2m}$$

and compute $\phi_{yxx}(k_1, k_2)$ using Eq. (6.20) for $i = m+1, \ldots, 2m$. These are partial values of $\phi_{yxx}(k_1, k_2)$. Next, we save the last half of records x, y that are in core and read in the next m points of each record, to obtain (in core)

$$y_{m+1}, \ldots, y_{2m}, y_{2m+1}, \ldots, y_{3m}$$

$$x_{m+1}, \ldots, x_{2m}, x_{2m+1}, \ldots, x_{3m}$$

Again we compute $\phi_{yxx}(k_1, k_2)$ using m points and accumulate the results with those previously computed. The same procedure is continued until the end of the records is reached (Fig. 6.4).

If there is not enough space to hold all values of $\phi_{yxx}(k_1, k_2)$ in core [$(m^2+m)/2$ of them] then the kernel may be computed along its diagonal

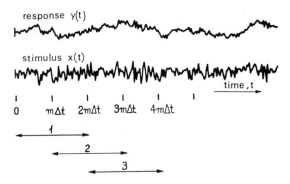

Fig. 6.4. Segmentation of stimulus–response data for computation of crosscorrelation (long records).

first and then along the lines parallel to it in a fashion similar to that shown in Fig. 6.3. In any case, more than $2m$ data points may be brought into core each time if there is room, thus reducing the number of "read" operations from auxiliary storage. It should also be noted that the method of the previous section (saving of intermediate products) may be utilized at each step of this procedure in order to reduce the number of multiplications required.

6.2.3. Quantization of the Input Signal

Suppose that the input white-noise signal is quantized into, say, three levels for positive and negative excursions (Fig. 6.5). Thus, x_i takes only the values $-3, -2, -1, 0, 1, 2, 3$. If the input signal is quantized, table look-ups can be used rather than multiplications in order to evaluate the product between any two values of x_i. For example, to compute the second-order kernel, Table 6.3 is formed. Notice its symmetry and the row and column of zeros. Taking advantage of these, the computation time of $\phi_{yxx}(k_1, k_2)$ [see Eq. (6.20)] can be greatly shortened. To multiply $x(i - k_1)$

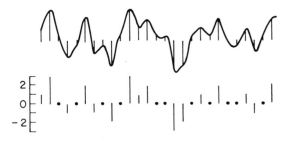

Fig. 6.5. Quantization of stimulus signal for kernel computation.

Table 6.3. Look-Up Table for Cross-Products of Seven-Level Signal

	−3	−2	−1	0	1	2	3
−3	9	6	3	0	−3	−6	−9
−2	6	4	2	0	−2	−4	−6
−1	3	2	1	0	−1	−2	−3
0	0	0	0	0	0	0	0
1	−3	−2	−1	0	1	2	3
2	−6	−4	−2	0	2	4	6
3	−9	−6	−3	0	3	6	9

by $x(i-k_2)$ all we do is look at the entry of the table appropriate to the quantized values of $x(i-k_1)$ and $x(i-k_2)$. Further computing-time savings can be realized by noting that the possible values of $x(i-k_1)x(i-k_2)$ are a few fixed ones, namely, 0, ±1, ±2, ±3, ±4, ±6, ±9. Therefore, they can be factored out, thus avoiding even the multiplication by $y(i)$. For example,

$$\phi_{yxx}(k_1, k_2) = 1[y(i)+\cdots-y(j)+\cdots]+2(\cdots)+\cdots+6(\cdots)+9(\cdots)$$

(6.21)

Thus, from the absolute value of the entry in the table of $x_i x_j$, the y_i are accumulated in separate sums. The result is that *no multiplications* are required for the computation of the second-order kernel (in fact, only 7).

We now turn our attention to the errors involved in approximating the continuous GWN signal by its quantized version. Since we are interested in the estimation of system kernels by crosscorrelation, the important aspect of this approximation is its effect on the autocorrelation functions of the input GWN. In particular, we will be interested in the effect of second-, third-, and fourth-order autocorrelations on the estimation of the first- and second-order kernels. Consider the case of binary quantization of $x(t)$, i.e.,

$$x'(t) = \begin{cases} +1 & \text{if } x(t) \geq 0 \\ -1 & \text{if } x(t) < 0 \end{cases}$$

(6.22)

Obviously, in this case the multiplication operation is reduced to logical conjunction of signs. This is an extremely fast operation on a digital machine. Thus, the various products $x_i x_j \cdots x_k$ are simply +1 or −1. Then, the values of y_i can be simply added with the proper sign to obtain the kernels. The question arises: what is the error introduced? It has been shown (cf. Otnes and Enochson, 1972) that for the first-order correlation (kernel)

$$\phi_{yx}(\tau) = (\tfrac{1}{2}\pi)^{1/2}\phi_{xx}(0)\phi_{yx'}(\tau)$$

(6.23)

where $x'(t)$ is the binary version of $x(t)$.

It is expected that the approximation of the GWN $x(t)$ by its quantized version should introduce an increase in the statistical variance of the kernel estimates. Therefore, in order to achieve the same statistical accuracy [as that resulting from use of the continuous $x(t)$] we may be forced to increase the length of the stimulus–response records (i.e., the length of the white-noise experiment). This, in the case of physiological systems, is usually an undesirable proposition. It can be shown (Otnes and Enochson, 1972) that the variance of an autocorrelation function estimate is increased by a maximum factor of roughly $\pi^2/4 \simeq 2.5$. As shown in Chapter 7, this variance is inversely proportional to the record length. Thus, if the variance is to be kept constant, record lengths two or three times as long as unquantized records are required. It has been shown that wide-band signals (highly uncorrelated data points) in their binary quantized version exhibit a larger variance than narrow-band signals. The theoretical 2.5-fold increase in variance assumes very-wide-band data samples. For narrow-band data an increase of about 1.3–1.5 times is more typical.

6.2.4. Monte Carlo Methods for Kernel Computation

Monte Carlo methods can prove very effective in the reduction of the computational requirements of high-order kernels. This can be accomplished in two related ways. First the evaluation of higher-order crosscorrelations is essentially the estimation of an integral whose integrand is a product of a number of Gaussian variables and another variable (the response of the system). Monte Carlo techniques are applicable in the evaluation of such integrals. Second, the estimation of the kernel involves essentially the evaluation of a *multidimensional* function; it can be carried out by Monte Carlo methods of evaluating the kernel in "randomly" selected regions, rather than by exhaustive computations over the entire domain of the arguments $(\tau_1, \tau_2, \ldots, \tau_n)$ of this function.

6.3. Frequency-Domain Approach: Use of the Fast Fourier Transform Algorithm

The introduction, in 1965, of algorithms for the fast digital computation of Fourier transforms (FFT) has had an impact on the computation of crosscorrelation (and convolution) (cf. Cooley and Tukey, 1965; French and Butz, 1973).

6.3.1. Frequency-Domain Formulation and Procedure

If, as in Chapter 2 (see Sec. 2.4.2), we define the Fourier transform (FT) of a function $f(t)$ by

$$F(\omega) = \mathscr{F}[f(t)] = \int_{-\infty}^{\infty} f(t)\, e^{-i\omega t}\, dt \tag{6.24}$$

and the inverse transform by

$$f(t) = \mathcal{F}^{-1}[F(\omega)] = \frac{1}{2\pi} \int_{-\infty}^{\infty} F(\omega) e^{i\omega t} \, d\omega \qquad (6.25)$$

then, the FT of the crosscorrelation $\phi_{yx}(\tau)$ is (for ergodic processes)

$$\Phi_{yx}(\omega) = \mathcal{F}[\phi_{yx}(\tau)] = \mathcal{F}[E[y(t)x(t-\tau)]] = Y(\omega)X^*(\omega) \qquad (6.26)$$

where $Y(\omega)$, $X(\omega)$ are the FT of $y(t)$ and $x(t)$, respectively, and $X^*(\omega)$ is the complex conjugate of $X(\omega)$. Thus, to compute the crosscorrelation $\phi_{yx}(\tau)$, or, effectively, the kernel $h_1(\tau)$, we compute $Y(\omega)$ and $X(\omega)$ via the FFT, then multiply, and use the FFT to invert back to the time domain. The steps would be as follows:

(1) Compute $Y(\omega)$ and $X(\omega)$ via the FFT.

(2) Form the product $Y(\omega)X^*(\omega) = \Phi_{yx}(\omega)$.

(3) Compute $(1/P)\phi_{yx}(\tau) = h_1(\tau)$ through FFT of $\Phi_{yx}(\omega)$.

Similarly, we may define the two-dimensional FT $F(\omega_1, \omega_2)$ of a function $f(t_1, t_2)$

$$F(\omega_1, \omega_2) = \int\int_{-\infty}^{\infty} f(t_1, t_2) \exp[-i(\omega_1 t_1 + \omega_2 t_2)] \, dt_1 \, dt_2 \qquad (6.27)$$

and the inverse two-dimensional transform

$$f(t_1, t_2) = \frac{1}{(2\pi)^2} \int\int_{-\infty}^{\infty} F(\omega_1, \omega_2) \exp[i(\omega_1 t_1 + \omega_2 t_2)] \, d\omega_1 \, d\omega_2 \qquad (6.28)$$

Then the FT $\Phi_{yxx}(\omega_1, \omega_2)$ of $\phi_{yxx}(\tau_1, \tau_2)$ is given by

$$\Phi_{yxx}(\omega_1, \omega_2) = \mathcal{F}[E[y(t)x(t-\tau_1)x(t-\tau_2)]]$$

$$= \int\int\int_{-\infty}^{+\infty} y(t)x(t-\tau_1)x(t-\tau_2) \exp[-i(\omega_1 \tau_1 + \omega_2 \tau_2)] \, d\tau_1 \, d\tau_2 \, dt$$

$$= \int\int_{-\infty}^{+\infty} y(t)x(t-\tau_1) \exp(-i\omega_1 \tau_1)$$

$$\times \left[\int_{-\infty}^{+\infty} x(t-\tau_2) \exp(-i\omega_2 \tau_2) \, d\tau_2 \right] d\tau_1 \, dt$$

$$= -X^*(\omega_2) \int\int_{-\infty}^{+\infty} y(t)x(t-\tau_1) \exp(-i\omega_1 \tau_1) \exp(-i\omega_2 t) \, d\tau_1 \, dt$$

$$= X^*(\omega_2)X^*(\omega_1) \int_{-\infty}^{+\infty} y(t) \exp(-i\omega_1 t - i\omega_2 t)\, dt$$

$$= X^*(\omega_2)X^*(\omega_1)Y(\omega_1 + \omega_2) \tag{6.29}$$

Therefore the FT of $h_2(\tau_1, \tau_2)$ would be [according to Eq. (4.106) of Sec. 4.3],

$$H_2(\omega_1, \omega_2) = (1/2P^2)Y_0(\omega_1 + \omega_2)X^*(\omega_1)X^*(\omega_2) \tag{6.30}$$

assuming the constant h_0 has been subtracted from $y(t)$ to give $y_0(t)$. Therefore, the steps involved in the estimation of $h_2(\tau_1, \tau_2)$ are as follows:

(1) Compute $Y_0(\omega)$ and $X(\omega)$ via the FFT.
(2) Form the product $Y_0(\omega_1 + \omega_2)X^*(\omega_1)X^*(\omega_2)$.
(3) Obtain the time-domain inverse of this product by FFT.

The whole procedure for obtaining $h_1(\tau)$ and $h_2(\tau_1, \tau_2)$, as well as their frequency domain representation $H_1(\omega)$ and $H_2(\omega_1, \omega_2)$, is outlined in Fig. 6.6.

It should be noted that convolution integrals can also be computed by a similar procedure employing the FFT. Specifically, to compute

$$\int_{-\infty}^{+\infty} h_1(\tau)x(t-\tau)\, d\tau$$

we compute (via FFT)

$$H_1(\omega)X(\omega)$$

and invert (via FFT) back to the time domain. To compute

$$G_2(t) = \iint_{-\infty}^{+\infty} h_2(\tau_1, \tau_2)x(t-\tau_1)x(t-\tau_2)\, d\tau_1\, d\tau_2 \tag{6.31}$$

we need to compute (via FFT) its FT

$$\mathscr{F}[G_2(t)] = H_2(\omega_1, \omega_2)X(\omega_1)X(\omega_2) \tag{6.32}$$

This is easily shown. Let

$$u(t) = v(t, t) \tag{6.33}$$

where

$$v(t_1, t_2) = \iint_{-\infty}^{\infty} h_2(\tau_1, \tau_2)x(t_1-\tau_1)x(t_2-\tau_2)\, d\tau_1\, d\tau_2 \tag{6.34}$$

Taking the two-dimensional FT of this we obtain

$$V(\omega_1, \omega_2) = H_2(\omega_1, \omega_2)X(\omega_1)X(\omega_2) \tag{6.35}$$

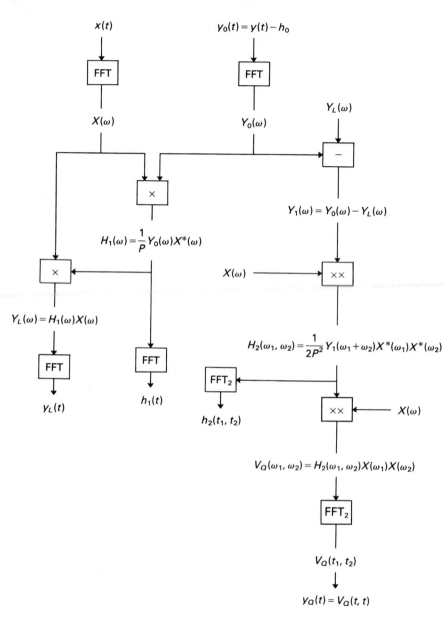

Fig. 6.6. Outline of kernel and model response computation in the frequency domain (via FFT).

Inverting back (via FFT) we obtain $v(t_1, t_2)$ and from this $u(t)$, according to Eq. (6.33).

Thus, the steps for computing the second-order nonlinear term are as follows:

(1) Compute (via FFT) $H_2(\omega_1, \omega_2)$ and $X(\omega)$.
(2) Form the product $H_2(\omega_1, \omega_2)X(\omega_1)X(\omega_2) = V(\omega_1, \omega_2)$.
(3) Invert (FFT) $V(\omega_1, \omega_2)$ to obtain $v(t_1, t_2)$.
(4) Obtain the desired $u(t) = v(t, t)$.

Figure 6.7 shows a nonlinear system having only the first two kernels. A GWN input is applied to this system and, from the resulting stimulus–response data, the FTs of the first- and second-order kernels, $H_1(\omega)$ and $H_2(\omega_1, \omega_2)$, respectively, are computed using Eqs. (6.26) and (6.30). The results are shown in Fig. 6.7. Inversion of $H_1(\omega)$ and $H_2(\omega_1, \omega_2)$ from the frequency domain back to the time domain gives the kernel estimate $\hat{h}_1(\tau)$ and $\hat{h}_2(\tau_1, \tau_2)$ shown in the figure.

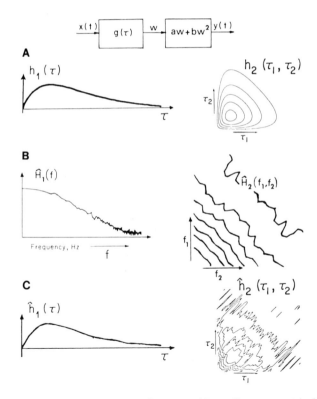

Fig. 6.7. Computation of $h_1(\tau)$ and $h_2(\tau_1, \tau_2)$ for a specific nonlinear system via the frequency domain. (A) The system kernels. (B) The Fourier transforms of the kernel estimates. (C) The kernel estimates.

Higher-order kernels can be obtained similarly. For example, it can be shown easily that

$$H_3(\omega_1, \omega_2, \omega_3) = (1/3!P^3)Y_2(\omega_1 + \omega_2 + \omega_3)X^*(\omega_1)X^*(\omega_2)X^*(\omega_3) \tag{6.36}$$

where $Y_2(\omega)$ is the FT of $y_2(t)$ and

$$y_2(t) = y(t) - h_0 - y_L(t) - y_Q(t) \tag{6.37}$$

Terms $y_L(t)$ and $y_Q(t)$ are the linear and quadratic responses, respectively, to white-noise stimulus $x(t)$, given by

$$y_L(t) = \int_{-\infty}^{+\infty} h_1(\tau)x(t - \tau) \, d\tau \tag{6.38}$$

and

$$y_Q(t) = \int\int_{-\infty}^{+\infty} h_2(\tau_1, \tau_2)x(t - \tau_1)x(t - \tau_2) \, d\tau_1 \, d\tau_2 - P \int_{-\infty}^{+\infty} h_2(\tau, \tau) \, d\tau \tag{6.39}$$

The reason for this is to avoid contributions of these lower-order terms to the estimate of $h_3(\ )$, as has been discussed in Chapter 4.

The cross-kernel in the case of a two-input system can be computed in a similar fashion. Let the two independent inputs be $x(t)$ and $u(t)$ and the output $y(t)$. Then, it can be shown that

$$H_{2xu}(\omega_1, \omega_2) = (1/P_xP_u)Y_0(\omega_1 + \omega_2)X^*(\omega_1)U^*(\omega_2) \tag{6.40}$$

where $y_0(t) = y(t) - h_0$ and $X(\omega)$, $U(\omega)$ are the FTs of $x(t)$ and $u(t)$, respectively. Similarly, the convolution (second-order) integral arising from this kernel can be computed. The quantity

$$v(t_1, t_2) = \int\int_{-\infty}^{+\infty} h_{2xu}(\tau_1, \tau_2)x(t_1 - \tau_1)u(t_2 - \tau_2) \, d\tau_1 \, d\tau_2 \tag{6.41}$$

has a FT

$$V(\omega_1, \omega_2) = H_{2xu}(\omega_1, \omega_2)X(\omega_1)U(\omega_2) \tag{6.42}$$

which can be computed using the FT of the inputs and the cross-kernel. Inverting $V(\omega_1, \omega_2)$ through FFT we obtain $v(t_1, t_2)$, and from that

$$v(t, t) = \int\int_{-\infty}^{+\infty} h_{2xu}(\tau_1, \tau_2)x(t - \tau_1)u(t - \tau_2) \, d\tau_1 \, d\tau_2 \tag{6.43}$$

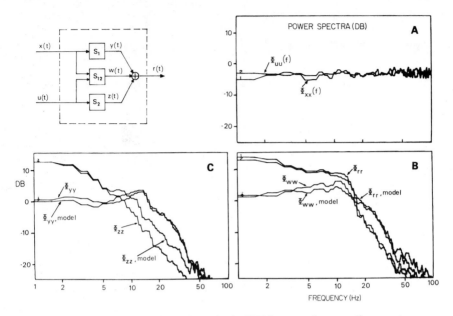

Fig. 6.8. Component spectra obtained via the FFT for a two-input nonlinear system.

Figure 6.8 shows estimates of the power spectra from an experiment of finite length R, for (A) the input stimuli, $\Phi_{xx}(\omega)$, $\Phi_{uu}(\omega)$, (B) the response components $\Phi_{rr}(\omega)$, $\Phi_{ww}(\omega)$, and (C) the components $\Phi_{zz}(\omega)$, $\Phi_{yy}(\omega)$, as well as the spectra of the model responses. These latter were computed using Eq. (6.46) as shown below. In this respect it should be noted that for a nonlinear system

$$y(t) = \int_{-\infty}^{+\infty} g_1(\tau)x(t-\tau)\,d\tau + \int\!\!\int_{-\infty}^{+\infty} g_2(\tau_1, \tau_2)x(t-\tau_1)x(t-\tau_2)\,d\tau_1\,d\tau_2 + \cdots$$

$$(6.44)$$

the FT of the response $y(t)$ is

$$Y(\omega) = G_1(\omega)X(\omega) + \int_{-\infty}^{\infty} G_2(\omega, \omega-\omega_1)X(\omega)X(\omega-\omega_1)\,d\omega_1 + \cdots \quad (6.45)$$

Thus, for example, to estimate the power spectrum $\Phi_{yy}(\omega)$ we use Eq. (6.45) for $Y(\omega)$, where $G_1(\omega) = H_{1x}(\omega)$ and $G_2(\omega_1, \omega_2) = H_{2xx}(\omega_1, \omega_2)$, and then

$$\Phi_{yy}(\omega) = Y(\omega)Y^*(\omega) \quad (6.46)$$

Similar procedures apply to the computation of the other spectra shown in Fig. 6.8.

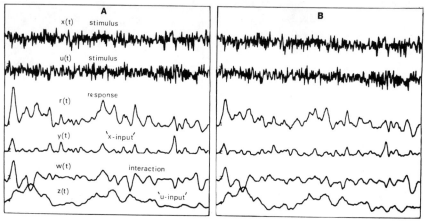

Fig. 6.9. Responses obtained via the frequency domain for the two-input system. (A) System responses. (B) Kernel-predicted responses.

To compute the kernel-predicted responses we must evaluate convolution integrals of the form shown in Eq. (6.44). This we can do conveniently through frequency-domain manipulation as indicated previously. Figure 6.9 shows model responses computed in this fashion from the estimated kernels of the system in Fig. 6.8, as well as the actual responses.

The saving in computing time using the FFT approach compared to the time-domain approach can be considerable. This is discussed in the next section, where examples are also given.

There is one inconvenience in using the FFT algorithm: Whether we desire them or not, the algorithm produces all Fourier coefficients obtainable from a given record. Thus, if we are interested only in a small number of them (e.g., in computing crosscorrelations with maximum lag that is 1/10 of the total record length), the procedure may be inefficient. We discuss this problem further below and suggest a remedy. Along similar lines of argument, note that the procedure gives us $v(t_1, t_2)$, see Eq. (6.41) above, while we only need $v(t, t)$, i.e., only the diagonal. In short, in some cases, the FFT procedure may give us more than we need with a corresponding decrease in efficiency.

6.3.2. Analysis of Kernel Computation via the Frequency Domain

In Sec. 6.1 it was shown that the number of multiplications necessary to compute the nth-order kernel (in a straightforward manner) is

$$n\left(N - \frac{m}{2}\right)\left[\frac{(m+n-1)(m+n-2)\cdots m}{n!}\right]$$

We wish to compare this number with the number of multiplications required if the FFT route of computing the kernels is chosen.

The computation of the FT of stimulus $x(t)$ and response $y(t)$ required $N \log_2 N$ complex multiplications for each (Cooley and Tukey, 1965), where N is the number of samples in each record. Thus, since $x(t)$ and $y(t)$ exist only from $t=0$ to $t=T$ and we can take them to be zero outside this interval, we have for the FT of $x(t)$

$$X(f) = \int_0^T x(t) \exp(-i2\pi ft) \, dt \qquad (6.47)$$

The records $x(t)$ and $y(t)$ are sampled every Δt sec, where Δt is made small enough to represent the highest frequencies present and to avoid aliasing (cf. Sec. 2.9). So we have

$$x(t) = \sum_{n=0}^{N-1} x_n \Delta t \, \delta(t - n\Delta t)$$

where $x_n = x(n\Delta t)$ and $N = T/\Delta t$ is the total number of samples. Then, Eq. (6.47) becomes

$$X(f) = \sum_{n=0}^{N-1} x_n \exp(-i2\pi fn\Delta t) \, \Delta t \qquad (6.48)$$

The fundamental frequency of a Fourier series expansion of $x(t)$ in the interval $[0, T]$ is $f_0 = 1/T$. Thus, the Fourier coefficients X_K of $x(t)$ are found for the discrete frequencies $f_K = K(1/T) = K(1/N\Delta t)$ to be

$$X_K = \Delta t \sum_{n=0}^{N-1} x_n \exp\left(-i2\pi \frac{Kn}{N}\right), \qquad K = 0, 1, 2, \ldots, N-1 \qquad (6.49)$$

It should be noted here that if the data are sampled every Δt, then we can only measure reliably the frequencies up to $1/(2\Delta t)$, according to the Nyquist sampling theorem. That is, the Fourier coefficients X_K have no aliasing only up to $K = N/2$, since that frequency $f_{N/2} = (N/2)(1/N\Delta t) = 1/2\Delta t$ is the Nyquist folding frequency, above which the X_K's are aliased (cf. Sec. 2.9). From a different point of view, since the original data have only N independent values, it is expected that the Fourier transformation cannot produce more than N independent outputs. This is manifested also by the presence of a certain symmetry in the real and imaginary parts of the complex quantities X_K as K goes from 0 to $N-1$.

To compute the FT using Eq. (6.49), we need to perform about N^2 operations, where complex multiplication is the most time-consuming part of each operation. The FFT algorithm produces *all* the complex Fourier coefficients X_K ($K = 0, 1, \ldots, N-1$), requiring only about $N \log_2 N$ complex multiplications. The fact that the FFT procedure produces *all* X_K

$(K = 0, 1, \ldots, N-1)$, whether we want all of them or only a part, is an inflexibility that often reduces the efficiency of the FFT in practice (e.g., if only a few frequency values are needed).

The inverse FT can be computed by the same procedure (algorithm) of FFT. We have

$$x(t) = \int_{-\infty}^{\infty} X(f) \exp(i2\pi ft)\, df \qquad (6.50)$$

which becomes, in the sampled version,

$$x_n = \frac{1}{N} \sum_{K=0}^{N-1} X_K \exp(i2\pi Kn/N), \qquad n = 0, 1, \ldots, N-1 \qquad (6.51)$$

where X_K $(K = 0, \ldots, N-1)$ are the Fourier coefficients computed by the FFT algorithm. From this equation it is obvious that the same algorithm can be used to compute the inverse FT.

The First-Order Kernel

These considerations suggest the following procedure for the calculation of the first-order kernel:

(1) Compute the FFT of $x(n\Delta t)$ to get X_K; $n, K = 0, 1, \ldots, N-1$.
(2) Compute the FFT of $y(n\Delta t)$ to get Y_K; $n, K = 0, 1, \ldots, N-1$.
(3) Form the product $\Phi_{yx}(K) = Y_K X_K^*$, $K = 0, 1, 2, \ldots, N-1$.
(4) Compute the inverse FFT of $\Phi_{yx}(K)$ to obtain the crosscorrelation $\phi_{yx}(j\Delta t)$, $j = 0, 1, \ldots, N-1$.

Steps 1 and 2 above can be carried out with a single application of the FFT algorithm, since $x(n)\,[=x(n\Delta t)]$ and $y(n)$ are real arrays. Specifically, if $x(n)$ is inserted as the real part and $y(n)$ is inserted as the imaginary part of a complex array $z(n)$, the FT of $z(n)$ is related to the FT of $x(n)$ and $y(n)$ by

$$\left. \begin{array}{l} X_K = (1/2)(Z_K + Z_{N-K}^*) \\[4pt] Y_K = (1/2i)(Z_K - Z_{N-K}^*) \end{array} \right\} \quad K = 0, 1, \ldots, N-1 \qquad \begin{array}{l} (6.52) \\[4pt] (6.53) \end{array}$$

Therefore, by taking the FFT of $z(n)$ we find the FFT of both $x(n)$ and $y(n)$ with no additional multiplication required.

However, in computing the crosscorrelation between $y(n)$ and $x(n)$ via the FFT route, a circularity effect takes place due to the fact that the signals, as represented by their Fourier series, are periodic. This circularity is shown in Fig. 6.10 for a shift of $x(n)$ by j positions in order to compute $\phi_{yx}(j\Delta t)$. Then, it can be shown that the computed "circular" crosscorrelation is given by

$$\phi_{yx}^c(j\Delta t) = \frac{N-j}{N}\{\phi_{yx}(j\Delta t) + \phi_{xy}[(N-j)\Delta t]\} \qquad (6.54)$$

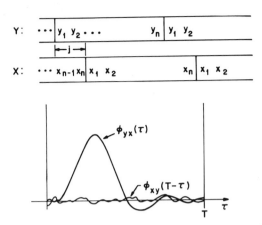

Fig. 6.10. Circularity in the computation of the crosscorrelation.

However, in computing system kernels, $\phi_{xy}(\tau)$ $(\tau > 0)$ is small—nearly zero— since x is the system input and y is the output, which has to *follow* it in time (causality). In practice, however, $\phi_{xy}(\tau)$ is nonzero and measured by the statistical variance of the estimate of $\phi_{xy}(\tau)$ from the stimulus–response records. Therefore, the resulting crosscorrelation will be the sum of two components, as shown in Fig. 6.10. If $\phi_{xy}(\tau)$ is sufficiently small then no major correction, except for the weighting factor $(N-j)/N$, need be made. However, if we want to avoid the error due to $\phi_{xy}(\tau)$, we must augment the y and x arrays by N zeros (either in the front or in the back) prior to computing their FFTs and following steps 1–4 above. Then, as illustrated in Fig. 6.11, the circular effect is nullified because, as x is shifted to the right, the "circulating" x's are multiplied by zeros in the y positions, thus not contributing anything. It should be noted that this "circulation" is nothing else but the previous (or next) period of the waveform as represented by the Fourier series. Thus, if the arrays are augmented by N zeros, as shown in Fig. 6.11A, then the resulting crosscorrelation ϕ_{yx} is as shown in Fig. 6.11B.

Now let us estimate the number of multiplications necessary for the estimation of the first-order kernel. The computation of each FFT of N points requires approximately $N \log_2 N$ complex multiplications (1 complex multiplication = 4 real multiplications). However, since x and y are real, a single FFT can be used to compute the FT of both x and y, as explained above. Therefore, to compute X_K and Y_K we need

$$4(N \log_2 N) \text{ multiplications}$$

To compute the product $Y_K X_K^*$ $(K = 0, 1, 2, \ldots, N-1)$ we require

$$N \text{ complex multiplications} = 4N \text{ multiplications}$$

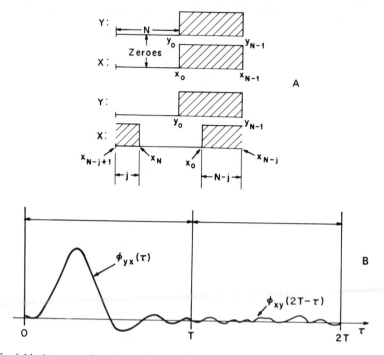

Fig. 6.11. Augmentation of arrays by zeros in order to take care of effects of circularity.

To compute the inverse FFT of $Y_K X_K^*$ we need

$$4(N \log_2 N) \text{ multiplications}$$

We thus need a total of

$$8N \log_2 N + 4N \cong 8N \log_2 N$$

multiplications. By use of efficient programming this number can be reduced somewhat. As seen in Sec. 6.2, the straightforward way requires

$$(N - \tfrac{1}{2}m)m \text{ multiplications}$$

where m is the extent (number of points) to which the kernels are computed. Therefore, the computing-time ratio for h_1 is

$$\text{efficiency ratio} = \frac{(N - \tfrac{1}{2}m)m}{8N \log_2 N} \tag{6.55}$$

For typical values of N and m (as would be encountered in experimental situations) we obtain Table 6.4 for the efficiency ratio. We note that no substantial savings result from this approach, for the computation of the first-order kernel, if m is substantially smaller than N. The reason for this lack of great savings is that the FFT route gives the kernel values for all τ up to T while we are usually interested in no more than the first $1/10$ of them (as determined by the memory extent of the kernel). In this respect, some of the other methods discussed in this chapter are superior to the FFT method. However, it should be noted that once the FFTs of x and y are computed, they can also be used for the computation of the other (higher-order) kernels.

Most physiology laboratories are equipped with small computers whose core memory does not allow the whole x and y arrays to be stored at one time. Then we are forced to process the data (compute the kernels) by bringing them into core in segments. If these segment lengths are close to m (the number of points at which the kernel is computed), then substantial savings will result if the FFT route is used to compute the kernels.

Figure 6.12A shows the y and x arrays segmented into K equal parts. The x array should be shifted to the right by i positions (to multiply and average) for the computation of $\phi_{yx}(i)$. We are interested only in the first m points of the crosscorrelation (where $m \Delta t = \mu$ is the system memory). Therefore, to achieve maximum efficiency via the FFT, we section the stimulus and response arrays into segments of length m each. Then we crosscorrelate these segments and add the results from each, forming the final crosscorrelation estimate.

For example, consider the first segment as shown below. We append m zeros to the y and x segments in order to avoid the effects of circularity, as discussed above. Then, for the ith position we have the configuration shown in Fig. 6.12B. Notice that the segment length on which we work is $2m$.

Then steps 1–3 above are used to compute $Y(\omega)X^*(\omega)$ for this segment. We now proceed to compute this same quantity—the frequency-domain representation of $\phi_{yx}(\tau)$ for the segment—for all segments, add these partial results, and transform the sum back to the time domain to

Table 6.4. *Efficiency Ratios of First-Order Kernel Computation through FFT*[a]

		m		
N	64	128	256	512
512	0.83	1.6	2.7	3.6
1024	0.77	1.5	2.8	4.8
2048	0.71	1.4	2.7	5.1
4096	0.66	1.3	2.6	5.0
8192	0.61	1.2	2.4	4.8

[a]N and m are as defined in Table 6.1.

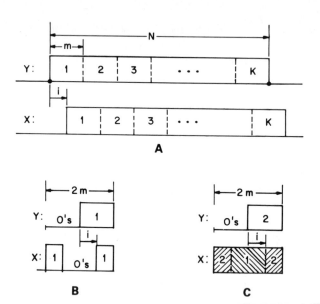

Fig. 6.12. Computation of first-order kernel.

obtain $\phi_{yx}(\tau)$. We can do this summation of the segments in the frequency domain (before inverting to the time domain) because the Fourier transform is a linear transformation.

For the second segment, the first m positions of x must be filled with the *previous* segment of x, i.e., #1, and last m positions with the current— #2 segment—values of x. For the y segment, the first m positions are again filled by zeros and the last m by the values of the second segment. Thus, we have the configuration shown in Fig. 6.12C. Notice that we need to have the previous section of x as well as the current one, as shown above, in order to pick up the correlation of the x values of the #1 section with those of the #2 y values. Again, steps 1–3 above are used to compute $Y(\omega)X^*(\omega)$ for this segment. The result is added (accumulated) to the previous values of the $Y(\omega)X^*(\omega)$ quantity. This procedure is repeated until all sections have been used for the computation of $Y(\omega)X^*(\omega)$. If the last section has less than m points, zeros are filled in to make its length equal to m. Finally, the result is inverted to the time domain using the FFT.

We now consider the computing time involved if this segmenting procedure is followed. At each stage (i.e., for each section) we have to correlate two real arrays of $2m$ points each, without, however, performing the last step (#4), which takes about half the time. Therefore according to what was previously discussed,

$$4(2m)\log_2 2m \text{ multiplications}$$

are required. Since there are K sections, where $N \simeq Km$, the total number of multiplications required is

$$K \cdot 4 \cdot (2m) \log_2 2m = 8N \log_2 2m$$

Then the ratio of computing times of the "straightforward" way to the FFT (with sectioning) way becomes

$$\text{efficiency ratio} = \frac{(N - \frac{1}{2}m)m}{8N \log_2 2m} \tag{6.56}$$

Therefore, in following this method of segmentation—a fact of life imposed on us because of small core size of the typical laboratory computer—we achieve a savings ratio in the number of multiplications equal to

$$\frac{\log_2 N}{\log_2 2m}$$

For typical values of N and m, such as those of Table 6.4, this savings ratio varies from about 1 to about 2. However, this savings, in practice, is usually countered by the additional time required to shuffle the data segments in and out of core.

The Second-Order Kernel

We consider now the second-order kernel $h_2(\tau_1, \tau_2)$. The computational steps involved here (assuming X_K and Y_K have already been computed for the first-order kernel) are as follows:

(1) Form the product $V(\omega_1, \omega_2) = Y(\omega_1 + \omega_2) X^*(\omega_1) X^*(\omega_2)$. Since $V(\omega_1, \omega_2) = V(\omega_2, \omega_1)$ only half of the entries for $V(\omega_1, \omega_2)$ need be computed and the other half can be filled in by symmetry. Noting that X_K and Y_K are uniquely defined only up to $K = N/2$, then $Y_{K_1+K_2}$ is uniquely defined only for $K_1 + K_2 \leq N/2$ (cf. Fig. 6.13).

(2) Compute the inverse FFT of $V(\omega_1, \omega_2)$ to obtain $\phi_{yxx}(\tau_1, \tau_2)$. Computation of $V(\omega_1, \omega_2)$ for each unique (ω_1, ω_2) entry of step 1 involves

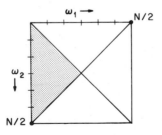

Fig. 6.13. Symmetry of second-order kernel transform.

Table 6.5. Efficiency Ratios of Second-Order Kernel Computation through FFT^a

		m		
N	64	128	256	512
512	0.11	0.44	1.8	7.1
1024	0.05	0.20	0.8	3.2
2048	0.02	0.09	0.4	1.9
4096	0.01	0.04	0.2	0.7
8192	0.004	0.02	0.1	0.3

^{a}N and m are as defined in Table 6.1.

two complex multiplications. Therefore, the number of necessary operations is

$$4(2 \cdot \tfrac{1}{2}N^2) = 4N^2$$

Step 2 above involves the computation of a two-dimensional (inverse) Fourier transform. This requires approximately

$$N^2 \log_2 N^2 \text{ complex multiplications} = 8N^2 \log_2 N \text{ multiplications}$$

Therefore, the total number of multiplications required is

$$4N^2 + 8N^2 \log_2 N \simeq 8N^2 \log_2 N$$

If $h_2(\tau_1, \tau_2)$ is computed in a straightforward manner

$$2\left(N - \frac{m}{2}\right)\frac{(m+1)m}{2} \simeq N(m^2 + m) \text{ multiplications}$$

are needed. The ratio of computing times is

$$\frac{\text{time of "straightforward" way}}{\text{time of FFT way}} \simeq \frac{m^2 + m}{8N \log_2 N} \qquad (6.57)$$

Table 6.5 lists the "efficiency ratio" for typical values (as encountered in practice) of N and m. Again, it is evident that savings in computing time, via the FFT, result only if the extent m of the kernel arguments is close to N. This suggests segmentation of the data to sections of length m, as was done for the first-order kernel. This segmentation often occurs naturally anyway, since the computer memory does not accommodate whole arrays and the data are brought in from auxiliary storage in segments. For the computation of $\phi_{yxx}(\tau_1, \tau_2)$, at each stage the quantity $Y(\omega_1 + \omega_2)X^*(\omega_1)X^*(\omega_2)$ is computed and accumulated with that of the previous stages. At the end, the two-dimensional inverse FFT is used to compute $\phi_{yxx}(\tau_1, \tau_2)$. Since at each stage we deal with arrays of length $2m$, the following number of multiplications are needed:

To compute the FFTs of the y and x segments we need

$$4(2m)\log_2 2m = 8m\log_2 2m$$

To form the product $Y(\omega_1+\omega_2)X^*(\omega_1)X^*(\omega_2)$ we need

$$4\left[2\frac{(2m)^2}{2}\right] = 16m^2$$

Therefore, the total number of multiplications at each step is

$$8m\log_2 2m + 16m^2$$

It should be noted here that if the first-order *and* the second-order kernels are to be computed the computation of the FFTs of x and y for each segment need only be done once. If that is the case, the number of operations is $16m^2$. This procedure is repeated for all K segments. The result is a $2m \times 2m$ complex matrix, which we invert—via FFT—to obtain $\phi_{yxx}(\tau_1, \tau_2)$. This requires

$$4(2m)^2\log_2(2m)^2 = 32m^2\log_2 2m \quad \text{multiplications}$$

Therefore, the total number of multiplications is

$$32m^2\log_2 2m + K(8m\log_2 2m + 16m^2)$$

$$\approx 32m^2\log_2 2m + 8N\log_2 2m + 16Nm$$

or

$$32m^2\log_2 2m + 16Nm$$

if we assume that the FFTs of the x and y segments have already been computed for the first-order kernel. Taking the worst case, we have for the ratio of "straightforward" to FFT ways

$$\text{efficiency ratio} = \frac{(N-\frac{1}{2}m)(m^2+m)}{32m^2\log_2 2m + 8N\log_2 2m + 16Nm} \tag{6.58}$$

For typical values of N and m, encountered in practice, we obtain the efficiency ratios shown in Table 6.6.

The nth-Order Kernel

Generalizing these results, the multiplications needed in step 1 above for an nth-order kernel (assuming the FT of the x and y segments have already been computed) are approximately

$$4\left[n\frac{(2m)^n}{n!}\right] = \frac{2^{n+2}m^n}{(n-1)!}$$

Table 6.6. *Efficiency Ratios of Second-Order Kernel*
Computation through Segmentation and FFT[a]

N	m			
	64	128	256	512
512	1.3	1.4	1.2	0.8
1024	2.0	2.5	2.5	2.2
2048	2.7	3.9	4.6	4.7
4096	3.2	5.2	7.3	8.6
8192	3.5	6.2	10.0	13.8

[a]N and m are as defined in Table 6.1.

for the method of segmenting the records. For step 2, the required number of multiplications is

$$4(2m)^n \log_2 (2m)^n = n \cdot 2^{n+2} \cdot m^n \log_2 2m$$

Thus, the total number of multiplications is

$$2^{n+2} m^n \left[\frac{1}{(n-1)!} + n \log_2 2m \right] \approx n 2^{n+2} m^n \log_2 2m$$

Thus, the ratio of the computing times (straightforward vs FFT way) is, for the nth-order kernel,

$$\text{(efficiency ratio)}_n = \frac{(N - \frac{1}{2}m)[(m+n-1)(m+n-2) \cdots m]}{n! 2^{n+2} m^n \log_2 2m} \qquad (6.59)$$

Examples. Figure 6.14 shows the exact and estimated (via frequency-domain computation) kernels of a nonlinear system. For the estimation of the linear kernel, 2048 points of stimulus–response samples were used and 128 values of $h_1(\tau)$ were estimated, i.e., $N = 2048$ and $m = 128$. The computation was carried out on an IBM 360/68, taking 9 sec in the straightforward manner of computation (i.e., by shifting and multiplying the stimulus–response arrays) and 7 sec using the FFT method. For the computation of the second-order kernel $\hat{h}_2(\tau_1, \tau_2)$ a larger number of stimulus–response samples was used and a smaller number of lags for (τ_1, τ_2): $N = 8192$ and $m = 64$. Computing in the straightforward manner took 4 min, while computing via the FFT through segmentation took 1.4 min.

Figures 6.15 and 6.16 show the kernel estimates for a two-input system obtained by calculation in the frequency domain. The computing times required for each first- or second-order kernel were the same as those for the first- and second-order kernels of the one-input system.

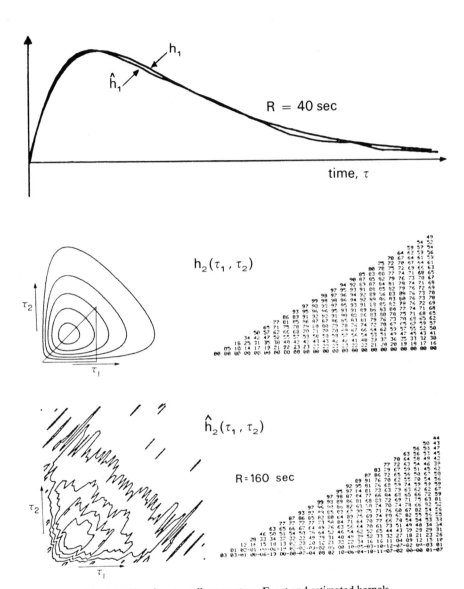

Fig. 6.14. One-input nonlinear system. Exact and estimated kernels.

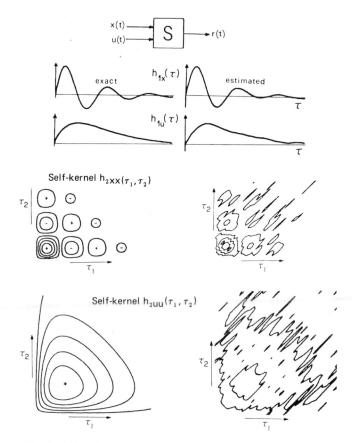

Fig. 6.15. Two-input nonlinear system. Exact and estimated kernels.

6.4. Special Cases of Kernel Computation

Significant simplifications in the computation of kernels occur in the cases of binary and ternary input or spike train output. These special cases are discussed separately in this section because of the increasing use that they receive in actual applications.

6.4.1. The Use of Binary and Ternary Inputs

A binary signal is one that assumes only two values, e.g., +1 and −1 (Fig. 6.17). A ternary signal is one that assumes only three values, e.g., +1, 0, and −1 (Fig. 6.18). The principal virtue of the use of these signals is computational. They allow the substitution of a chain of floating-point multiplications by a logical conjunction and an addition during the

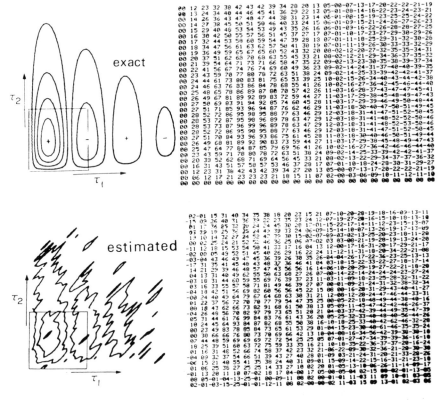

Fig. 6.16. Cross-kernels (exact and estimated).

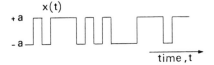

Fig. 6.17. Binary signal.

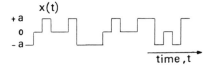

Fig. 6.18. Ternary signal.

computation of a crosscorrelation by a digital computer. The resulting reduction in computational time becomes appreciable when proper hardware and/or software is used.

Another significant advantage in the use of binary and ternary signals is the simple way of generating and applying them in the laboratory. It must be noted that even when the signal is not very steep at the switching times (i.e., finite transition time) the autocorrelation properties are not seriously affected (cf. Godfrey *et al.*, 1966; V. Z. Marmarelis, 1976). For reasonably small response time of the digital-to-analog transducer (as compared to the system bandwidth) this kind of error is negligible for all practical purposes. However, it is expedient in practice to design the transducer so that the pattern of upward transition is similar to the one of downward transition.

An important theoretical point that ought to be emphasized in connection with the use of binary and ternary pseudorandom and random test signals is that the functional series that correspond to these signals are slightly modified from the original Wiener series. Consequently, the set of kernel estimates that are obtained are somewhat different from the Wiener kernels but still provide a legitimate model of the system under study. It must be noted that, if the step length Δt of the binary or ternary input signal is very small, then the kernel estimates are very close to the Wiener kernels of the system except at the diagonal points. This is illustrated through examples at the end of this section.

Evidently, binary and ternary quasiwhite test signals can be either random or pseudorandom according to the discussion in Chapter 5. The relative advantages and disadvantages of these two categories are discussed extensively in Chapter 5; however, a brief review of the most important points is again given below for the convenience of the reader.

Both the random and pseudorandom binary and ternary signals possess autocorrelation properties that allow their use in nonlinear systems identification through the crosscorrelation technique. Still, the random signals exhibit imperfections, due to their random nature, i.e., the values of their autocorrelation functions are random variables and therefore deviations occur due to statistical variance. This variance decreases monotonically with the record length, and therefore for sufficiently long records these deviations become practically negligible. On the other hand, pseudorandom signals have imperfections that are associated with their deterministic structure. These imperfections appear in the form of spikes in the even-order autocorrelation functions of order higher than 2. These "anomalies" cannot be eliminated by increasing the record length or by any other means. They are inherent and characteristic of the m sequences.

Clearly, pseudorandom signals are much shorter than the random signals for comparable experiments, and therefore their computational merits are greater. However, if the system under test has significant higher-order nonlinearities then the presence of anomalies might cause significant errors in the kernel estimates. The power of random signals lies in the fact that their autocorrelation properties are uniformly good. They require, of course, longer records, but the kernel estimates we obtain are free from errors induced by higher-order nonlinearities. On the other hand exploitation of the computational advantages provided by the form of binary and ternary signals makes the computational burden more bearable.

Although random signals have some redundancy (being random) and consequently require longer records, they give kernel estimates that are free from systematic error. Pseudorandom signals have a very sophisticated and efficient structure, requiring much shorter records, but they give kernel estimates contaminated with systematic error when the system under test contains higher-order nonlinearities.

As an illustration of the use of binary input, consider the cascade of a linear filter and a zero-memory nonlinearity, shown in Fig. 6.19. The exact Wiener kernels of the cascade system are shown in Fig. 6.19, along with the kernel estimates obtained through the use of a binary random input. Portions of the binary stimulus, the system response, and the

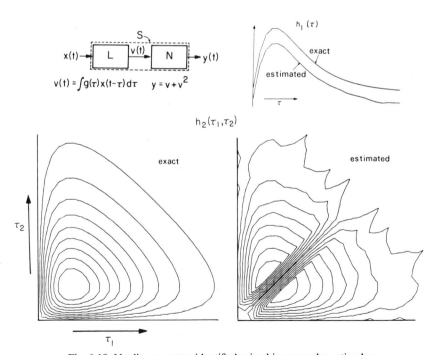

Fig. 6.19. Nonlinear system identified using binary random stimulus.

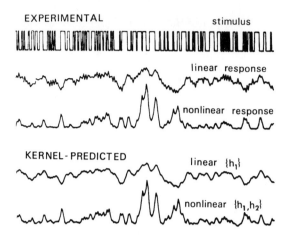

Fig. 6.20. Comparison of system and model responses in the case of binary random stimulus.

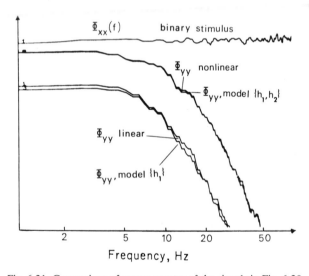

Fig. 6.21. Comparison of power spectra of the signals in Fig. 6.20.

model-predicted response are shown in Fig. 6.20 (for both the linear and nonlinear components of the system). Comparison of the model-predicted response with the actual system response is also made through their respective power spectra in Fig. 6.21.

The same is shown for a different linear subsystem and a ternary pseudorandom stimulus, in Figs. 6.22–6.24.

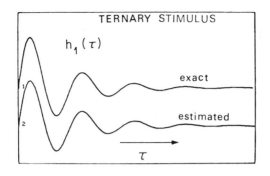

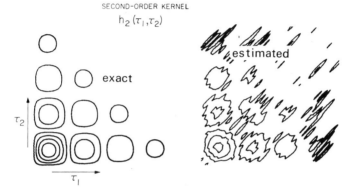

Fig. 6.22. Exact and estimated kernels using pseudorandom ternary stimulus.

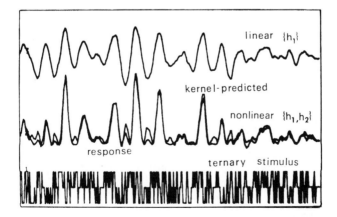

Fig. 6.23. Comparison of system and model responses in the case of pseudorandom ternary stimulus.

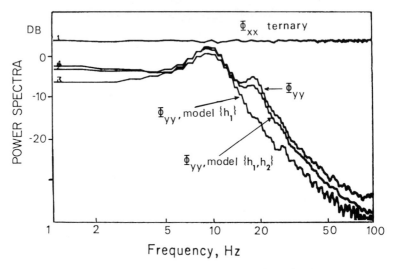

Fig. 6.24. Comparison of power spectra of the signals in Fig. 6.23.

6.4.2. Spike Train Output

In some physiological systems the output has the form of an impulse train, while the input to the system is continuous. This special form of the output signal allows the employment of delta functions to represent each one of the impulses. This has a simplifying effect on the computation of the system kernels, because of the deconvolution properties of a delta function, namely, that

$$\int_{-\infty}^{\infty} f(t)\delta(t-t_0)\, dt = f(t_0) \tag{6.60}$$

Thus, in the case of an impulse (spike) train output, we can denote the system response as

$$y(t) = \sum_{i=1}^{N} \delta(t-t_i) \tag{6.61}$$

where t_i are the times of spike occurrence. Evaluation of the nth-order system kernel is then simplified as

$$\hat{h}_n(\tau_1, \ldots, \tau_n) = \frac{1}{n! P^n} \frac{1}{T} \int_0^T y(t)x(t-\tau_1)\cdots x(t-\tau_n)\, dt$$

$$= \frac{1}{n! P^n} \frac{1}{T} \sum_{i=1}^{N} x(t_i-\tau_1)\cdots x(t_i-\tau_n) \tag{6.62}$$

where $x(t)$ is the continuous white-noise input of the system.

Under this formulation the kernel estimate appears to be an average waveform preceding the occurrence of a spike event (cf. Moore *et al.*, 1975; Bryant and Segundo, 1976). In that regard, this special case of kernel computation introduces an interesting physiological content to the mathematical notion of system kernels.

6.5. Analog (Hybrid) Methods for the Computation of Kernels

There are basically three reasons for the computation of kernels by analog or hybrid machinery. First, the digital computer is basically a serial processing machine and therefore only one point of the correlation can be computed at a time. Second, multiplication is a time-consuming operation for a digital machine. Third, since the correlations are computed from the sampled x and y signals, the averages that they represent have a larger statistical variance than if the continuous signals are used.

Let us consider the case of the first-order kernel h_1. We need to compute the following correlation function:

$$\phi_{yx}(\tau) = \frac{1}{T} \int_0^T y(t)x(t-\tau)\,dt \qquad (6.63)$$

In computing this by analog means the following operations are involved:

(1) Delaying the input signal $x(t)$ by τ sec.
(2) Multiplying the response signal $y(t)$ with the delayed signal $x(t)$ and averaging this product.

This must be done for all delayed times τ from 0 to μ, the memory of the system. The block diagram of this procedure is shown in Fig. 6.25. There are several ways to produce the delay time τ. It can be done using a tape recorder, or it can be done using delay lines. Recently the introduction of certain solid state devices (bucket brigades) perhaps offers the best alternative. However, it is desirable that this equipment be compatible with systems having widely varying bandwidths and therefore widely varying ranges of the delay τ. For this reason a better arrangement would be to first digitize the signals, normalize their bandwidths, and then generate their analog forms in this bandwidth. This is discussed later in this section. The

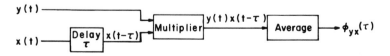

Fig. 6.25. Diagram of hybrid computation of crosscorrelation.

multiplication operation can now be performed by solid state devices recently made available. The integrating device (operational amplifier with feedback capacitor) computes the average value of the product of the signals for any time T (duration of record).

We need, of course, to compute the crosscorrelation for different lag values of τ. This can be done in two different ways. In one, we set the lag time τ to a specific value and then measure the crosscorrelation. Then we change to a new time lag and again measure the corresponding correlation. We repeat this procedure until the correlation for all lags of interest has been computed. This is basically a serial computation. We can do the same thing, however, in a parallel fashion. This will entail the employment of as many multipliers, averages, and delays as we have lags of interest. The employment of a tapped bucket-brigade delay circuit is suitable for this purpose, as shown in Fig. 6.26. The interval between the delays σ_1 and σ_2 is a measure of the resolution with which the correlation is computed. This resolution is a function of the frequency present in the data as required by the Nyquist sampling theorem. Clearly then, this frequency must be less than $1/2\Delta\tau$, where $\Delta\tau$ is the difference between adjacent lag values, for which the crosscorrelation function is computed.

The addition of a second multiplier for multiplying each (τ_1, τ_2) pair of delayed $x(t)$ terms puts the device in a form suitable for computing the second-order self-kernels. Alternately, this can be accomplished with switches and no additional multipliers, as shown in Fig. 6.27. Extension of this method for computing higher-order kernels column by column is accomplished with an additional multiplier set (or input) for each additional order of kernel. Extension of the system to handle mutual kernels representing multiple inputs requires one additional delay-line sequence for each additional input.

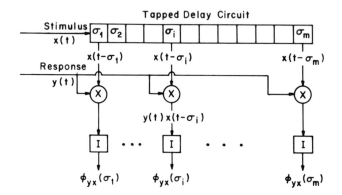

Fig. 6.26. Diagram of parallel computation of crosscorrelation.

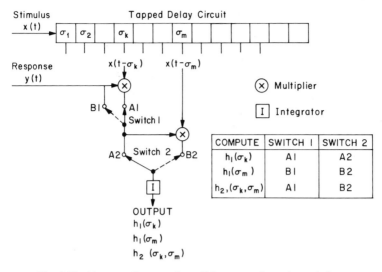

Fig. 6.27. Alternate diagram of parallel computation using switches.

There are several variations of this general scheme. One is to eliminate the analog delays and compute the appropriate delayed inputs to the multipliers using a digital computer. In any case, it appears advantageous to have only one value of analog unit delay and one actual frequency bandwidth for the system. Stimulus and response data are first digitized, smoothed, and converted in the digital computer to the fixed frequency range of the analog device. They are converted back into analog form for the kernel calculations. This is illustrated in Fig. 6.28. White-noise signals varying with variables other than time (space, light wavelength, etc.) are converted to equivalent time-domain variables.

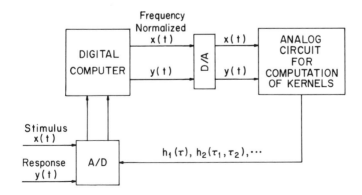

Fig. 6.28. Alternate diagram of kernel computation using D/A converters.

An additional consideration is the possibility that this type of device will give greater statistical accuracy than direct digital computation methods. This is due to the fact that the variance of the estimates becomes considerably smaller since a very great number of samples (resulting if one considers an analog signal as the extension of a digital signal sampled at a very high rate) is used for the estimation of any one average in the crosscorrelation. The achievement of the same statistical effect by the digital computation of kernels greatly increases the computational time and requires more memory. Convolutions (at least of first order) can also be performed by the same analog hardware.

6.6. Evaluation of the System Kernels

The methods discussed in this chapter for estimating system kernels have one problem in common, namely, the problem of weighting the kernels. This amounts to determining the relative magnitudes of the linear and nonlinear kernels. To illustrate this problem we consider the computation of the kernels through the crosscorrelation technique, the main approach in the practical evaluation of kernels. If the stimulus employed in the experiment were perfect Gaussian white noise then the linear and nonlinear kernels would be weighted by the factors $1/P$ and $1/2P^2$, respectively, that is,

$$h_1(\tau) = (1/P)\phi_{yx}(\tau) \tag{6.64}$$

$$h_2(\tau_1, \tau_2) = (1/2P^2)\phi_{yxx}(\tau_1, \tau_2) \tag{6.65}$$

However, since the stimulus is not perfect white noise (that is, the autocorrelation functions of the stimulus are not perfect delta functions of specified power P), problems may arise if the linear or the nonlinear kernel is weighted too much or too little. Admittedly, this is only a relative scale factor between the linear and nonlinear components of the system response. However, it may be very important in certain cases wherein quantitative assessment of the nonlinearity of the system is of importance. We discuss this point here and suggest remedies for its rectification.

Let us first consider a linear system. Computing the crosscorrelation between the stimulus and response signals—$x(t)$ and $y(t)$, respectively—we obtain

$$\phi_{yx}(\sigma) = \int_0^\infty h(\tau)\phi_{xx}(\sigma - \tau)\, d\tau \tag{6.66}$$

This integral is shown graphically in Fig. 6.29. It indicates that the value of $h(\tau)$ at $\tau = \sigma$ is "sampled" by $\phi_{xx}(\tau - \sigma)$. Hence, it is easily seen why it would be exactly equal to $h(\sigma)$ if $\phi_{xx}(\tau - \sigma) = \delta(\tau - \sigma)$. However, in prac-

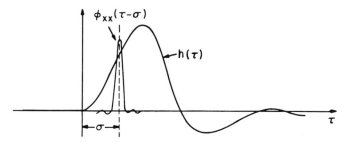

Fig. 6.29. Convolution for kernel estimation.

tice $\phi_{xx}(\tau)$ has a finite width, thus *smearing* its sample of $h(\tau)$. Now let us consider the sampled versions of all quantities involved:

$$\phi_{yx}(\tau): \quad \phi_{yx}(0), \phi_{yx}(1), \phi_{yx}(2), \ldots, \phi_{yx}(m)$$

$$\phi_{xx}(\tau): \quad \phi_{xx}(0), \phi_{xx}(1), \phi_{xx}(2), \ldots, \phi_{xx}(l)$$

$$h(\tau): \quad h(0), h(1), h(2), \ldots, h(m)$$

It should be noted that $\phi_{yx}(i)=0$, $h(i)=0$ for $i<0$ and that l is a rather small integer as compared to m [i.e., the bandwidth of $x(t)$ is wider than the bandwidth of the system). Also, $\phi_{xx}(i)$ is symmetric around $i=0$. Then we have approximately (for a sampling interval Δt)

$$\phi_{yx}(k) = \sum_{i=0}^{m} h(i)\phi_{xx}(i-k)\Delta t, \qquad k = 0, 1, \ldots, m \qquad (6.67)$$

For example, let us assume that $\phi_{xx}(j)$ is effectively zero for $j \geqslant 3$ (Fig. 6.30). Then Eq. (6.67) becomes

$$\phi_{yx}(k) = \sum_{i=k-2}^{k+2} h(i)\phi_{xx}(i-k)\Delta t, \qquad k = 0, 1, \ldots, m \qquad (6.68)$$

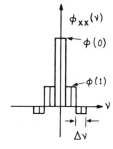

Fig. 6.30. Digitalized autocorrelation function.

or in matrix form, noting that $\phi(-i) = \phi(i)$ [denoting $\Delta t \phi_{xx}(\tau)$ by $\phi(\tau)$],

$$
\begin{bmatrix}
\phi(0) & \phi(1) & \phi(2) & 0 & 0 & \cdots & 0 & 0 \\
\phi(1) & \phi(0) & \phi(1) & \phi(2) & 0 & \cdots & 0 & 0 \\
\phi(2) & \phi(1) & \phi(0) & \phi(1) & \phi(2) & \cdots & 0 & 0 \\
0 & \phi(2) & \phi(1) & \phi(0) & \phi(1) & \cdots & 0 & 0 \\
\vdots & \vdots & \vdots & \vdots & \vdots & & \vdots & \vdots \\
0 & 0 & 0 & 0 & 0 & \cdots & \phi(1) & \phi(0)
\end{bmatrix}
\begin{bmatrix}
h(0) \\
h(1) \\
h(2) \\
h(3) \\
\vdots \\
h(m)
\end{bmatrix}
=
\begin{bmatrix}
\phi_{yx}(0) \\
\phi_{yx}(1) \\
\phi_{yx}(2) \\
\phi_{yx}(3) \\
\vdots \\
\phi_{yx}(m)
\end{bmatrix}
$$

$$\tag{6.69}$$

resulting in a so-called symmetric *band* matrix. Such matrix equations are easily solved without much demand on computer time or memory size. The solution for $h(k)$ is automatically scaled in this case. The same automatic scaling results if "deconvolution" in the frequency domain is employed. That is, taking the FT of Eq. (6.66) we have

$$\Phi_{yx}(\omega) = H(\omega)\Phi_{xx}(\omega) \tag{6.70}$$

However, this method may have considerable problems associated with its numerical accuracy. To counter these problems it may be necessary to filter the high frequencies considerably, before inverting back to the time domain. Similar formulas may be derived for the higher-order (nonlinear) kernels.

In the study of physiological systems, however, such accuracy (as afforded by the above methods) is usually not warranted since other error sources tend to be considerably greater. Therefore, we need a method which, even though less accurate computationally, is more stable than the frequency-domain deconvolution and the inversion of the matrix solution approach, especially for the higher-order kernels. From Eq. (6.68) we have

$$\phi_{yx}(k) = \Delta t\{h(k)\phi_{xx}(0) + \phi_{xx}(1)[h(k-1) + h(k+1)]$$
$$+ \phi_{xx}(2)[h(k-2) + h(k+2)]\} \tag{6.71}$$

assuming again that $\phi_{xx}(i) \approx 0$ for $i \geq 3$. We may now use the following approximation, if we assume that $h(k)$ does not change rapidly over the interval $[(k-2)\Delta t, (k+2)\Delta t]$:

$$h(k) = \frac{\phi_{yx}(k)}{\Delta t[\phi_{xx}(0) + 2\phi_{xx}(1) + 2\phi_{xx}(2)]} \tag{6.72}$$

Note that the denominator is simply the area under $\phi_{xx}(\tau)$ as approximated by a rectangular rule of integration. Other, more accurate, schemes of estimating this area may be employed.

We proceed now to the estimation of the second-order kernel. We first rewrite the Wiener series so that the resulting functionals are orthogonal with respect to the stimulus $x(t)$, which is no longer ideal white noise. However, the signal is Gaussian, and therefore the autocorrelation functions still have some of the desired properties, e.g., $\phi_{xxx}(\ ) = 0$. The orthogonal functionals with respect to this Gaussian, finite-bandwidth white noise will be

$$G_0 = h_0 \tag{6.73}$$

$$G_1(t) = \int_0^\infty h_1(\tau)x(t-\tau)\,d\tau \tag{6.74}$$

$$G_2(t) = \int\int_0^\infty h_2(\tau_1, \tau_2)x(t-\tau_1)x(t-\tau_2)\,d\tau_1\,d\tau_2$$

$$-\int\int_0^\infty h_2(\tau_1, \tau_2)\phi_{xx}(\tau_1-\tau_2)\,d\tau_1\,d\tau_2 \tag{6.75}$$

Thus, the second-order crosscorrelation yields

$$\phi_{yxx}(\sigma_1, \sigma_2) = \int\int_0^\infty h_2(\tau_1, \tau_2)[\phi_{xx}(\tau_1-\tau_2)\phi_{xx}(\sigma_1-\sigma_2)$$

$$+ \phi_{xx}(\tau_1-\sigma_1)\phi_{xx}(\tau_2-\sigma_2)$$
$$+ \phi_{xx}(\tau_2-\sigma_1)\phi_{xx}(\tau_1-\sigma_2)]\,d\tau_1\,d\tau_2$$

$$- \phi_{xx}(\sigma_1-\sigma_2)\int\int_0^\infty h_2(\tau_1, \tau_2)\phi_{xx}(\tau_1-\tau_2)\,d\tau_1\,d\tau_2$$

$$= 2\int\int_0^\infty h_2(\tau_1, \tau_2)\phi_{xx}(\tau_1-\sigma_1)\phi_{xx}(\tau_2-\sigma_2)\,d\tau_1\,d\tau_2 \tag{6.76}$$

Thus, assuming again that $\phi(i) \simeq 0$ for $i \geq 3$, we have

$$\phi_{yxx}(k_1, k_2) \simeq 2\sum_{j=k_2-2}^{k_2+2}\sum_{i=k_1-2}^{k_1+2} h_2(i, j)\phi(i-k_1)\phi(j-k_2) \tag{6.77}$$

which, after some manipulation, and, recalling that $h_2(i, j) = h_2(j, i)$, gives us approximately

$$\phi_{yxx}(k_1, k_2) \simeq 2h_2(k_1, k_2)[\phi(0)+2\phi(1)+2\phi(2)]^2 \tag{6.78}$$

Here, of course, it is assumed that $h_2(\tau_1, \tau_2)$ is fairly smooth, i.e., does not change appreciably within the square $\tau_1 = [t_1 - 2\Delta t, t_1 + 2\Delta t]$, $\tau_2 = [t_2 - 2\Delta t, t_2 + 2\Delta t]$. Therefore, we obtain for $h_2(k_1, k_2)$

$$h_2(k_1, k_2) \approx \frac{1}{2} \frac{\phi_{yxx}(k_1, k_2)}{[\phi(0) + 2\phi(1) + 2\phi(2)]^2} \tag{6.79}$$

Notice again that $[\phi(0) + 2\phi(1) + 2\phi(2)]$ is the area under the autocorrelation curve of the stimulus $x(t)$.

The sequence used in weighting the kernels h_1 and h_2 is, therefore, as follows:

(1) Compute the autocorrelation $\phi_{xx}(\tau)$.

(2) Compute the "area" under it,

$$\int_{-a}^{a} \phi_{xx}(\tau)\, d\tau = A_x \tag{6.80}$$

for a big enough a so that $\phi_{xx}(a) \approx 0$.

(3) Compute crosscorrelations $\phi_{yx}(\sigma)$ and $\phi_{yxx}(\sigma_1, \sigma_2)$.

(4) Use Eqs. (6.72) and (6.79) to compute kernels h_1, h_2.

There is an alternative way of estimating the relative weights of kernels h_1 and h_2. This way, however, involves considerably more computation but it may yield slightly more accurate results in certain cases. The procedure to be used is approximately the following: The stimulus record is multiplied by a constant in order to normalize the power level P over the flat portion of the input spectrum to a value around 1 (0 db). The exact value of P is picked after the kernels have been computed with $P = 1$ in the following way: The model responses to the GWN input are computed with P as a variable and then the value of P is found using a variational technique that minimizes the mean-square error between model and experimental responses to the white-noise stimulus used in the identifying experiment. Of course, the entire record, or a considerable part of it, is used for this purpose. This procedure is outlined below.

(1) Estimate the area A_x under the autocorrelation curve $\phi_{xx}(\tau)$.

(2) Compute the kernels h_1' and h_2', using formulas (6.72) and (6.79).

(3) Using h_1' and h_2' compute the model response to $x(t)$ (to all or part of the record):

$$y_{m1}(t) = \int_0^{\infty} h_1'(\tau) x(t - \tau)\, d\tau \tag{6.81}$$

$$y_{m2}(t) = \int\int_0^{\infty} h_2'(\tau_1, \tau_2) x(t - \tau_1) x(t - \tau_2)\, d\tau_1\, d\tau_2 \tag{6.82}$$

for $t = 0$ to $t = t_0$.

(4) Find constants C_0, C_1, C_2 that minimize the squared error:

$$\varepsilon^2(C_0, C_1, C_2) = \int_0^{t_o} [y(t) - C_0 - C_1 y_{m1}(t) - C_2 y_{m2}(t)]^2 \, dt \qquad (6.83)$$

by solving the following system:

$$\left\{ \frac{\partial \varepsilon^2}{\partial C_0} = 0, \ \frac{\partial \varepsilon^2}{\partial C_1} = 0, \ \frac{\partial \varepsilon^2}{\partial C_2} = 0 \right\} \qquad (6.84)$$

(5) The correctly weighted kernels are then

$$h_1(\tau) = C_1 h_1'(\tau) \qquad (6.85)$$

$$h_2(\tau_1, \tau_2) = C_2 h_2'(\tau_1, \tau_2) \qquad (6.86)$$

The disadvantage of this procedure is that a lot of computing time is required in carrying out step 3. In certain cases, it may be necessary to constrain C_1 and C_2 by the relationship derived from

$$C_1 = 1/P \qquad (6.87)$$

$$C_2 = 1/2P^2 \qquad (6.88)$$

This produces

$$C_1^2 = 2C_2 \qquad (6.89)$$

Again, a similar minimization procedure can be followed.

A similar procedure may be used in the case of a system with more than one input. Assume that we have a system with two inputs x and u and one output y. The procedure is as follows:

1. Evaluate the area under the autocorrelation curve of each input, $x(t)$ and $u(t)$, using integrals as in Eq. (6.80).

2. Compute the self-kernels $h_{1x}'(\tau)$, $h_{1u}'(\tau)$, $h_{2xx}'(\tau_1, \tau_2)$, $h_{2uu}'(\tau_1, \tau_2)$ using formulas (6.72) and (6.79) above. Compute the cross-kernel $h_{2xu}'(\tau_1, \tau_2)$ using

$$h_{2xu}'(\tau_1, \tau_2) = \frac{1}{A_x A_u} \phi_{yxu}(\tau_1, \tau_2) \qquad (6.90)$$

where A_x, A_u are the areas under the autocorrelation curves of $x(t)$, $u(t)$.

3. Using these kernel estimates we estimate the various response contributions to $y(t)$ using all or part of the record:

$$y_x(t) = \int_0^\infty h_{1x}'(\tau) x(t - \tau) \, d\tau \qquad (6.91)$$

$$y_{xx}(t) = \int_0^\infty \int h_{2xx}'(\tau_1, \tau_2) x(t - \tau_1) x(t - \tau_2) \, d\tau_1 \, d\tau_2 \qquad (6.92)$$

$$y_{xu}(t) = \int\limits_0^\infty \int h'_{2xu}(\tau_1, \tau_2) x(t-\tau_1) u(t-\tau_2)\, d\tau_1\, d\tau_2 \tag{6.93}$$

etc., for $t = 0$ to $t = t_0$.

4. Find constants C_0, C_{1x}, C_{2x}, C_{1u}, C_{2u}, C_{xu} that minimize the square error

$$\varepsilon^2 = \int_0^{t_0} [y(t) - C_0 - C_{1x}y_x(t) - C_{2x}y_{xx}(t) - C_{1u}y_u(t) - C_{2u}y_{uu}(t)$$

$$- C_{xu}y_{xu}(t)]^2\, dt \tag{6.94}$$

5. The correctly weighted kernels are then

$$h_{1x}(\tau) = C_{1x}h'_{1x}(\tau) \tag{6.95}$$

$$h_{2xx}(\tau_1, \tau_2) = C_{2x}h'_{2xx}(\tau_1, \tau_2) \tag{6.96}$$

etc.

6.7. Evaluation of Results of Experiment

After the system characterization has been obtained in terms of the measured kernels, the question arises: How good is this characterization? There are several ways in which one can compare the actual system with the derived characterization. However, most would tend to measure the degree of agreement only of certain specific features or over a limited area of the stimulus–response space. In contrast, Wiener argued that two systems are equivalent if and only if they respond identically to a white-noise input. Consequently, the criterion of "goodness" of the functional identification and predictability of the measured kernels is how well the "model" response mimics the actual experimental response to the same white-noise stimulus. This comparison of the experimental and functional "model" system (manifested by the measured system kernels) is carried out, in this study, by quantifying the agreement in wave shape of the two responses in terms of the mean-square deviation. The "model" responses (linear, nonlinear, due to a particular input, etc.) are computed by evaluating the integrals indicated by Eqs. (6.81) and (6.82) using the measured kernels.

6.7.1. One-Input System

Consider, for example, the case of a one-input system. The zero-order model (h_0) is a constant equal to the average value of the response over the entire record. The mean-square error for this model is computed and normalized to 100 (arbitrary) units. The response, as predicted by $h_1(\tau)$, is

$$y_L(t) = \int_0^\infty h_1(\tau)x(t-\tau)\,d\tau \tag{6.97}$$

and it is computed [with $x(t)$ the white-noise signal used in the experiment] and its mean-square deviation from the experimental response is measured and normalized in the same units. This number gives a measure of "goodness" of the linear representation of the system as a percentage (since the error to the zeroth model is 100 units). The smaller this number, the better is the agreement. Subsequently, the second-order nonlinear response term

$$y_N(t) = \int\int_0^\infty h_2(\tau_1, \tau_2)x(t-\tau_1)x(t-\tau_2)\,d\tau_1\,d\tau_2 - P\int_0^\infty h_2(\tau, \tau)\,d\tau \tag{6.98}$$

is computed. Then the mean-square deviation from the experimental response of this nonlinear model

$$\varepsilon^2 = \frac{1}{T}\int_0^T [y(t) - y_N(t) - y_L(t) - h_0]^2\,dt \tag{6.99}$$

is computed and normalized in the same units. In addition to assessing the predictive capacity of the characterization at each (linear, nonlinear) stage, a quantitative measure of the system nonlinearity is also obtained by comparing the reduction in MSE for the various models.

Figure 6.31 shows a nonlinear system whose kernels were estimated from a record length of 80 sec. The exact system kernels are also shown for comparison. To judge the "goodness" of the identification, model responses (linear and nonlinear) were computed and compared to the actual system response (Fig. 6.32). The MSE reduction is as follows:

Characterization:	$\{h_0\}$	$\{h_1(\tau)\}$	$\{h_1(\tau), h_2(\tau_1, \tau_2)\}$
MSE:	100	22	3

Since this was a second-order nonlinear system and both $\hat{h}_1(\tau)$ and $\hat{h}_2(\tau_1, \tau_2)$ were estimated and used to compute the model responses, the remaining error of 3% is due solely to the finite record length of the data. In this respect it should be noted that although $\hat{h}_2(\tau_1, \tau_2)$ looks "noisy" in Fig. 6.31 it performs quite well in predicting the system response [obviously, one reason for this performance is that an *integral* computation usually smoothes the response].

Another measure of "goodness" of the characterization is the comparison of the predicted response frequency spectra (linear and nonlinear) with the spectrum of the actual system response, as shown in

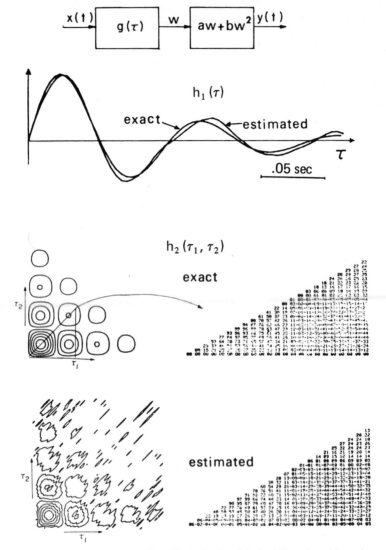

Fig. 6.31. Nonlinear system identified using band-limited Gaussian white noise.

Fig. 6.33. Note the secondary peak, around 18 Hz, in the nonlinear model response (and actual system reponse) which is absent in the linear model response. This peak is expected since this is a *second-order nonlinear* system and the linear part exhibits a peak around 9 Hz.

SYSTEM RESPONSE

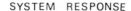

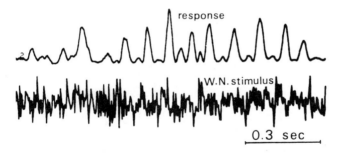

response

W.N. stimulus

0.3 sec

KERNEL-PREDICTED RESPONSES

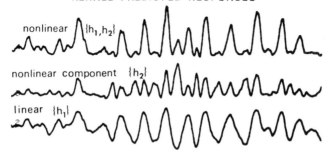

nonlinear $\{h_1, h_2\}$

nonlinear component $\{h_2\}$

linear $\{h_1\}$

Fig. 6.32. Comparison of system and model responses in the case of band-limited Gaussian white-noise stimulus.

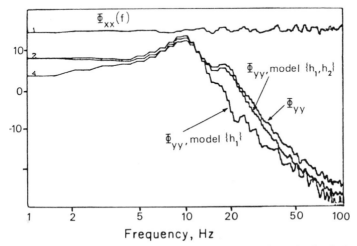

Fig. 6.33. Comparison of power spectra (in db) of the signals in Fig. 6.32.

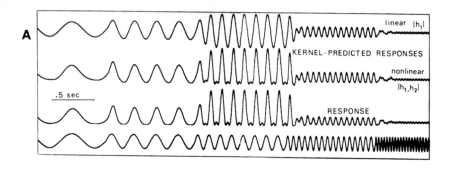

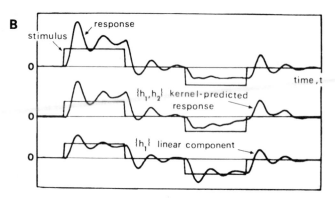

Fig. 6.34. System and model responses to specific deterministic stimuli: (A) sine waves, (B) pulses.

Since the system is second order, the second-order Wiener model is a complete model of the system and the model should predict accurately the system response to any arbitrary stimulus. This is illustrated in Fig. 6.34 for sinusoidal and pulse stimuli.

6.7.2. Two-Input System

A similar analysis of goodness of the characterization can be carried out in the case of multi-input systems. This analysis is simplified by the fact that the terms due to each input are mutually orthogonal. Figure 6.8 shows a two-input system, and frequency spectra of the various model response components as compared to actual response components (the latter are obtainable because this system was synthesized from known components simulated on a digital computer). Figure 6.9 shows portions of actual response components and the corresponding kernel-predicted response components. The MSE reduction is shown in Table 6.7. It should be noted

*Table 6.7. Percentage MSE of Responses
Predicted by Various Models of a Two-Input
System*

Characterization	MSE
$\{h_0\}$	100
$\{h_{1x}, h_{2xx}\}$	54
$\{h_{1u}, h_{2uu}\}$	47
$\{h_{2xu}\}$	62
$\{h_{1x}, h_{2xx}, h_{1u}, h_{2uu}, h_{2xu}\}$	11

that in this case, in addition to assessing the predictive capability of the model, the MSE gives an indication of the relative contribution of each input component.

For example, knowing the MSE for the spot and annular inputs for a retinal neuron cell it is possible to estimate the relative contribution of each input to its response with reference to the MSE of the zeroth-order model. Also, the MSE (or, more exactly, the difference between the MSEs of the linear and nonlinear characterizations) can be used to indicate the degree of nonlinearity involved in the generation of responses from a given class of neurons. These two measures—relative contribution of each input and degree of nonlinearity—have been used to characterize and classify the neurons in a vertebrate retina using the results of about 150 two-input GWN experiments (cf. Naka *et al.*, 1975).

6.7.3. Physical Units of Kernels

Another matter of concern here may be that of converting the units of the kernels to the physical units that they represent. It is easily seen that if the units of the stimulus are u_x and the units of the response are u_y, then

units of h_1: $\quad u_y/(u_x \cdot \sec)$

units of h_2: $\quad u_y/(u_x \cdot \sec)^2$

These units can easily be interpreted. Consider, for example, a neural system where the stimulus is current injected intracellularly (measured in amperes) and the response is a membrane potential measured in volts. Then, the first-order kernel h_1 denotes the response in volts to an impulse of strength one (amp·sec) of a linear system that is the best MSE representation of the system under study. Similarly, the second-order kernel h_2 can be interpreted as a voltage correction (or nonlinear response cross talk) to the linear representation, when two impulses, each of strength one (amp·sec) are delivered to the system (cf. Sec. 4.2).

In determining the actual physical units of the kernels estimated for a particular system, care must be taken to compensate for the various scaling factors introduced by the procedures outlined above. If the system is linear these units are affected only by a constant of proportionality. If, however, the system is nonlinear, then the relative magnitudes of the linear and nonlinear kernels affected by this scaling must be determined carefully. According to the kernel-computation procedure discussed above, the stimulus signal is scaled twice, once by the transducer and recording equipment (amplifiers, etc.) and once to normalize the power level:

$$x \xrightarrow[\text{amplifiers etc.}]{\text{transducer}} C_1 x \xrightarrow[\text{power level}]{\text{normalize}} C_n C_1 x = x' \qquad (6.100)$$

The response signal is scaled only once—by the transducer:

$$y \xrightarrow{\text{transducer}} C_2 y = y' \qquad (6.101)$$

The estimated first-order kernel h_1' relates *these* signals x' and y'

$$y'(t) = \int_0^\infty h_1'(\tau) x'(t - \tau)\, d\tau \qquad (6.102)$$

Considering the scaling operations we find the relationship between the unscaled signals (in their physical units):

$$y(t) = \frac{C_n C_1}{C_2} \int_0^\infty h_1(\tau) x(t - \tau)\, d\tau \qquad (6.103)$$

Therefore, the real magnitude of the first-order kernel $h_1(\tau)$ is related to the estimated one $h_1'(\tau)$ by

$$h_1(\tau) = \frac{C_n C_1}{C_2} h_1'(\tau) \qquad (6.104)$$

Similarly, we find for the second-order nonlinear kernel that

$$h_2(\tau_1, \tau_2) = \frac{C_n^2 C_1^2}{C_2} h_2'(\tau_1, \tau_2) \qquad (6.105)$$

These two relations, (6.105) and (6.104), yield the magnitudes of the linear and nonlinear kernels in their unscaled physical units and indicate the physical proportion of these kernels to each other.

Errors in the Estimation of System Kernels

Introduction

Estimation of kernels with the crosscorrelation technique is associated with a variety of errors. The most important of these errors are due to the finite bandwidth and the finite record length of the quasiwhite stimulus signal, since the white-noise method and the crosscorrelation technique are theoretically designed for a white stimulus signal of infinite bandwidth and record length. It is important for the user of the white-noise method to have a quantitative idea of the estimation error that is committed using any of the quasiwhite test signals that have been previously discussed (Chapter 5).

In this chapter, we discuss these estimation errors for each of the families of quasiwhite test signals (GWN, PRS, CSRS).

7.1. Estimation Errors Using GWN Stimulus

The types of error that are encountered using GWN include those due to finite record length, finite stimulus bandwidth, and the amplitude truncation of the Gaussian distribution.

7.1.1. Errors Due to the Finite Record Length

The system kernels are computed as crosscorrelations from stimulus–response records of finite length R. Therefore there is some statistical error associated with the kernel estimates due to the finite number of samples used in computing the averages that these crosscorrelations represent.

Linear System: Variance of the Linear Kernel Estimate

To simplify the discussion, let us assume initially that the system is linear, i.e., $h_n(\tau_1, \ldots, \tau_n) \equiv 0$ for $n \geq 2$.

We have

$$\hat{h}(\tau) = K_1 \cdot \hat{\phi}_{yx}(\tau)$$

$$= K_1 \frac{1}{R} \int_0^R y(t)x(t-\tau)\, dt \qquad (7.1)$$

The statistically unbiased expression for the crosscorrelation would require

$$\hat{\phi}_{yx}(\tau) = \frac{1}{R-\tau} \int_\tau^R y(t)x(t-\tau)\, dt \qquad (7.2)$$

However, it can be shown that the estimate derived from Eq. (7.1), although biased, is more accurate statistically (smaller variance) than the one in Eq. (7.2) as long as τ is less than about $\frac{1}{10}R$. For the present discussion we will follow (7.1) (which, in fact, can be made an unbiased estimate if the data exist for a record of length $R + \tau$). The statistical error in the kernel estimate, for any τ, is given by the variance

$$\text{Var}\,[\hat{h}(\tau)] = E[[K_1\hat{\phi}_{yx}(\tau)]^2] - [E[K_1\hat{\phi}_{yx}(\tau)]]^2$$

$$= \frac{K_1^2}{R^2}\Bigg[\int\int_0^R E[y(\mu)x(\mu-\tau)y(\nu)x(\nu-\tau)]\, d\mu\, d\nu$$

$$- \int\int_0^R E[y(\mu)x(\mu-\tau)]E[y(\nu)x(\nu-\tau)]\, d\mu\, d\nu\Bigg] \qquad (7.3)$$

Given that the system is linear, $y(t)$ is a Gaussian process since $x(t)$ is Gaussian. However, even if $y(t)$ were not Gaussian the present analysis would hold in most cases if certain weak integrability conditions on the non-Gaussian components are satisfied, conditions almost always realized in practice. Then we have

$$E[y(\mu)x(\mu-\tau)y(\nu)x(\nu-\tau)]$$

$$= \phi_{yx}^2(\tau) + \phi_{yy}(\mu-\nu)\phi_{xx}(\mu-\nu) + \phi_{yx}(\mu-\nu+\tau)\phi_{yx}(\nu-\mu+\tau) \qquad (7.4)$$

and Eq. (7.3) becomes

$$\text{Var}\,[\hat{h}(\tau)] = \frac{K_1^2}{R^2}\int\int_0^R [\phi_{yy}(\mu-\nu)\phi_{xx}(\mu-\nu)$$

$$+ \phi_{yx}(\mu-\nu+\tau)\phi_{yx}(\nu-\mu+\tau)]\, d\mu\, d\nu \qquad (7.5)$$

In this expression, we observe that the several correlation functions depend on $(\mu-\nu)$ and not on μ and ν separately. Setting $\xi = \mu - \nu$, we see from

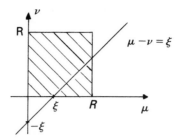

Fig. 7.1. Change of integration variable.

Fig. 7.1 that the range of integration for ξ is from $-R$ to R, and knowing that the integrand is an even function with respect to ξ, the integration over the variable μ for given ξ will give $(R - |\xi|)$. After this change of variable the variance of the estimate becomes

$$\text{Var}\,[\hat{h}(\tau)] = \frac{K_1^2}{R} \int_{-R}^{R} \left(1 - \frac{|\xi|}{R}\right)[\phi_{yy}(\xi)\phi_{xx}(\xi) + \phi_{yx}(\tau+\xi)\phi_{yx}(\tau-\xi)]\,d\xi \quad (7.6)$$

Note that, since $y(t)$ is the causal system output to input $x(t)$, $\phi_{yx}(u)=0$ for $u<0$. The various functions involved in the evaluation of the variance in Eq. (7.6) are shown graphically in Fig. 7.2. The weighing function $1-|\xi|/R$ is a triangle as shown. The autocorrelation of the input GWN $\phi_{xx}(\nu)$ is comparatively narrow since its bandwidth is chosen to be larger than the system bandwidth. In practice the response autocorrelogram $\phi_{yy}(\nu)$ becomes negligible for $\nu > \mu$ (the system memory). The same is true for the crosscorrelogram $\phi_{yx}(\nu)$, i.e., it is very close to zero for ν equal to the system memory.

Taking into consideration all these facts, the expression in Eq. (7.6) becomes approximately:

$$\text{Var}\,[\hat{h}(\tau)] \cong \frac{2K_1^2}{R}\left[\int_0^\mu \phi_{yy}(\xi)\phi_{xx}(\xi)\,d\xi + \int_0^\tau \phi_{yx}(\tau+\xi)\phi_{yx}(\tau-\xi)\,d\xi\right]$$

$$(7.7)$$

From this equation we conclude that the statistical error in the kernel estimate decreases with the record length R as $1/R^{1/2}$.

For an ideal white-noise stimulus, i.e., $\phi_{xx}(\xi) = (1/K_1)\delta(\xi)$, the variance of the kernel estimate becomes, from Eq. (7.6)

$$\text{Var}\,[\hat{h}(\tau)] = \frac{1}{R}\int_0^R h^2(\xi)\,d\xi + \frac{2}{R}\int_0^\tau \left(1 - \frac{\xi}{R}\right)h(\tau+\xi)h(\tau-\xi)\,d\xi \quad (7.8)$$

which clearly decreases with increasing record length R, depending on the specific system under identification and the specific argument τ. Note also

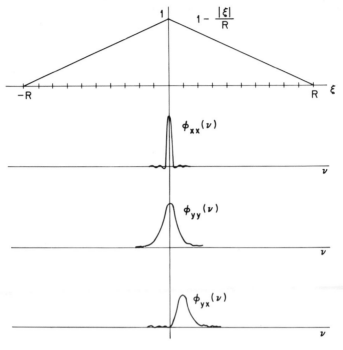

Fig. 7.2. Correlation functions.

that the above relation (7.8) is an exact formula, free of approximations, and expresses clearly the fact that the variance of $\hat{h}(\tau)$ has one term independent of τ and one dependent on τ.

Nonlinear System: Variance of Linear Kernel Estimate

In estimating the best (in the MSE sense for a GWN stimulus) linear kernel of a nonlinear system we must account for the additional variance due to the nonlinearity. To see this, let us consider a second-order nonlinear system described by

$$y(t) = \int_0^\infty h_1(\tau)x(t-\tau)\,d\tau + \int_0^\infty \int_0^\infty h_2(\tau_1, \tau_2)x(t-\tau_1)x(t-\tau_2)\,d\tau_1\,d\tau_2$$

$$= y_L(t) + y_N(t) \tag{7.9}$$

where $y_L(t)$ is the linear component (due to h_1) and $y_N(t)$ is the nonlinear component (due to h_2). Then proceeding as above to estimate the linear kernel we have

$$\hat{h}_1(\tau) = K_1 \hat{\phi}_{yx}(\tau)$$

$$= \frac{K_1}{R} \int_0^R [y_L(t) + y_N(t)] x(t-\tau) \, dt$$

$$= \frac{K_1}{R} \int_0^R y_L(t) x(t-\tau) \, dt + \frac{K_1}{R} \int_0^R y_N(t) x(t-\tau) \, dt$$

$$= r_1(\tau) + r_2(\tau) \tag{7.10}$$

where r_1 and r_2 are the two terms of $\hat{h}_1(\tau)$ due to the linear—$y_L(t)$—and nonlinear—$y_N(t)$—components of the response. For the variance of $\hat{h}_1(\tau)$ we have

$$\text{Var}\,[\![\hat{h}_1(\tau)]\!] = \text{Var}\,[\![r_1 + r_2]\!]$$

$$= E[\![(r_1 + r_2)^2]\!] - (E[\![r_1 + r_2]\!])^2$$

$$= E[\![r_1^2]\!] + E[\![r_2^2]\!] + 2E[\![r_1 r_2]\!] - (E[\![r_1]\!])^2 - (E[\![r_2]\!])^2 - 2E[\![r_1]\!]E[\![r_2]\!]$$

$$\tag{7.11}$$

We have, however, that

$$E[\![r_2]\!] = \frac{K_1}{R} \int_0^R \int_0^\infty \int_0^\infty h_2(\nu_1, \nu_2) E[\![x(t-\nu_1)x(t-\nu_2)x(t-\tau)]\!] \, d\nu_1 \, d\nu_2 \, dt$$

$$= 0 \tag{7.12}$$

since $x(t)$ is a Gaussian process with zero mean. By a similar argument we find that $E[\![r_1 r_2]\!] = 0$—since it involves the expected value of five Gaussian variables of zero mean. Thus, Eq. (7.11) finally becomes

$$\text{Var}\,[\![\hat{h}_1(\tau)]\!] = \text{Var}\,[\![r_1(\tau)]\!] + \text{Var}\,[\![r_2(\tau)]\!] \tag{7.13}$$

It should be noted that Var $[\![r_1]\!]$ is simply that given by Eq. (7.7) in the case of a linear system. Also, if $y_N(t)$ is nearly Gaussian, or if it satisfies certain weak integrability conditions (in essence, if it is "concentrated" enough around the mean), then a similar expression can be derived for Var $[\![r_2]\!]$. Noting, however, that $\phi_{y_N x}(u) = 0$, this variance is given by

$$\text{Var}\,[\![r_2]\!] \cong \frac{2K_1^2}{R} \int_0^\mu \phi_{y_N y_N}(\xi) \phi_{xx}(\xi) \, d\xi \tag{7.14}$$

Again, we note that it is a quantity that decreases in proportion to the record length R.

Let us estimate it in terms of the kernel $h_2(\tau_1, \tau_2)$. We find

$$\phi_{y_N y_N}(\zeta) = \int_0^\infty \int_0^\infty \int_0^\infty \int_0^\infty h_2(\tau_1, \tau_2) h_2(\tau_1', \tau_2')$$

$$\times [\phi_{xx}(\tau_1 - \tau_2)\phi_{xx}(\tau_1' - \tau_2') + \phi_{xx}(\zeta - \tau_1' + \tau_1)\phi_{xx}(\zeta - \tau_2' + \tau_2)$$

$$+ \phi_{xx}(\zeta - \tau_2' + \tau_1)\phi_{xx}(\zeta - \tau_1' + \tau_2)]\, d\tau_1\, d\tau_2\, d\tau_1'\, d\tau_2' \qquad (7.15)$$

If the input $x(t)$ is ideal white noise, i.e., $\phi_{xx}(u) = (1/K_1)\delta(u)$, we find that

$$\phi_{y_N y_N}(\zeta) = \frac{1}{K_1^2}\left[\int_0^\infty h_2(\tau_1, \tau_1)\, d\tau_1\right]^2$$

$$+ \frac{2}{K_1^2}\int_0^\infty \int_0^\infty h_2(\tau_1, \tau_2) h_2(\tau_1 + \zeta, \tau_2 + \zeta)\, d\tau_1\, d\tau_2 \qquad (7.16)$$

and the additional variance due to the nonlinearity becomes

$$K_1\text{Var}\,[\![r_2]\!] = \frac{2}{R}\left[\int_0^\infty h_2(\tau_1, \tau_1)\, d\tau_1\right]^2 + \frac{4}{R}\int_0^\infty \int_0^\infty h_2^2(\tau_1, \tau_2)\, d\tau_1\, d\tau_2 \qquad (7.17)$$

This expression gives explicitly the variance of the linear kernel due to the presence of nonlinearity manifested by $h_2(\tau_1, \tau_2)$. It should be noted that if the average of the response $y(t)$ to the GWN stimulus is subtracted before $\phi_{yx}(\tau)$ is estimated, then the first term of Var $[\![r_2]\!]$ is eliminated. This can be derived easily by noting that

$$E[\![y(t)]\!] = \int_0^\infty h_2(\tau_1, \tau_1)\, d\tau_1 \qquad (7.18)$$

To summarize, the total variance of the linear kernel of a second-order nonlinear system for an ideal GWN input is given by

$$\text{Var}\,[\![\hat{h}_1(\tau)]\!] = \frac{1}{R}\int_0^\infty h_1^2(\xi)\, d\xi + \frac{2}{R}\int_0^\tau \left(1 - \frac{\xi}{R}\right)h_1(\tau + \xi)h_1(\tau - \xi)\, d\xi$$

$$+ \frac{2}{K_1 R}\left[\int_0^\infty h_2(\tau_1, \tau_1)\, d\tau_1\right]^2$$

$$+ \frac{4}{K_1 R}\int_0^\infty \int_0^\infty h_2^2(\tau_1, \tau_2)\, d\tau_1\, d\tau_2 \qquad (7.19)$$

where the third term can be eliminated if the response average is subtracted before the crosscorrelation $\phi_{yx}(\tau)$ is computed.

Figure 7.3 shows kernel estimates for various record lengths and various degrees of nonlinearity (the exact kernels are also shown for comparison). As expected, we note that the estimates improve faster with record length R for the case where the degree of nonlinearity is smaller.

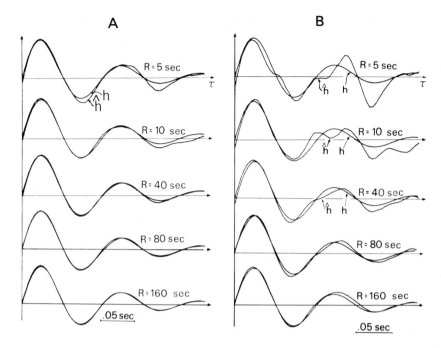

Fig. 7.3. Linear kernel estimates for two nonlinear systems with different degrees of nonlinearity. In both cases the system is a cascade of a linear filter followed by a nonlinearity of the form $aw + bw^2$. In A: $a = 1$, $b = 0.04$ and in B: $a = 1$, $b = 0.20$.

Variance of Nonlinear Kernel Estimate

The nonlinear second-order kernel is estimated as

$$\hat{h}_2(\tau_1, \tau_2) = K_2 \hat{\phi}_{yxx}(\tau_1, \tau_2)$$

$$= \frac{K_2}{R} \int_0^R y(t) x(t - \tau_1) x(t - \tau_2)\, dt \qquad (7.20)$$

where $K_2 = 1/(2P^2)$ and P is the power level of the GWN stimulus.

We have for the variance of this kernel estimate

$$\text{Var}\,[\![\hat{h}_2(\tau_1, \tau_2)]\!] = K_2^2\, E[\![\hat{\phi}_{yxx}(\tau_1, \tau_2)]^2]\! - [E[\![\hat{\phi}_{yxx}(\tau_1, \tau_2)]\!]]^2$$

$$= \frac{K_2^2}{R^2}\left[\int\!\!\int_0^R E[\![y(\mu)x(\mu - \tau_1)x(\mu - \tau_2)y(\nu)x(\nu - \tau_1)x(\nu - \tau_2)]\!]\, d\mu\, d\nu \right.$$

$$- \int\!\!\int_0^R E[\![y(\mu)x(\mu - \tau_1)x(\mu - \tau_2)]\!]$$

$$\left. \times E[\![y(\nu)x(\nu - \tau_1)x(\nu - \tau_2)]\!]\, d\mu\, d\nu \right] \qquad (7.21)$$

To simplify matters let us consider, as an example, a system that has no linear part but is described entirely by the nonlinear kernel $h_2(\tau_1, \tau_2)$; i.e., we have

$$y(t) = \int\limits_0^\infty\!\!\int h_2(v_1, v_2)x(t-v_1)x(t-v_2)\,dv_1\,dv_2 \tag{7.22}$$

Then

$$E[\![y(\mu)x(\mu-\tau_1)x(\mu-\tau_2)y(\nu)x(\nu-\tau_1)x(\nu-\tau_2)]\!]$$

$$= \int\limits_0^\infty\!\!\int\!\!\int\!\!\int h_2(u_1, u_2)h_2(v_1, v_2)$$

$$\times E[\![x(\mu-u_1)x(\mu-u_2)x(\mu-\tau_1)x(\mu-\tau_2)x(\nu-\tau_1)x(\nu-\tau_2)$$

$$\times x(\nu-v_1)x(\nu-v_2)]\!]\,du_1\,du_2\,dv_1\,dv_2 \tag{7.23}$$

and

$$E[\![y(\mu)x(\mu-\tau_1)x(\mu-\tau_2)]\!]$$

$$= \int\limits_0^\infty\!\!\int h_2(u_1, u_2)E[\![x(\mu-u_1)x(\mu-u_2)x(\mu-\tau_1)x(\mu-\tau_2)]\!]\,du_1\,du_2$$

$$\tag{7.24}$$

It can be shown that for Gaussian random variables (cf. Laning and Battin, 1956)

$$E[\![x_1x_2\cdots x_{2N}]\!] = \sum\prod E[\![x_ix_j]\!] \tag{7.25}$$

where, as in Chapter 2 (Sec. 2.5.1), $\sum\prod$ denotes the sum of products of $E[\![x_ix_j]\!]$, where the pairs x_ix_j are formed in all conceivable distinct ways of partitioning $x_1, x_2, \ldots, x_{2N}$ into pairs. There are $(2N)!/N!2^N$ such ways. Utilizing this fact the integrands of Eqs. (7.23) and (7.24) can be expanded. The expansion allows, in principle, the evaluation of expression (7.21), since each one of the $E[\![x_ix_j]\!]$ terms is approximately a delta function [for a sufficiently broadband signal $x(t)$]. However, the number of terms of the sum in which the expansion results is very large (105 in this case), and, therefore, the evaluation is fairly burdensome. For this reason it is not carried out here, but we simply remark that the variance of the second-order kernel estimate is also inversely proportional to the record length.

Figures 7.4 and 7.5 show second-order nonlinear kernel estimates for various record lengths R. Note that longer records are required for a certain accuracy of the second-order kernel estimate than in the first-order case.

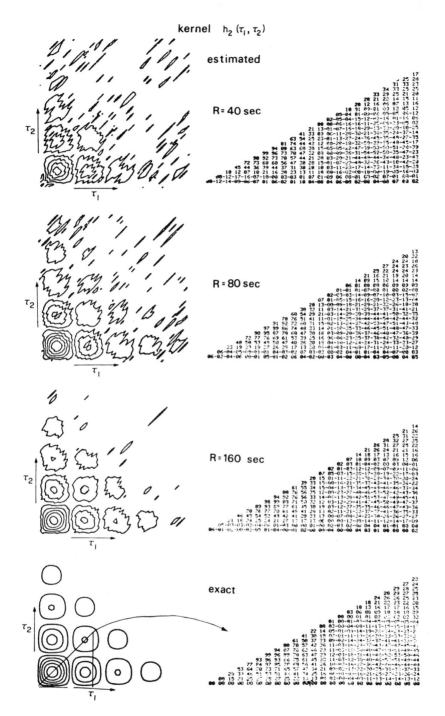

Fig. 7.4. Effect of record length on variance of second-order kernel estimates (underdamped system).

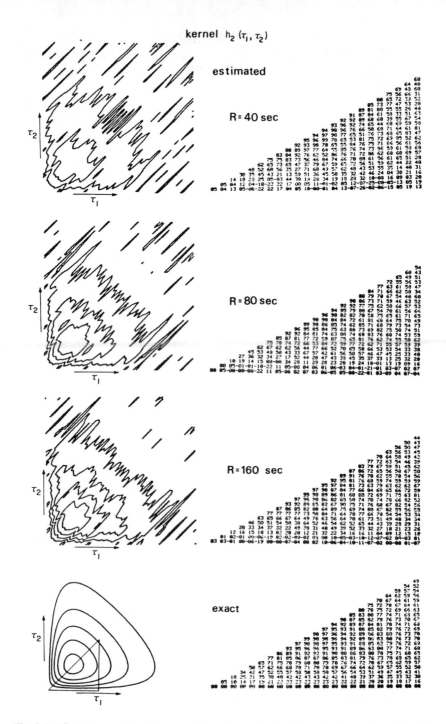

Fig. 7.5. Effect of record length on variance of second-order kernel estimates (overdamped system).

7.1.2. *Errors Due to the Finite Stimulus Bandwidth*

Consider the case of a linear system tested with band-limited white noise with power level P and cutoff frequency B. The estimate of the system impulse response (linear kernel) is

$$\hat{h}(\sigma) = \frac{1}{P} \hat{\phi}_{yx}(\sigma)$$

$$= \frac{1}{PT} \int_0^T y(t) x(t-\sigma)\, dt$$

$$= \frac{1}{PT} \int_0^T dt \int_0^\infty h(\tau) x(t-\tau) x(t-\sigma)\, d\tau \qquad (7.26)$$

Thus,

$$E[\hat{h}(\sigma)] = \frac{1}{P} \int_0^\infty h(\tau) \phi_{xx}(\sigma-\tau)\, d\tau \qquad (7.27)$$

where ϕ_{xx} is the expected value of

$$\hat{\phi}_{xx}(\sigma-\tau) = \frac{1}{T} \int_0^T x(t-\tau) x(t-\sigma)\, dt \qquad (7.28)$$

Clearly, our estimate is unbiased only in the case of ideal white noise; otherwise it is biased and the bias is greater as ϕ_{xx} deviates more from an impulse (delta) function. The bias amounts to a loss of high frequencies in the kernel estimate resulting from the smoothing effect of the convolution integral. The extent of this smoothing is determined by the cutoff frequency B.

As a first approximation, let us approximate $\phi_{xx}(\lambda)$ with a pulse of height BP, extended from $\lambda = -1/2B$ to $\lambda = 1/2B$. Then Eq. (7.27) becomes

$$E[\hat{h}(\sigma)] = B \int_{\sigma-1/2B}^{\sigma+1/2B} h(\tau)\, d\tau \qquad (7.29)$$

which means that each value of the kernel estimate is the average of the actual kernel values within a symmetric neighborhood of width $1/B$. Obviously a better estimate is obtained as B becomes large in comparison to the system bandwidth. Significant estimation errors may occur in the initial region of the kernel ($0 \leqslant \sigma < 1/2B$) due to its possible nonalyticity at the origin.

A more elaborate mathematical analysis of this error can be based on a Taylor-series expansion of the kernel. Thus, consider the basic relation that gives the expected value of the estimate of the first-order Wiener kernel of a nonlinear system:

$$E[\hat{h}_1(\sigma)] = \frac{1}{P} \int_0^\infty h_1(\tau)\phi_2(\sigma - \tau)\, d\tau$$

$$= \frac{1}{P} \int_0^\infty h_1(\tau) 2PB \frac{\sin\left[2\pi B(\sigma - \tau)\right]}{2\pi B(\sigma - \tau)}\, d\tau \tag{7.30}$$

We expand $h_1(\tau)$ in a Taylor series about σ:

$$h_1(\tau) = h_1(\sigma) + h_1^{(1)}(\sigma)(\tau - \sigma) + h_1^{(2)}(\sigma)\frac{(\tau - \sigma)^2}{2} + h_1^{(3)}(\sigma)\frac{(\tau - \sigma)^3}{6} + \cdots$$

$$\tag{7.31}$$

Since ϕ_2 is an even function, the integration over a symmetric interval around σ will eliminate the odd-order terms of the Taylor expansion. Thus, considering a symmetric interval around σ we have approximately that

$$E[\hat{h}_1(\sigma)] \cong \frac{1}{\pi} \int_{\sigma - R}^{\sigma + R} h_1(\tau) \frac{\sin\left[2\pi B(\sigma - \tau)\right]}{\sigma - \tau}\, d\tau \tag{7.32}$$

where R is an arbitrary constant considerably larger than $1/B$, but still within the range of validity of the Taylor expansion (analytic region).

Finally,

$$E[\hat{h}_1(\sigma)] \cong \frac{1}{\pi} \sum_{n=0}^\infty \frac{h_1^{(2n)}(\sigma)}{2n!} \int_{-R}^R \xi^{2n-1} \sin(2\pi B\xi)\, d\xi$$

$$\cong h_1(\sigma) + \frac{2}{\pi} \sum_{n=1}^\infty C_n \frac{h_1^{(2n)}(\sigma)}{2n!} \tag{7.33}$$

where

$$C_n = \int_0^R \xi^{2n-1} \sin(2\pi B\xi)\, d\xi$$

$$= -\sum_{k=0}^{2n-1} k! \binom{2n-1}{k} \frac{R^{2n-k-1}}{(2\pi B)^{k+1}} \cos\left(2\pi BR + k\frac{\pi}{2}\right) \tag{7.34}$$

Clearly, the deconvolution error that we commit because of the finite stimulus bandwidth is

$$E[\hat{h}_1(\sigma)] - h_1(\sigma) \cong \frac{2}{\pi} \sum_{n=1}^\infty C_n \frac{h_1^{(2n)}(\sigma)}{2n!} \tag{7.35}$$

where the coefficients C_n decrease rapidly as the bandwidth B of the GWN increases [Eq. (7.34)]. Consequently, the deconvolution error can become negligible for a sufficiently broad stimulus bandwidth.

For example, consider only the first term of the deconvolution error:

$$r_1(\sigma) = -\frac{1}{\pi} h_1^{(2)}(\sigma) \left[\frac{R}{2\pi B} \cos(2\pi BR) + \frac{1}{(2\pi B)^2} \cos\left(2\pi BR + \frac{\pi}{2}\right) \right]$$

$$\cong -\frac{1}{\pi} h_1^{(2)}(\sigma) \frac{R}{2\pi B} \cos(2\pi BR) \qquad (7.36)$$

It depends on the second derivative of the kernel and vanishes when B approaches infinity. Similar arguments hold for higher-order kernel estimates, but the analytical expressions that describe them are much more complex.

In conclusion, the deconvolution error, which is due to the finite stimulus bandwidth, can become practically negligible if a stimulus bandwidth broad with respect to the system bandwidth is used. It must be emphasized, however, that in practice we cannot extend the stimulus bandwidth without some loss, because even though the increase in stimulus bandwidth reduces the deconvolution error, it also increases, in general, the statistical fluctuation error.

To illustrate the effect of the GWN bandwidth on the statistical fluctuation error, we will study the variance of a single sample, $s_1(t, \sigma)$, of the crosscorrelation in the first-order kernel case:

$$s_1(t, \sigma) = \int_0^\infty h_1(\tau) x(t-\tau) x(t-\sigma) \, d\tau \qquad (7.37)$$

The kernel estimate is obtained as a time average over these samples:

$$\hat{h}_1(\sigma) = \frac{1}{PT} \int_0^T s_1(t, \sigma) \, dt \qquad (7.38)$$

The derivations below are valid for $x(t)$ being band–limited Gaussian white noise of bandwidth B:

$$\text{Var}\,[s_1(t, \sigma)] = \int_0^\infty \int_0^\infty h_1(\tau) h_1(\tau') E[x(t-\tau) x(t-\sigma) x(t-\tau') x(t-\sigma)] \, d\tau \, d\tau'$$

$$- \left\{ \int_0^\infty h_1(\tau) E[x(t-\tau) x(t-\sigma)] \, d\tau \right\}^2$$

$$= \int_0^\infty \int_0^\infty h_1(\tau) h_1(\tau') [\phi_2(\tau-\sigma)\phi_2(\tau'-\sigma) + \phi_2(0)\phi_2(\tau-\tau')$$

$$+ \phi_2(\tau-\sigma)\phi_2(\tau'-\sigma)] \, d\tau \, d\tau'$$

$$- \int_0^\infty \int_0^\infty h_1(\tau) h_1(\tau') \phi_2(\tau-\sigma)\phi_2(\tau'-\sigma) \, d\tau \, d\tau'$$

$$= \phi_2(0) \int_0^\infty \int_0^\infty h_1(\tau) h_1(\tau') \phi_2(\tau - \tau') \, d\tau \, d\tau'$$

$$+ \left[\int_0^\infty h_1(\tau) \phi_2(\sigma - \tau) \, d\tau \right]^2 \tag{7.39}$$

Consider now the Fourier transforms H_1 and Φ_2 of h_1 and ϕ_2, respectively. Then, the expression for the variance becomes

$$\text{Var} \left[\!\!\left[s_1(t, \sigma) \right]\!\!\right] = 2BP^2 \int_{-B}^{B} |H_1(f)|^2 \, df + P^2 \left[\int_{-B}^{B} H_1(f) \, e^{j2\pi f \sigma} \, df \right]^2 \tag{7.40}$$

given that

$$\Phi_2(f) = \begin{cases} P & \text{for } -B \leqslant f \leqslant B \\ 0 & \text{for } |f| > B \end{cases} \tag{7.41}$$

Recalling that the estimation of $h_1(\sigma)$ requires the normalization of the first-order crosscorrelation by $1/P$, we get (disregarding for the moment the dependence on T)

$$\text{Var} \left[\!\!\left[\hat{h}_1(\sigma) \right]\!\!\right] \sim 2B \int_{-B}^{B} |H_1(f)|^2 \, df + \left[\int_{-B}^{B} H_1(f) \, e^{j2\pi f \sigma} \, df \right]^2 \tag{7.42}$$

The first term of this expression is clearly increasing with B and it is independent of σ. The second term depends on σ, and no general statement can be made on the way it depends on B. If the GWN bandwidth B is broad enough with respect to the system bandwidth, it is reasonable to expect that the first term of the expression for the variance [Eq. (7.42)] will be much more sensitive to changes of B than the second term. Consequently, the pattern of dependence of the kernel estimate variance upon the GWN bandwidth will be predominantly determined by the first term, which indicates a monotonically increasing pattern. Notice also that the first term is an upper bound of the second term for every value of σ, which means that the first term is also dominant in the formation of the variance of the kernel estimate.

Considering Eqs. (7.34) and (7.42), which describe the dependence of the deconvolution and the statistical fluctuation estimation errors on the GWN bandwidth, we come to the important realization that the overall effect of B upon the kernel estimation error is not monotonic. Unlike the effect of the record length, a change of the bandwidth triggers two antagonistic error-producing mechanisms: the one relating to the statistical fluctuation error [cf. Eq. (7.42)] and the other relating to the deconvolution error [cf. Eq. (7.34)].

The existence of these two antagonistic mechanisms leads us to the expectation of an optimum value of B, for which the overall estimation error becomes minimum. Unfortunately, we cannot suggest, at present, a systematic optimization procedure with which the optimum values of the test parameters can be determined, because of the great complexity of the relevant expressions, especially in the higher-order kernel cases. Of course, a procedure of successive trials can always be followed to determine approximately these optimum values. Notice, however, that a complete analysis is feasible in the case of the CSRS and an optimization procedure for the test parameters can be practicably designed, as discussed in Sec. 8.8.

Figure 7.6 shows kernel estimates of a linear system for different bandwidths of the stimulus GWN. The increase in variance of the high stimulus bandwidth is evident in the expanded scale inset of this figure.

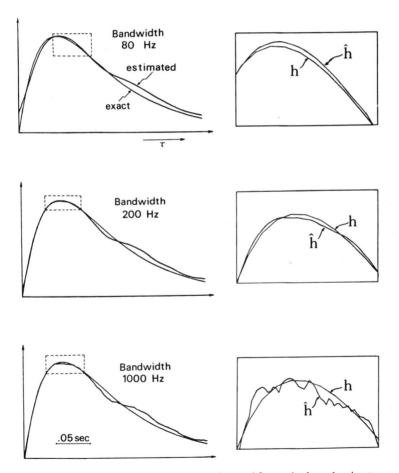

Fig. 7.6. Effect of stimulus bandwidth on variance of first-order kernel estimates.

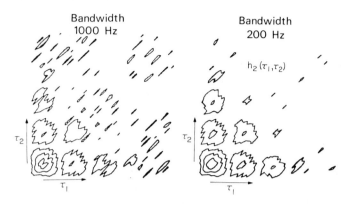

Fig. 7.7. Effect of stimulus bandwidth on variance of second-order kernel estimates.

A similar analysis can be carried out for the variance of the second-order kernel as affected by the stimulus bandwidth. An example is shown in Fig. 7.7, where it is clearly indicated that the estimate obtained from stimulation at the lower bandwidth has less variance (both estimates were obtained from data of equal record length).

7.1.3. Errors Due to Experimental Limitations

An example of an error that occurs naturally during a white-noise experiment is the error introduced by the truncation of the Gaussian distribution of the GWN signal amplitudes at very low and very high levels. This, of course, is a physical necessity in all cases. If we are studying a system that at some stage contains a nonlinearity of the form shown in Fig. 7.8, then clearly, if the system is tested with a GWN stimulus of small amplitude, i.e., whose Gaussian amplitude distribution has a small variance, the characterization will be nearly linear since the nonlinear satura-

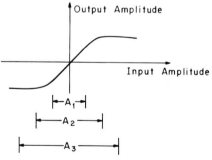

Fig. 7.8. Nonlinear characteristic. Notice that the nature of the nonlinearity depends on the stimulus range.

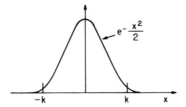

Fig. 7.9. Truncation of Gaussian amplitude distribution.

tion and cutoff portions are rarely tested by such a signal. However, if the variance of the Gaussian amplitudes of the GWN stimulus is large, then the system will be operating in the nonlinear regions more often, and the characterization, since it is a statistical average, will be strongly nonlinear. Again, stressing that the method gives a *statistical average* characterization based on the GWN stimulus–response records, we can easily see that, in practice (e.g., a finite duration of experiment) the characterization of the system is valid only for amplitude ranges within some range around the mean of the GWN stimulus. Therefore, since the tails of the Gaussian amplitude distribution are ineffective in characterizing the system in practice, it may be desirable to increase the gain of the instrument producing the GWN stimulus in the laboratory in order to obtain a statistically valid characterization for the whole range of amplitudes that the instrument is capable of producing.

Faced with GWN stimuli that have been truncated (Fig. 7.9), what is the effect of this truncation on the kernel estimates? The experimental signal $x^*(t)$ has an amplitude probability distribution given by (Fig. 7.9)

$$\Pr\{x^*\} = \begin{cases} [C_k/(2\pi)^{1/2}]\, e^{-x^{*2}/2}, & |x^*| \leq k \\ 0, & |x^*| > k \end{cases} \tag{7.43}$$

where C_k is a scaling correction making the area under the probability density equal to unity. A usual alternative truncation is $x^*(t) = x(t) + \varepsilon(t)$, where $x(t)$ is ideally Gaussian and

$$\varepsilon(t) = \begin{cases} 0, & |x(t)| < k \\ k - x(t), & x(t) > k \\ -k - x(t), & x(t) < -k \end{cases} \tag{7.44}$$

The truncation signal $\varepsilon(t)$ represents noise at the input; formulas for its effect on the kernels are derived in Sec. 7.4. Notice that it is a case of input noise that goes through the system. Therefore, with regard to the linear kernel, the error is

$$\text{error} = \frac{1}{P} \int_0^\infty h_1(\nu)[\phi_{x\varepsilon}(\tau - \nu) + \phi_{\varepsilon x}(\tau - \nu) + \phi_{\varepsilon\varepsilon}(\tau - \nu)]\, d\nu \tag{7.45}$$

Now, in order to compute $\phi_{x\varepsilon}$, $\phi_{\varepsilon x}$, and $\phi_{\varepsilon\varepsilon}$ we must utilize the joint probability density $p_{x\varepsilon}$ [of $x(t)$ and $\varepsilon(t+\tau)$] and $p_{\varepsilon\varepsilon}$ [of $\varepsilon(t)$ and $\varepsilon(t+\tau)$]. Then we have

$$\phi_{x\varepsilon}(\tau) = \int\int_{-\infty}^{\infty} x\varepsilon p_{x\varepsilon}(x, \varepsilon; \tau)\, dx\, d\varepsilon$$

$$= \delta(\tau)\int\int_{-\infty}^{\infty} x\varepsilon p_{x\varepsilon}(x, \varepsilon)\, dx\, d\varepsilon \qquad (7.46)$$

which, in view of Eq. (7.44), becomes

$$\phi_{x\varepsilon}(\tau) = \frac{\delta(\tau)}{(2\pi)^{1/2}}\left[\int_{-\infty}^{-k} x(-k-x)\, e^{-x^2/2}\, dx + \int_{k}^{\infty} x(k-x)\, e^{-x^2/2}\, dx\right]$$

$$= \frac{2\delta(\tau)}{(2\pi)^{1/2}}\int_{k}^{\infty} (kx-x^2)\, e^{-x^2/2}\, dx \qquad (7.47)$$

In this case, it is easily seen that $\phi_{x\varepsilon}(\tau) = \phi_{\varepsilon x}(\tau)$. We also have, similarly,

$$\phi_{\varepsilon\varepsilon}(\tau) = \delta(\tau)\int_{-\infty}^{\infty} \varepsilon^2 p_{\varepsilon\varepsilon}(\varepsilon)\, d\varepsilon$$

$$= \frac{\delta(\tau)}{(2\pi)^{1/2}}\left[\int_{-\infty}^{-k} (-k-x)^2\, e^{-x^2/2}\, dx + \int_{k}^{\infty} (k-x)^2\, e^{-x^2/2}\, dx\right]$$

$$= \frac{2\delta(\tau)}{(2\pi)^{1/2}}\int_{k}^{\infty} (k-x)^2\, e^{-x^2/2}\, dx \qquad (7.48)$$

Thus, finally we have from Eq. (7.45) that the error is (for $P=1$)

$$\text{error}\,(\tau, h_1(\nu), k) = \int_{0}^{\infty} h_1(\nu)\left[\delta(\tau-\nu)\frac{2}{(2\pi)^{1/2}}\int_{k}^{\infty} (k^2-x^2)\, e^{-x^2/2}\, dx\right] d\nu$$

$$= h_1(\tau)\frac{2}{(2\pi)^{1/2}}\int_{k}^{\infty} (k^2-x^2)\, e^{-x^2/2}\, dx$$

$$= h_1(\tau)F(k) \qquad (7.49)$$

Notice that the error function $F(k)$ is negative since $x^2 > k^2$, i.e., we would tend to underestimate $h_1(\tau)$. Therefore, the kernel estimate is

$$\hat{h}_1(\tau) = h_1(\tau)[1+F(k)] \qquad (7.50)$$

and $F(k)$ indicates the percentage error. It should be noted, however, that knowledge of the truncation level k can correct for this error, simply by utilizing Eq. (7.49).

What is the effect of such truncation on the estimation of higher-order kernels? Intuitively we guess that this effect would probably be larger. As discussed in Chapter 5, estimation of a linear kernel, in the absence of nonlinear ones, requires only that the second-order autocorrelation function of the stimulus be close to an impulse function. However, if nonlinearities exist, the higher-order autocorrelation functions of the stimulus have an effect. Therefore, an indirect way of determining the effect of truncation on higher-order kernel estimates involves examining the effect of truncation on the higher-order autocorrelation functions of the stimulus.

In this respect, if the high and low truncation levels are not symmetric about the mean, the third-order autocorrelation of $x(t)$ is not zero. For example consider the following nonlinear system:

$$y(t) = \int_0^\infty h_1(\nu)x(t-\nu)\,d\nu + \int\int_0^\infty h_2(\nu_1, \nu_2)x(t-\nu_1)x(t-\nu_2)\,d\nu_1\,d\nu_2$$

$$(7.51)$$

To estimate the linear kernel $h_1(\tau)$ we compute

$$\phi_{yx}(\tau) = \int_0^\infty h_1(\nu)\phi_{xx}(\tau-\nu)\,d\nu + \int\int_0^\infty h_2(\nu_1, \nu_2)\phi_{xxx}(\tau-\nu_1, \tau-\nu_2)\,d\nu_1\,d\nu_2$$

$$(7.52)$$

which gives us, therefore, an additional error term, due to the nonzero ϕ_{xxx}:

$$\text{error} = \int\int_0^\infty h_2(\nu_1, \nu_2)\phi_{xxx}(\tau-\nu_1, \tau-\nu_2)\,d\nu_1\,d\nu_2 \qquad (7.53)$$

Similar expressions can be found in the case of higher-order kernel estimation. The explicit relations are rather unwieldy and, for this reason, are not presented here.

7.1.4. Dependence of Kernel Estimate Accuracy on the Degree of System Nonlinearity

Can a general statement be made about the relative magnitudes of the linear kernel variance versus the nonlinear kernel variance? In practice it often seems that the estimation of the nonlinear kernels is less accurate—i.e., the estimate appears to have a greater variance—and, therefore, one may be tempted to generalize this observation. However, it appears to depend critically on the specific system under study.

Consider a system that has only a linear kernel $h_1(\tau)$ and a second-order nonlinear kernel $h_2(\tau_1, \tau_2)$. The response of this system to a GWN stimulus has two components: One arises from h_1 and the other from h_2. Recall, now, that the estimation of any kernel by crosscorrelation depends on the orthogonality of the terms of the Wiener series. This latter fact suggests, for example, that the estimation of the linear kernel h_1 depends on certain averages involving h_2—and the response arising from h_2—becoming zero. Thus, in practice, where finite record lengths are used to estimate the crosscorrelations, the response arising from h_2 acts as "contaminating noise" as far as the estimation of h_1 is concerned. (Of course, this "contaminating noise" is orthogonal and therefore not detrimental, when long records are considered.) Therefore, the variance of h_1, under these circumstances, depends on the relative magnitude of the nonlinear response component as compared to the linear response component (one may wish to think of a signal-to-noise ratio where the "signal" is the response arising from h_1 and "noise" is the response arising from h_2). Similar arguments, of course, hold for the estimation of the nonlinear kernel h_2, as it would be affected by the magnitude of the linear response component.

Figure 7.10 shows estimates of the first-order kernel of a nonlinear system for several degrees of nonlinearity and two different record lengths.

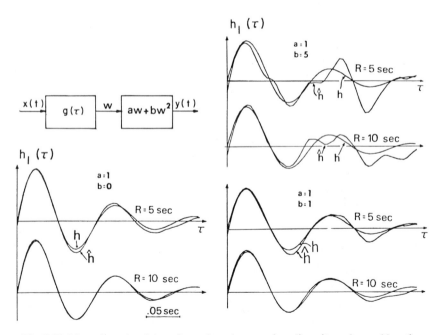

Fig. 7.10. Linear kernel estimates for various degrees of nonlinearity and record lengths.

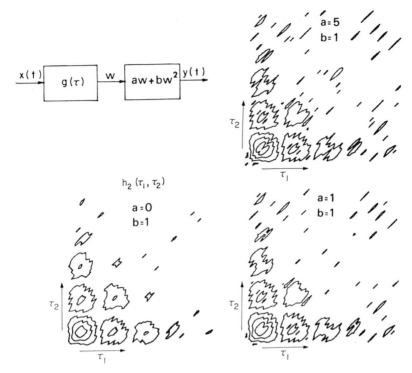

Fig. 7.11. Nonlinear kernel estimates for various degrees of nonlinearity.

Figure 7.11 shows estimates of the second-order kernel of a nonlinear system for several degrees of nonlinearity.

7.1.5. Effect of Kernel Memory Truncation on Frequency Response Estimate

Consider a fairly general linear system with impulse response given by

$$g(\tau) = \sum_i A_i e^{-\alpha_i \tau} \tag{7.54}$$

a sum of exponentials. In the conduct of a white-noise identification experiment, this $g(\tau)$ is calculated for lags only up to $\tau = \tau_m$. That is, the estimated kernel $\hat{g}(\tau)$ is

$$\hat{g}(\tau) = \begin{cases} g(\tau), & \tau \leq \tau_m \\ 0, & \tau > \tau_m \end{cases} \tag{7.55}$$

as shown in Fig. 7.12. What is the error at each frequency due to this truncation of the kernel? The Laplace transform of $g(\tau)$ is

$$G(s)=\sum_i \frac{A_i}{s+\alpha_i} \qquad (7.56)$$

and that of $\hat{g}(\tau)$ can easily be shown to be

$$\hat{G}(s)=\sum_i \frac{A_i}{s+\alpha_i}(1-e^{-\tau_m(s+\alpha_i)}) \qquad (7.57)$$

Thus we note that each $1/(s+\alpha_i)$ term of the transfer function is affected, both in gain and phase, by a factor $1-e^{-\tau_m(s+\alpha_i)}$. To examine this effect, we let $s=i\omega$, where ω is the frequency in rad/sec, obtaining

$$1-e^{-\tau_m(i\omega+\alpha)}=1-e^{-\alpha\tau_m}\cos\omega\tau_m+ie^{-\alpha\tau_m}\sin\omega\tau_m \qquad (7.58)$$

We plot this in the complex plane with ω as a parameter. We have

$$x=1-e^{-\alpha\tau_m}\cos\omega\tau_m \qquad (7.59)$$

$$y=e^{-\alpha\tau_m}\sin\omega\tau_m \qquad (7.60)$$

and hence

$$(x-1)^2+y^2=e^{-2\alpha\tau_m} \qquad (7.61)$$

i.e., a circle centered at $(1,0)$ and of radius $e^{-\alpha\tau_m}$, as shown in Fig. 7.13. The vector drawn from the origin of this plane to the circle depicts the correction both in gain and phase due to the truncation of the kernel at $\tau=\tau_m$. Notice in Fig. 7.13 that as the frequency increases the vector travels around the circle, thus adding an extra phase shift and introducing a "modulating" error factor for the gain. Thus, the graph in Fig. 7.13 can be used to determine the error in the frequency response behavior that is due to the necessary truncation of the kernel at $\tau=\tau_m$.

Continuing with the same linear system let us take τ_m to be four time constants, i.e., $\tau_m=4/\alpha$. Then, the radius of the circle is $e^{-4}\approx0.018$, which is indeed small compared to 1. At frequencies near $\omega=0$, the gain is underestimated by a factor of $(1-0.018)$ and the phase is affected at most by about 1°. Near the corner frequency $\omega=\alpha$ the gain is overestimated by

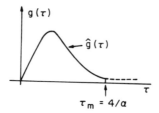

Fig. 7.12. Truncated kernel.

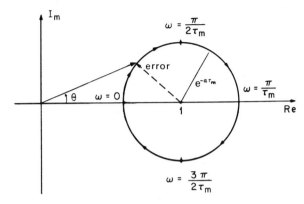

Fig. 7.13. Effect of truncation in the frequency domain.

a factor of $(1+0.018)$ and the phase is affected little. All these results are conveniently read from the graph in Fig. 7.13.

The effect of this truncation on the nonlinear kernels can be studied similarly. For example, consider a linear system followed by a square law device, the kernel of the linear system being $g(\tau)=e^{-\alpha\tau}$. This system has a second-order (nonlinear) kernel $h_2(\tau_1, \tau_2)=g(\tau_1)g(\tau_2)$. The truncated estimate is

$$\hat{h}_2(\tau_1, \tau_2)=\begin{cases} g(\tau_1)g(\tau_2), & \tau_1, \tau_2 \leq \tau_m \\ 0, & \tau_1, \tau_2 > \tau_m \end{cases} \tag{7.62}$$

Taking the two-dimensional Laplace transform we have

$$\hat{G}_2(s_1, s_2)= G_2(s_1, s_2)(1-e^{-\tau_m(s_1+\alpha)})(1-e^{-\tau_m(s_2+\alpha)}) \tag{7.63}$$

Proceeding as above for the linear kernel, we find the correction factor from the magnitude and phases of a vector moving as (ω_1, ω_2) go from low to high frequencies. We note that for $\tau_m \approx 4/\alpha$, the effect of the truncation is indeed small.

7.1.6. Errors Due to the Presence of Other Inputs in the Multi-Input Case

In the case of a system with more than one input, there are additional statistical error terms. Consider, for example, a system with two inputs, $u(t)$ and $x(t)$, and one output $y(t)$. To simplify matters, let us disregard the nonlinear kernels. We have

$$y(t)= \int_0^\infty h_x(\nu)x(t-\nu)\, d\nu + \int_0^\infty h_u(\nu)u(t-\nu)\, d\nu$$

$$= y_x(t)+y_u(t) \tag{7.64}$$

and, if excited by independent white-noise signals, the system kernels can be estimated from the crosscorrelations:

$$\hat{h}_x(\tau) = (1/P_x)\hat{\phi}_{yx}(\tau) \tag{7.65}$$

$$\hat{h}_u(\tau) = (1/P_u)\hat{\phi}_{yu}(\tau) \tag{7.66}$$

We pursue here the estimation of $h_x(\tau)$—analogous results holding, of course, for the estimation of $h_u(\tau)$. We have

$$\hat{\phi}_{yx}(\tau) = \frac{1}{R} \int_0^R y(t)x(t-\tau) \, dt$$

$$= \hat{\phi}_{y_xx}(\tau) + \hat{\phi}_{y_ux}(\tau) \tag{7.67}$$

In order to study the dependence of the kernel estimate variance on the record length, we assume (for the time being) infinite bandwidth for $x(t)$ and $u(t)$. Then,

$$\mathrm{Var}\,[\hat{h}_x(\tau)] = \mathrm{Var}\left[\frac{1}{P_x}\hat{\phi}_{y_xx}(\tau)\right] + \mathrm{Var}\left[\frac{1}{P_x}\hat{\phi}_{y_ux}(\tau)\right] \tag{7.68}$$

since $\hat{\phi}_{y_xx}(\tau)$ and $\hat{\phi}_{y_ux}(\tau)$ are uncorrelated because of the statistical independence of $x(t)$ and $u(t)$. After some analytical manipulation we derive

$$\mathrm{Var}[\hat{h}_x(\tau)] = \frac{1}{R} \int_0^R h_x^2(\lambda) \, d\lambda + \frac{2}{R} \int_0^R \left(1 - \frac{\lambda}{R}\right) h_x(\tau+\lambda)h_x(\tau-\lambda) \, d\lambda$$

$$+ \frac{P_u}{P_x} \frac{1}{R} \int_0^R h_u^2(\lambda) \, d\lambda \tag{7.69}$$

We see that the variance of the estimate of $h_x(\tau)$ is roughly proportional to $1/R$, and depends on the square integral (which is a Euclidean measure) of both kernels h_x and h_u in a relative way that is determined by the ratio of the power levels of the two inputs. A similar relation holds for the variance of $\hat{h}_u(\tau)$.

Fig. 7.14 shows the effect on the kernel estimate variance of the power level of the second input (for a two-input system). Notice how the waveform of the kernel of the second input affects the estimate.

Figures 7.15–7.18 show linear and nonlinear kernel estimates of a two-input nonlinear system for various record lengths R. The exact kernels are also shown for comparison.

7.2. Estimation Errors Using PRS Stimuli

The PRS are periodic deterministic signals. Consequently, they do not exhibit any kind of statistical estimation error. However, they exhibit several other kinds of estimation error:

(1) *Deconvolution error*, i.e., the error due to the finite stimulus bandwidth, which results in some loss of high frequencies during the deconvolution process. Because of the stairlike form of PRS, the principal lobes of the even-order autocorrelation functions have a curvipyramidal form (cf. Sec. 5.2.2). Thus, if we expand the corresponding kernel into a

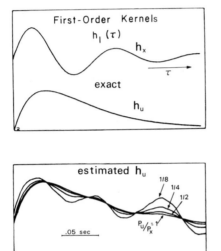

Fig. 7.14. Effect of power of "other" input on kernel estimate. The ratios indicate the relative powers of the two input signals.

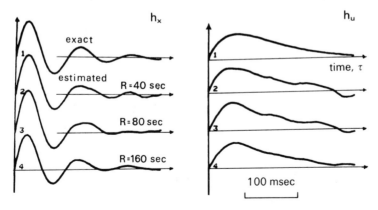

Fig. 7.15. Linear kernel estimates of two-input nonlinear system as a function of record length.

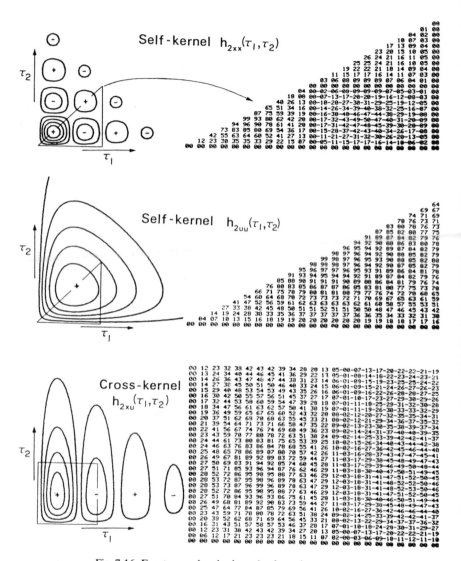

Fig. 7.16. Exact second-order kernels of two-input system.

(2) *The "statistical fluctuation" error*: This is due to the finite
length and the random nature of the CSRS. It contributes some ra[ndom]
deviations in the kernel estimates.

(3) *The "approximate orthogonality" error*: This refers to the [ap]-
proximate orthogonality of the CSRS functional series, because of th[e]
finite stimulus bandwidth and the finite record length. The finite stimulus
bandwidth makes the CSRS functional series only approximately orthogonal, while the finite record length makes the *estimated* functionals only
approximately orthogonal to one another.

(4) *The "erroneous power level" error*: This is due to erroneous estimation of the power level (and consequently of the normalizing factors)
and amounts to scalar distortion (disproportionality) of the kernel estimates.

(5) *The "finite transition time" error*: This is due to the finite response
time of the stimulus transducer, and it usually results in a small change of
the actual power level.

(6) *"Computational" errors*: These are due to the finite capacity of a
digital computer and the digital processing of continuous data. They usually result in negligible deviations in the kernel estimates, if proper operational procedures are followed.

In the following, the mechanisms that produce each of these kinds of
estimation errors will be studied, suggesting the optimum procedure that
ought to be followed in every case in order to maximize the accuracy of the
resulting system model.

The Deconvolution Error (θ Error)

In order to study the mechanism that is producing the deconvolution
estimation error, we first have to review the general deconvolution procedure with which the kernels are estimated from the crosscorrelation
functions.

For instance, consider the estimation of the first-order kernel from the
first-order crosscorrelation (to simplify derivations, assume here an infinite
record length):

$$\psi_1(\sigma) = E[\![y(t)x(t-\sigma)]\!]$$

$$= \int_0^\infty h_1(\tau) E[\![x(t-\tau)x(t-\sigma)]\!]\, d\tau$$

$$= \int_0^\infty h_1(\tau)\phi_2(\sigma-\tau)\, d\tau$$

$$= m_2 \int_{\sigma-\Delta t}^{\sigma+\Delta t} h_1(\tau)(1-|\sigma-\tau|/\Delta t)\, d\tau \tag{7.71}$$

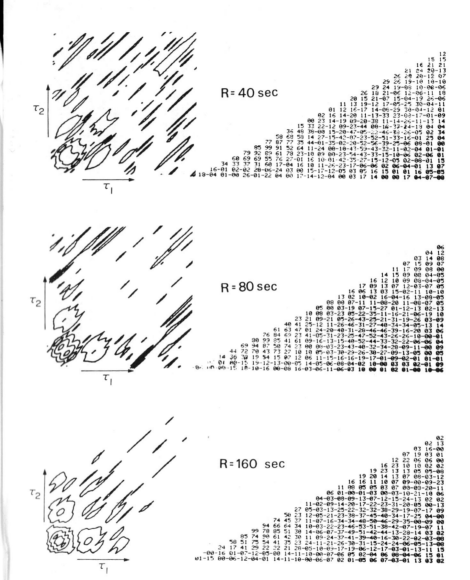

Fig. 7.17. Kernel estimates of second-order self-kernel $h_{2xx}(\tau_1, \tau_2)$ as a function of record length.

multidimensional Taylor series we can analytically evaluate th
volution error $\theta_n(\sigma_1, \ldots, \sigma_n)$ for the nth-order kernel estimate:

$$\theta_n(\sigma_1, \ldots, \sigma_n) = \sum_{m=1}^{\infty} \frac{\Delta t^{2m}}{2m!} \sum_{j_1,\ldots,j_m=1}^{n} C_m(j_1, \ldots, j_m) \frac{\partial^{2m} h_n(\sigma_1, \ldots,)}{\partial \sigma_{j_1}^2 \cdots \partial \sigma}$$

$$(\sigma_k \geq \Delta t; \quad k = 1, 2, \ldots,)$$

where $C_m(j_1, \ldots, j_m)$ is given by Eq. (7.79) below, and Δt is
tary step length of the PRS (cf. Sec. 5.2). More details on
evaluation of this error are given in Sec. 7.3, in the analogou
CSRS. This deconvolution error apparently becomes n
sufficiently small Δt (as compared to the system bandwidth)

(2) *Autocorrelation anomalies error*, i.e. the error in
anomalies present in the higher even-order autocorrelati
discussed in Sec. 5.2. It is presently very laborious to dete
magnitude of this error, and consequently it remains an i
in each specific case. It is definitely the most serious kind
of PRS and the most significant drawback in their use i
identification. Several methods to reduce the effect of th
been suggested (Barker *et al.*, 1972) and others can be
less, the overall appreciation of the situation is still a m
personal judgement.

(3) *Finite transition time error*, i.e. the error due
(rise) time of the input transducer. This subject
Godfrey *et al.*, (1966) for the case of a pseudorandc
study suggests that the resulting estimation error i
transitions (i.e., when the patterns of upward and d
similar) and for reasonably small response tim
compared to the system bandwidth) is negligible.
be taken in the design of the transducer in order f
negligible.

(4) Finally, there are *approximate orthogon*
GWN, which are usually negligible for all p
roneous power level and computational errors
ble under some easily implemented provisions
CSRS (cf. Sec. 7.3).

7.3. Estimation Errors Using CSRS Sti

In this section we discuss several erro
use of the CSRS. The principal estimation

(1) *The "deconvolution" error*, due t
which results in a loss of high frequencies

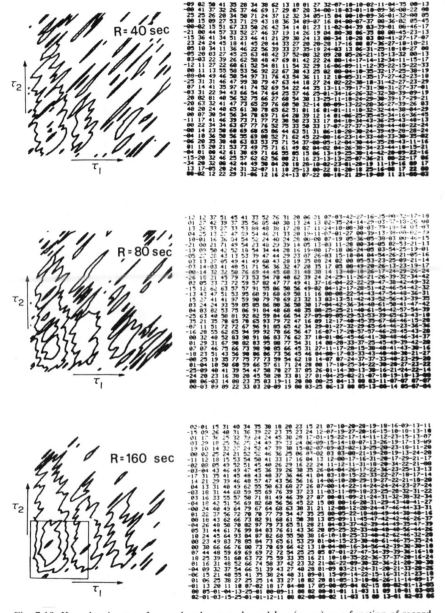

Fig. 7.18. Kernel estimates of second-order cross-kernel $h_{2xu}(\tau_1, \tau_2)$ as a function of record
length.

Thus, the crosscorrelation expression takes the form of a convolution integral, where one of the convolving functions has its significant values highly concentrated in a narrow area, approaching the form of an impulse function with the ability to deconvolve the integral:

$$\psi_1(\sigma) \cong (m_2 \Delta t) h_1(\sigma) \tag{7.72}$$

The deconvolution error that we intend to study here is the deviation of this approximation. To evaluate this error, we evaluate the exact convolution integral of Eq. (7.71). Assuming $h_1(\tau)$ is analytic in the neighborhood of σ, we expand it in a Taylor series:

$$\psi_1(\sigma) = m_2 \int_{\sigma - \Delta t}^{\sigma + \Delta t} \left[h_1(\sigma) + h_1^{(1)}(\sigma)(\tau - \sigma) + \frac{h^{(2)}(\sigma)}{2}(\tau - \sigma)^2 + \cdots \right]$$

$$\times \left(1 - \frac{|\tau - \sigma|}{\Delta t} \right) d\tau$$

$$= (m_2 \Delta t) \sum_{n=0}^{\infty} \frac{\Delta t^{2n}}{2n!(2n+1)(n+1)} h_1^{(2n)}(\sigma) \tag{7.73}$$

Therefore,

$$\hat{h}_1(\sigma) = \frac{1}{(m_2 \Delta t)} \psi_1(\sigma) = \sum_{n=0}^{\infty} \frac{\Delta t^{2n}}{2n!(2n+1)(n+1)} h_1^{(2n)}(\sigma) \tag{7.74}$$

Notice that since ϕ_2 is an even function, all the odd-order terms vanish so long as the kernel h_1 is analytic within the interval $[\sigma - \Delta t, \sigma + \Delta t]$.

In some cases the kernel $h_1(\tau)$ is not analytic at $\tau = 0$. In these cases, ϕ_2 is not symmetric in the area of analyticity of $h_1(\tau)$, and the odd-order terms of the Taylor-series expansion do not vanish with the integration. More specifically, this is the case where $0 \leq \sigma < \Delta t$, and the convolution integral gives then the estimate

$$\hat{h}_1(\sigma) = \sum_{n=0}^{\infty} \alpha_n(\lambda) \frac{\Delta t^n}{n!} h_1^{(n)}(\sigma), \qquad 0 \leq \sigma < \Delta t \tag{7.75}$$

where

$$\alpha_n(\lambda) = \frac{1}{(n+1)(n+2)} + (-1)^n \frac{\lambda^{n+1}}{n+1} + (-1)^{n+1} \frac{\lambda^{n+2}}{n+2}, \qquad 0 \leq \lambda = \frac{\sigma}{\Delta t} < 1 \tag{7.76}$$

Therefore, special correctional procedures must be employed for the points of the initial region $(0 \leq \sigma_i < \Delta t)$ of the kernel estimates.

The expressions become more involved in higher-order kernel cases; nevertheless, some basic remarks can be made: (1) Because of the symmetry of the autocorrelation functions, only the even-order partial derivatives are included in the expressions (for the points outside the initial region); (2) for sufficiently small Δt, the higher-order terms decline very rapidly, and the second-order terms contribute the principal error, as

$$\hat{h}_n(\sigma_1, \ldots, \sigma_n) = h_n(\sigma_1, \ldots, \sigma_n) + \frac{\Delta t^2}{12} \cdot \sum_{i=1}^{n} \frac{\partial^2 h_n(\sigma_1, \ldots, \sigma_n)}{\partial \sigma_i^2} + O(\Delta t^4)$$

$$\text{for } \sigma_k \geqslant \Delta t, \ k = 1, 2, \ldots, n \qquad (7.77)$$

The complete expression for the deconvolution error of the nth-order kernel estimate is

$$\theta_n(\sigma_1, \ldots, \sigma_n) = \sum_{m=1}^{\infty} \frac{\Delta t^{2m}}{2m!} \sum_{j_1, \ldots, j_m = 1}^{n} C_m(j_1, \ldots, j_m) \frac{\partial^{2m} h_n(\sigma_1, \ldots, \sigma_n)}{\partial \sigma_{j_1}^2 \cdots \partial \sigma_{j_m}^2}$$

$$(\sigma_k \geqslant \Delta t, \ k = 1, 2, \ldots, n) \qquad (7.78)$$

where $C_m(j_1, \ldots, j_m)$ depends on the multiplicity of the set of indices $(j_1, \ldots, j_m)$. More specifically, if a certain combination $(j_1, \ldots, j_m)$ consists of M distinct groups of identical indices, and m_i is the population number of the ith group, then

$$C_m(j_1, \ldots, j_m) = \prod_{i=1}^{M} \frac{(2m!)^{1/M}}{(m_i + 1)(2m_i + 1)2m_i!} \qquad (7.79)$$

In first approximation, for Δt fairly small

$$\theta_n(\sigma_1, \ldots, \sigma_n) \cong \frac{\Delta t^2}{12} \sum_{i=1}^{n} \frac{\partial^2 h_n(\sigma_1, \ldots, \sigma_n)}{\partial \sigma_i^2} \qquad (\sigma_k \geqslant \Delta t, \ k = 1, 2, \ldots, n)$$

$$(7.80)$$

For later use, let us establish the notation

$$\theta_n(\sigma_1, \ldots, \sigma_n) = \Delta t^2 D_{h_n}(\Delta t, \sigma_1, \ldots, \sigma_n) \qquad (7.81)$$

where

$$D_{h_n}(\Delta t, \sigma_1, \ldots, \sigma_n) = \sum_{m=1}^{\infty} \frac{\Delta t^{2m-2}}{2m!} \sum_{j_1, \ldots, j_m = 1}^{n} C_m(j_1, \ldots, j_m) \frac{\partial^{2m} h_n(\sigma_1, \ldots, \sigma_n)}{\partial \sigma_{j_1}^2 \cdots \partial \sigma_{j_m}^2}$$

$$(7.82)$$

Clearly, D_{h_n} depends very little on Δt, when Δt is much smaller than unity. So, whenever Δt is very small, we accept the approximation

$$D_{h_n}(\sigma_1, \sigma_2, \ldots, \sigma_n) \cong \frac{1}{12} \sum_{j_1=1}^{n} \frac{\partial^2 h_n(\sigma_1, \ldots, \sigma_n)}{\partial \sigma_{j_1}^2} \qquad (7.83)$$

i.e., D_{h_n} is independent of Δt, for Δt in the range of values of practical interest.

Notice, however, that the initial region may disturb the square relation between Δt and θ_n. This is because in the initial region θ_n depends on Δt

according to a polynomial relation including all powers of Δt [cf. Eq. (7.75)]. For example, in the first-order kernel case the deconvolution error for the initial region $(0 \leqslant \sigma < \Delta t)$ is

$$\theta_1(\sigma) = [\alpha_0(\lambda) - 1]h_1(\sigma) + \alpha_1(\lambda)h^{(1)}(\sigma)\Delta t + \tfrac{1}{2}\alpha_2(\lambda)h^{(2)}(\sigma)\Delta t^2 + \cdots \tag{7.84}$$

where $\lambda = \sigma/\Delta t$. Thus,

$$D_{h_1}(\sigma) = \beta_0(\sigma) + \beta_1(\sigma)\Delta t + \beta_2(\sigma)\Delta t^2 + \beta_3(\sigma)\Delta t^3 + \beta_4(\sigma)\Delta t^4 + \cdots \tag{7.85}$$

where $\beta_0(\sigma)$, $\beta_1(\sigma)$, $\beta_3(\sigma)$, $\beta_5(\sigma)$, ... (and the rest of the odd-order terms) are nonzero only when $0 \leqslant \sigma < \Delta t$.

Therefore, the dependence of $\theta_1(\sigma)$ on Δt becomes analytically complicated if the initial region is to be included. For this reason, it is suggested in practice that we compute the deconvolution error over the space of the kernel outside the initial region (i.e., $\Delta t \leqslant \sigma_i \leqslant \mu$), in order to keep the analytical relation between θ_n and Δt in the simple form described by Eq. (7.81).

We illustrate this in Fig. 7.19 by plotting the deconvolution error of the first-order kernel estimate versus the second derivative of the kernel. The three plots A, B, and C correspond to kernel estimates obtained by using ternary equirandom test signals of half-operational range $A = 1$, record length $T = 8000\,\text{sec}$, and step lengths $\Delta t = 0.30$, 0.45, $0.60\,\text{sec}$, respectively.

The linear form of the plots validates the assumption of independence of D_{h_1} from Δt; and the slope of these lines demonstrates the square relation between θ_1 and Δt. Notice that the initial regions of the kernels have been excluded from these plots.

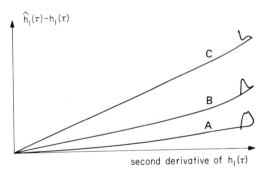

Fig. 7.19. Illustration of the dependence of deconvolution error on the kernel second derivative and on the stimulus step length; (A) $\Delta t = 0.15$, (B) $\Delta t = 0.30$, (C) $\Delta t = 0.45$.

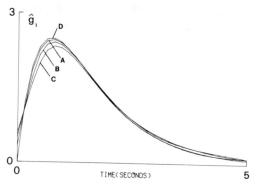

Fig. 7.20. Illustration of deconvolution error of first-order kernel estimates for three different step lengths (A) 0.15 sec, (B) 0.30 sec, (C) 0.45 sec, (D) exact.

The dependence of the deconvolution error upon the second derivative and the step length can also be seen in the actual kernel estimates. In Fig. 7.20, the previously discussed first-order kernel estimates are shown, along with the exact first-order kernel of the system. It can be seen that the deviation of the estimates from the exact kernel is positive or negative according to whether the second derivative is positive or negative. However, this is not true in the initial region ($\sigma < \Delta t$) because of the derivative discontinuity of the kernel at the origin. Thus, the deviation of the estimates within the initial region is positive even though the second derivative is negative.

7.3.2. The Statistical Fluctuation Error (ε Error)

In the previous section, autocorrelation functions were computed as statistical averages. However, in practice we have to compute the averages by integrating in time over finite time intervals, and we can only obtain an estimate of the autocorrelation functions, as

$$\hat{\phi}_n(\tau_1, \ldots, \tau_n) = \frac{1}{T - T_m} \int_{T_m}^{T} x(t - \tau_1) \cdots x(t - \tau_n) \, dt,$$

$$T_m = \max\{\tau_1, \ldots, \tau_n\} \tag{7.86}$$

Usually, the record length T is much longer than the memory of the system (and, consequently, much bigger than T_m), and therefore we can write

$$\hat{\phi}_n(\tau_1, \ldots, \tau_n) \simeq \frac{1}{T} \int_{0}^{T} x(t - \tau_1) \cdots x(t - \tau_n) \, dt \tag{7.87}$$

This autocorrelation estimate $\hat{\phi}_n$ is a random variable itself and, consequently, its convolution with a kernel will give a kernel estimate with random characteristics. Therefore, the kernel estimates that we obtain in practice by averaging over finite records are deviating randomly from the exact kernels. This random deviation of the kernel estimates constitutes the statistical fluctuation error, which we will try to evaluate. First, let us study the first-order kernel case:

$$\hat{h}_1(\sigma) = \frac{1}{(m_2 \Delta t)} \int_0^\infty h_1(\tau) \hat{\phi}_2(\sigma - \tau) \, d\tau \tag{7.88}$$

where

$$\hat{\phi}_2(\sigma - \tau) = \frac{1}{T - \max\{\tau, \sigma\}} \int_{\max\{\sigma, \tau\}}^T x(t - \tau) x(t - \sigma) \, dt$$

$$\cong \frac{1}{T} \int_0^T x(t - \tau) x(t - \sigma) \, dt \qquad \text{since } T \gg \sigma, \tau \tag{7.89}$$

Every value of $\hat{\phi}_2(\sigma - \tau)$ is a random variable with

$$E[\hat{\phi}_2(\sigma - \tau)] = \phi_2(\sigma - \tau) \tag{7.90}$$

$$\text{Var}\,[\hat{\phi}_2(\sigma - \tau)] = \frac{1}{T^2} \int_0^T \int_0^T E[x(t-\tau)x(t-\sigma)x(t'-\tau)x(t'-\sigma)] \, dt \, dt'$$

$$- \phi_2^2(\tau - \sigma)$$

$$= \begin{cases} (\Delta t/T)m_2^2 & \text{for } \tau \neq \sigma \\ (\Delta t/T)(m_4 - m_2^2) & \text{for } \tau = \sigma \end{cases} \tag{7.91}$$

These expressions for the variance refer only to the nodal points $(\sigma - \tau)$, and they are accurate under the condition that the memory of the system is much smaller than the record length T, and much bigger than the step length Δt $(\Delta t \ll \mu \ll T)$. From expression (7.91), we clearly see that the variance of the second-order autocorrelation estimate is inversely proportional to the number of steps of the stimulus signal. The same holds true for the higher-order autocorrelation estimates.

Consider now the "deviation function":

$$r_2(\sigma - \tau) = \hat{\phi}_2(\sigma - \tau) - \phi_2(\sigma - \tau) \tag{7.92}$$

which is the source of the statistical fluctuation error. Clearly,

$$\hat{h}_1(\sigma) = \frac{1}{m_2 \Delta t} \int_0^\infty h_1(\tau) \phi_2(\sigma - \tau) \, d\tau + \frac{1}{m_2 \Delta t} \int_0^\infty h_1(\tau) r_2(\sigma - \tau) \, d\tau$$

$$= [I_{p_1}(\sigma) + I_{s_1}(\sigma)]/(m_2 \Delta t) \tag{7.93}$$

We call these two integrals, the "principal" and the "side" part integral, respectively. The principal part integral is deterministic, while the side part integral is random in nature. In order to evaluate the statistical fluctuation

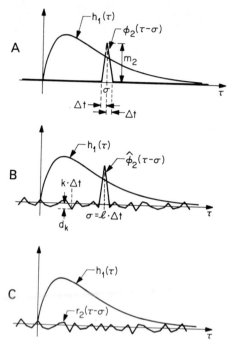

Fig. 7.21. Convolution of first-order kernel with (A) second-order CSRS autocorrelation function, (B) second-order CSRS autocorrelation estimate, (C) second-order CSRS deviation function.

error ε_1, we simply have to evaluate the side part integral I_{s_1}, which is the convolution of the deviation function r_2 with the kernel h_1 (see Fig. 7.21):

$$\varepsilon_1(\sigma) = \frac{I_{s_1}(\sigma)}{m_2 \Delta t} = \frac{1}{m_2 \Delta t} \int_0^\infty h_1(\tau) r_2(\sigma - \tau) \, d\tau \qquad (7.94)$$

First, we study the statistical structure of the deviation function r_2. For this purpose, notice that $\phi_2(\sigma - \tau)$ is computed as

$$\hat{\phi}_2[(i-j)DT] = \frac{DT}{T} \sum_{k=1}^N x[(k-i)DT]x[(k-j)DT] \qquad (7.95)$$

where DT is the sampling interval, not necessarily equal to the step length Δt (usually Δt is an integral multiple of DT). Of course, $x[(k-i)DT]$ and $x[(k-j)DT]$ are uncorrelated for any k, as long as $|(i-j)DT| \geq \Delta t$. Also, for a given pair (i, j), a great number of the products $\{x[(k-i)DT]x[(k-j)DT]\}$ are statistically independent. Consequently, the central limit theorem can be practically employed and the distribution of each value of $\hat{\phi}_2$ is found to be approximately Gaussian. In the case where $i = j$ (diagonal points), the same reasoning holds, and all the values $\hat{\phi}_2(kDT)$ are found to be approximately Gaussian random variables.

The several $\hat{\phi}_2(kDT)$ seem to be statistically dependent, since they are constructed with the same population of values $x(iDT)$. However, they are uncorrelated, since

$$E[\hat{\phi}_2(kDT)\hat{\phi}_2(lDT)] = \sum_i \sum_j E[x(iDT)x[(i+k)DT]x(jDT)x[(j+l)DT]]$$

$$= 0 \qquad \text{for } k \neq \pm l \qquad (7.96)$$

In conclusion, if we call d_k the values of the deviation function r_2 at the nodal points, then the several d_k (of one side of the symmetric deviation function) are found to be uncorrelated approximately Gaussian random variables with zero mean and variance m_2^2/N for $k \neq 0$ and $(m_4 - m_2^2)/N$ for $k = 0$ (for $N = T/\Delta t$ and $T \gg \mu$).

In the following analysis, we will consider that the variance of d_0 is the same as the variance of all other d_k. This approximation is not expected to cause significant errors, while it facilitates the derivations greatly.

Our analysis is based upon the following basic remark: The side part integral is the convolution of the kernel with the corresponding deviation function. The convolution integral is a linear operation. Consequently, the Gaussian statistical characteristics of the deviation function are going to be preserved. Thus, if the statistical characteristics of the deviation function depend in some way on a parameter, then the statistical characteristics of the convolution integral are going to depend on that parameter in the same way. This is more evident in the case where the random function does not have any directionality, i.e., when the statistical properties of the convolution of this random function with any unitary deterministic function, (i.e., a function whose integral of the square of the function is unity) are the same.

According to Eq. (7.94), the side part integral I_{s_1} clearly belongs in this category, since its Gaussian statistical properties are completely described by the first two moments, and these moments are independent of Δt.

Notice that this convolution integral is analogous to the inner product of a random and a deterministic unitary vector in a linear vector space of infinite dimensionality. In this sense, the "random vector" r_2 has spherical directionality, i.e., attains all directions with the same likelihood. The direct implication of this is that the inner product of the "random vector" r_2 with the diagonal vector (step function) can be used as a reliable indicator of the statistical behavior of the inner product of r_2 with any other deterministic unitary vector of the space. Thus, the parametric study of the statistical behavior of the side part integral can be interchanged, for the purposes of the present analysis, with the study of the statistical behavior of the integral of the deviation function (inner product with the step function).

For the first-order case this quantity (hereafter called the "integrated deviation") is

$$R_2 = \int_0^{\mu_1} r_2(\lambda)\, d\lambda \qquad (7.97)$$

where μ_1 is the first-order memory of the system and $r_2(\lambda)$ is taken to be symmetric about zero. Since r_2 is piecewise linear, the evaluation of the integral R_2 requires the evaluation of each linear portion:

$$U_k = \int_{k\Delta t}^{(k+1)\Delta t} r_2(\lambda)\, d\lambda, \qquad k = 0, 1, 2, \ldots, M_1 - 1;\ M_1 = \frac{\mu_1}{\Delta t} \qquad (7.98)$$

where

$$r_2(\lambda) = d_k\left[(k+1) - \frac{\lambda}{\Delta t}\right] - d_{k+1}\left(k - \frac{\lambda}{\Delta t}\right) \qquad \text{for } k\Delta t \leqslant \lambda \leqslant (k+1)\Delta t \qquad (7.99)$$

Evaluating the integral in Eq. (7.98) we obtain

$$U_k = \tfrac{1}{2}\Delta t(d_k + d_{k+1}) \qquad (7.100)$$

and the integrated deviation becomes

$$R_2 = \sum_{k=0}^{M_1-1} U_k \cong \sum_{k=1}^{M_1} \Delta t d_k \qquad (7.101)$$

Therefore, R_2 is a Gaussian random variable with

$$E[\![R_2]\!] = 0 \qquad (7.102)$$

$$\operatorname{Var}[\![R_2]\!] \cong \Delta t^2 \sigma_{d_1}^2 M_1$$

$$\cong (m_2\Delta t)^2 \mu_1/T \qquad (7.103)$$

Note that the integrated deviation must be normalized by the normalizing factor of the respective order of kernel. Thus, finally, we have

$$\operatorname{Var}[\![R_2]\!] = q_1^2(\sigma, \Delta t, T) \sim 1/T \qquad (7.104)$$

So, we conclude that the variance of the statistical fluctuation error of first order is independent of Δt.

This approach can be extended easily to the higher-order kernel cases.

Following the same basic steps, in the nth-order case the integrated deviation is

$$R_{2n} = \int_0^{\mu_n} \cdots \int_0^{\mu_n} r_{2n}(\lambda_1, \ldots, \lambda_n)\, d\lambda_1 \cdots d\lambda_n$$

$$\cong \sum_{k_1=1}^{M_n} \cdots \sum_{k_n=1}^{M_n} \Delta t^n d_{k_1 k_2 \cdots k_n}, \qquad M_n = \frac{\mu_n}{\Delta t} \qquad (7.105)$$

where μ_n is the nth-order memory of the system and $r_{2n}(\lambda_1, \lambda_2, \ldots, \lambda_n)$ a symmetric function with respect to the arguments $(\lambda_1, \lambda_2, \ldots, \lambda_n)$. From Eq. (7.105) follows that R_{2n} is a Gaussian random variable with

$$E[\![R_{2n}]\!] = 0 \tag{7.106}$$

$$\operatorname{Var}[\![R_{2n}]\!] = \Delta t^{2n} \sigma_{d_n}^2 M_n^n$$

$$\simeq (m_2 \Delta t)^{2n} \mu_n^n / T \Delta t^{n-1} \tag{7.107}$$

since,

$$\sigma_{d_n}^2 = m_2^{2n} \Delta t / T \tag{7.108}$$

Consequently, for each point $(\sigma_1, \ldots, \sigma_n)$ we have

$$\operatorname{Var}[\![R_{2n}]\!] = q_n^2(\sigma_1, \ldots, \sigma_n, \Delta t, T) \sim 1/T \Delta t^{n-1} \tag{7.109}$$

that is, the variance of the statistical fluctuation error, in the nth-order case, is inversely proportional to the record length T and to the $(n-1)$th power of the step length Δt.

Of course, this is an approximate result, which illustrates the principal pattern of dependence of the statistical fluctuation error on T and Δt, in the cases where $\Delta t \ll \mu \ll T$ (which are the cases of interest in practice). Evidently, the exact pattern of dependence of q_n^2 on Δt is related to the specific kernel (system) involved; however, this is of secondary importance for all practical purposes.

In general, it can be stated that the variance of the statistical fluctuation error in the nth-order kernel case and in all situations of practical interest $(\Delta t \ll \mu \ll T)$ is

$$q_n^2(\sigma_1, \ldots, \sigma_n, \Delta t, T) = \frac{C_{h_n}^2(\sigma_1, \ldots, \sigma_n, \Delta t)}{T \Delta t^{n-1}} \tag{7.110}$$

where the function $C_{h_n}^2(\sigma_1, \ldots, \sigma_n, \Delta t)$ depends very slightly on Δt.

In order to illustrate the dependence of the statistical fluctuation error upon the record length T, we compute the percentage MSE of the first- and second-order kernel estimates for several ternary equirandom stimuli with various record lengths.

More specifically, all the ternary equirandom stimuli used have half-operational range $A = 1$ and step length $\Delta t = 0.15$ sec. We compute the average percentage MSE using five estimates for each one of three different record lengths: 500, 1000, and 2000 sec. The results obtained are shown in Fig. 7.22. Some representative kernel estimates are shown in Figs. 7.23(A)–7.23(C) and they verify our expectations. Notice that the total estimation error can be approximately identified with the statistical fluctuation because of the rather small step length $\Delta t = 0.15$ sec.

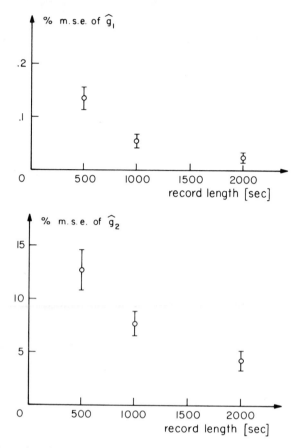

Fig. 7.22. Illustration of the dependence of the CSRS kernel estimation error on the record length.

   In order to illustrate the dependence of the statistical fluctuation error upon the step length, we use the following procedure: (a) We obtain four independent kernel estimates of first and second order for each one of four different step lengths: 0.15, 0.30, 0.45, and 0.60 sec, while keeping the length of each one of these records constant at 2000 sec. (b) We compute the integrated squared differences between any two of the four kernel estimates of the same order and step length. Notice that these integrated squared differences are quantities independent from the deconvolution error and they only depend on the statistical fluctuation error. (c) We compute the averages of these quantities for each group corresponding to a specific step length.
   The results obtained are shown in Fig. 7.24. Representative second-order kernel estimates are shown in Fig. 7.25 and they demonstrate the

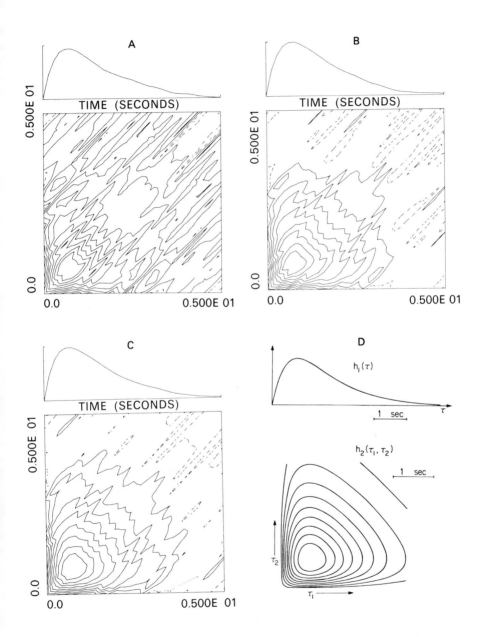

Fig. 7.23. First- and second-order kernel estimates obtained by use of records of various lengths: (A) 500 sec, (B) 1000 sec, (C) 2000 sec. The exact kernels of the system are shown in (D).

anticipated dependence of the statistical fluctuation error on the stimulus step length.

In conclusion, the ε error is due to random fluctuations of the estimates of the autocorrelation functions. The practical limitation that causes this error is the finite record length. The variance of the ε error monotonically decreases as the record length increases. However, the record length is not the only parameter affecting the ε error; the stimulus bandwidth is an even more crucial factor affecting this error in the higher-order kernel estimates. The degree of this dependence increases rapidly with the order of the kernel estimate under study.

The ε error at each point of the nth-order kernel estimate has been found to be a Gaussian random variable with zero mean and variance given by Eq. (7.110). The function $C^2_{h_n}(\sigma_1, \ldots, \sigma_n, \Delta t)$ that appears in Eq. (7.110) depends mainly on h_n and very slightly on Δt (for all cases of practical interest, where $\Delta t \ll \mu \ll T$).

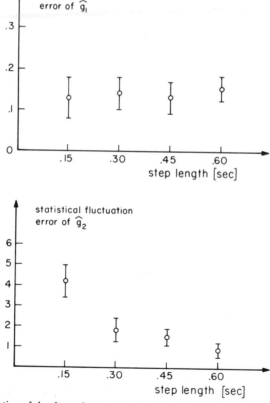

Fig. 7.24. Illustration of the dependence of the statistical fluctuation error on the step length.

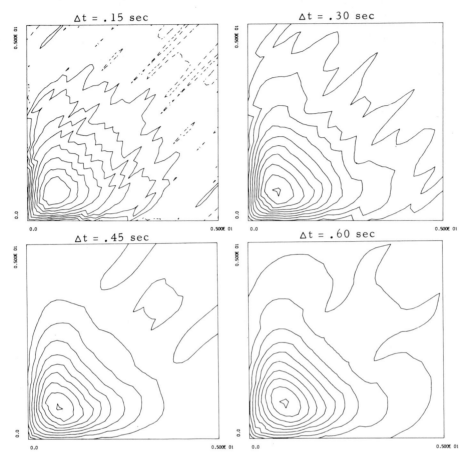

Fig. 7.25. Second-order CSRS kernel estimates obtained through stimuli of various step lengths.

We can obtain an expression of the mean-square ε error of the nth-order kernel estimate by integrating $q_n^2(\sigma_1, \ldots, \sigma_n, \Delta t)$ over the whole memory space of the kernel:

$$\overline{\varepsilon_n^2} = \int_0^{\mu_n} \cdots \int_0^{\mu_n} q_n^2(\sigma_1, \ldots, \sigma_n, \Delta t)\, d\sigma_1 \cdots d\sigma_n$$

$$= \frac{B_n(\Delta t)}{T \Delta t^{n-1}} \qquad\qquad (7.111)$$

where

$$B_n(\Delta t) = \int_0^{\mu_n} \cdots \int_0^{\mu_n} C_{h_n}^2(\sigma_1, \ldots, \sigma_n, \Delta t)\, d\sigma_1 \cdots d\sigma_n \qquad (7.112)$$

Clearly, $B_n(\Delta t)$ depends very slightly on Δt, in a way to be considered constant for all practical purposes, as long as Δt remains in the range of values of interest ($\Delta t \ll \mu_n$). Of course, B_n is characteristic of the kernel h_n, and it also depends on the specified memory extent μ_n.

7.3.3. The Approximate Orthogonality Errors

There are two kinds of approximate orthogonality errors. One refers to the approximate orthogonality of the G^* functionals as they are constructed (Sec. 5.3) and is due to the finite stimulus bandwidth (orthogonality error of the first kind). The other refers to the approximate orthogonality of the estimated G^* functionals, because of the finite records that are used in the estimation procedure (orthogonality error of the second kind).

(I) Orthogonality Error of First Kind

From the way that the G^* functionals are constructed, it is evident that their orthogonality is complete only when the stimulus bandwidth is infinite (ideal white noise). In practice, of course, the bandwidth of a quasiwhite signal is finite and the orthogonality of the G^* functionals (of order higher than unity) holds only approximately. This approximation improves as the stimulus bandwidth becomes broader with respect to the system bandwidth.

To illustrate this kind of error, let us consider the case of the second-order G^* functional:

$$G_2^*(t) = \int\limits_0^\infty\!\!\int g_2(\tau_1, \tau_2) x(t-\tau_1) x(t-\tau_2)\, d\tau_1\, d\tau_2 - (m_2 \Delta t) \int_0^\infty g_2(\tau, \tau)\, d\tau$$

$$(7.113)$$

The exact orthogonal form for the CSRS is

$$\widetilde{G_2^*}(t) = \int\limits_0^\infty\!\!\int g_2(\tau_1, \tau_2) x(t-\tau_1) x(t-\tau_2) d\tau_1\, d\tau_2$$

$$- \int\limits_0^\infty\!\!\int g_2(\tau_1, \tau_2) \phi_2(\tau_2 - \tau_1)\, d\tau_1\, d\tau_2 \qquad (7.114)$$

where ϕ_2 is the second-order autocorrelation function of the CSRS. Thus, $\widetilde{G_2^*}$ and G_2^* differ at the second integral term. The second integral term of

$\widetilde{G_2^*}$ can be written as

$$\int\int_0^\infty g_2(\tau_1, \tau_2)\phi_2(\tau_2 - \tau_1)\, d\tau_1\, d\tau_2 = \int_0^\infty d\tau \int_{-\Delta t}^{\Delta t} g_2(\tau, \tau + \lambda)m_2\left(1 - \frac{|\lambda|}{\Delta t}\right) d\lambda$$

$$= \int_0^\infty d\tau \int_{-\Delta t}^{\Delta t} \left\{ g_2(\tau, \tau) + \left[\frac{\partial g_2(\tau, \sigma)}{\partial \sigma}\right]_{\sigma=\tau} \lambda + \left[\frac{\partial^2 g_2(\tau, \sigma)}{\partial \sigma^2}\right]_{\sigma=\tau} \frac{\lambda^2}{2} \right.$$

$$\left. + \cdots \right\} m_2\left(1 - \frac{|\lambda|}{\Delta t}\right) d\lambda \tag{7.115}$$

if we expand $g_2(\tau, \tau + \lambda)$ in a Taylor series in the region of its analyticity. Since the interval of integration of λ is symmetric, the odd-power terms of λ will vanish with the integration, and therefore

$$\int\int_0^\infty g_2(\tau_1, \tau_2)\phi_2(\tau_2 - \tau_1)\, d\tau_1\, d\tau_2$$

$$= (m_2\Delta t) \int_0^\infty d\tau \sum_{n=0}^\infty \frac{\Delta t^{2n}}{2n!(2n+1)(n+1)} \left[\frac{\partial^{2n} g_2(\tau, \sigma)}{\partial \sigma^{2n}}\right]_{\sigma=\tau} \tag{7.116}$$

The orthogonality error of the first kind in the second-order case is

$$\xi_2 = G_2^* - \widetilde{G_2^*} = (m_2\Delta t) \sum_{n=1}^\infty \frac{\Delta t^{2n}}{2n!(2n+1)(n+1)} \int_0^\infty \left[\frac{\partial^{2n} g_2(\tau, \sigma)}{\partial \sigma^{2n}}\right]_{\sigma=\tau} d\tau \tag{7.117}$$

which obviously becomes negligible when Δt becomes very small (very broad stimulus bandwidth). Similar expressions can be derived for the higher-order G^* functionals.

(II) Orthogonality Error of Second Kind

The estimation of the G^* functionals through the crosscorrelation technique is based upon the orthogonality of these functionals, expressed as

$$E[G_m^* G_n^*] = 0 \qquad (m \neq n) \tag{7.118}$$

However, the statistical average is substituted, in practice, by a time average over a finite time period. This has as a result the incomplete formation of this average, and subsequently some estimation error occurs in terms of remnants from the incomplete implementation of the orthogonality. These remnants attain small nonzero values, which appear as estimation errors in the nth-order kernel estimates. The variance of these remnants is inversely proportional to the record length and becomes practically negligible for sufficiently long records.

7.3.4. The Erroneous Power Level Error

As discussed in Sec. 5.3, the normalizing factors of the crosscorrelation estimates depend upon the even moments and the step length of the respective CSRS or, in other words, upon the generalized power levels of the CSRS. Consequently, the evaluation of these normalizing factors requires knowledge of the appropriate even moments and of the step length.

This knowledge is either *a priori* or it must be estimated. In the case where it is accurately known *a priori* (for example, in computer simulations), there is no additional estimation error caused by the normalization procedure. However, in actual applications in the laboratory some test parameters are not accurately known and must be measured or estimated.

In that case, measurement or estimation errors in these parameters may induce a disproportionality estimation error in the kernel estimates due to the erroneous normalizing factors. An additional error may result from the fact that the G^* functionals of order higher than the first depend explicitly upon the generalized power levels, which may be erroneously estimated.

To illustrate these two kinds of error, consider the case where we are trying to estimate the first-order power level:

$$P_1 = m_2 \Delta t \tag{7.119}$$

in the laboratory. The step length Δt can usually be measured with high accuracy, because it is equal to the distance between two successive points of derivative discontinuity in the second-order autocorrelation function estimate. The measurement of the second moment m_2 usually involves more inaccuracies, since an estimate of it, obtained as the mean square of the signal samples, exhibits a variance of significant magnitude. More specifically

$$\hat{m}_2 = \frac{1}{N} \sum_{i=1}^{N} x_i^2, \qquad N = \frac{T}{\Delta t} \tag{7.120}$$

$$E[\hat{m}_2] = m_2 \tag{7.121}$$

$$\text{Var}[\hat{m}_2] = (\Delta t / T)(m_4 - m_2^2) \tag{7.122}$$

and $\hat{m}_2$ follows approximately a Gaussian distribution. Clearly, the accuracy of this estimate increases as the number of steps in the signal increases.

Another popular way of estimating the first-order power level is by computing the integral of the second-order autocorrelation function estimate from $\tau = -\mu_1$ to $\tau = +\mu_1$, where μ_1 is the first-order memory extent of the system. In this case the power level estimate is approximately a Gaussian random variable, with

$$E[\hat{P}_1] = m_2 \Delta t \qquad (7.123)$$

$$\text{Var}\,[\hat{P}_1] \cong (m_2 \Delta t)^2 4\mu_1 / T \qquad (7.124)$$

Notice that the accuracy of the estimate improves as the record length increases. The above integration may extend over part of the memory.

In the first method of estimation, the expected percentage error is

$$\varepsilon_1 = \left[\frac{\Delta t}{T} \left(\frac{m_4}{m_2^2} - 1 \right) \right]^{1/2} \qquad (7.125)$$

where we assume that Δt is measured with complete accuracy.

In the second method of estimation, the expected percentage error is

$$\varepsilon_2 = 2(\mu_1 / T)^{1/2} \qquad (7.126)$$

The disproportionality percentage error π_n in the nth-order kernel estimate (for the nondiagonal points), caused by a percentage error ε in the estimation of the first-order power level is

$$\pi_n = \frac{(1+\varepsilon)^n - 1}{(1+\varepsilon)^n} \qquad (7.127)$$

and, if $n\varepsilon \ll 1$ (which is usually the case in practice), then

$$\pi_n \cong n\varepsilon \qquad (7.128)$$

7.3.5. The Finite Transition Time Error

The generation of the stimulus signal in the laboratory comprises two basic steps. In the first step, a string of numbers corresponding to the values of the CSRS at each step is generated by the digital computer. In the second step, this sequence of numbers is fed into a digital-to-analog transducer, which, in turn, generates a continuous analog signal having physical dimensions required for the actual test of the system.

It must be expected that the response, or rise, time of the transducer will be finite, because of some inevitable inertia of the driving system. Of course, this finite response time can be reduced to an acceptable level by using appropriate hardware. The practical requirements concerning the response time of the transducer are set by the frequency bandwidth of the system under test.

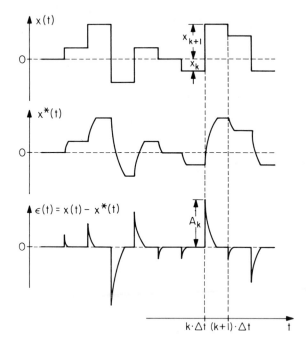

Fig. 7.26 Illustration of the error signal resulting from finite reversible transition time of the transducer.

In any case, the finite response time results in finite transition times at the switching points of the signal. The practical effect of this finite transition time is negligible if the inverse of the transition time is greater than the frequency bandwidth of the system under test. This is a practical requirement, which (in most cases) can be easily met, with the proper choice of hardware.

Nevertheless, we will study this effect for two general cases of practical interest: reversible and irreversible transitions. The reversibility of a transition is defined according to the patterns followed in an upward or a downward transition. If those patterns are the same the transition is called reversible, otherwise it is called irreversible.

Consider now the ideal (i.e., zero rise time) CSRS stimulus $x(t)$ and the actual output of a transducer $x^*(t)$, which has finite reversible transition times. Consider their difference as being an error signal (Fig. 7.26):

$$\varepsilon(t) = x(t) - x^*(t) \qquad (7.129)$$

Since the transition is assumed to be reversible, the operation of the transducer is described by the same differential equation both in upwards and downwards movements. This differential equation is usually linear with constant coefficients, and with all its roots on the negative real axis.

For illustrative purposes, let us consider the very simple case where the operation of the transducer is described by the first-order linear differential equation

$$T_r \frac{dx^*(t)}{dt} + x^*(t) = x(t) \qquad \text{for } k\Delta t \leqslant t < (k+1)\Delta t \qquad (7.130)$$

and T_r is the characteristic response time of the transducer, chosen to be much smaller than the step length Δt. The solution of the differential equation (7.130) for every step of the CSRS signal $x(t)$ is

$$x^*(t) = [x_k - x_{k+1}] \exp[-(t - k\Delta t)/T_r] + x_{k+1} \qquad \text{for } k\Delta t \leqslant t < (k+1)\Delta t \tag{7.131}$$

where x_k is the constant value of $x(t)$ for $(k-1)\Delta t < t \leqslant k\Delta t$. Notice that, since $T_r \ll \Delta t$, the error signal $\varepsilon(t)$ is practically zero most of the time.

Let us study the error signal:

$$\varepsilon(t) = [x_{k+1} - x_k] \exp[-(t - k\Delta t)/T_r]$$
$$= A_k \exp[-(t - k\Delta t)/T_r] \qquad \text{for } k\Delta t \leqslant t < (k+1)\Delta t \quad (7.132)$$

Clearly, $\varepsilon(t)$ is a sequence of random pulselike exponentials (see Fig. 7.26). Their random character is attributed to their random height A_k. From the generation mechanism of the CSRS family (namely, the statistical independence of each step and the symmetric amplitude probability density function) it follows directly that the random amplitude A_k is distributed according to a symmetric probability density function $q(A)$, which is the convolution integral of the amplitude probability density function $p(x)$ of the CSRS with itself. The mean of $q(A)$ is zero and the variance is double the variance of $p(x)$.

This brief analysis of the error signal $\varepsilon(t)$ will enable us to study its autocorrelation properties, as well as its crosscorrelation with the ideal CSRS $x(t)$. The study of these properties is necessary for the appreciation of the effect of the finite transition time on our kernel estimates, since we have to show that quasiwhiteness is preserved in $x^*(t)$ to an acceptable degree. We have

$$\phi_n^*(\tau_1, \ldots, \tau_n) = E[x^*(t - \tau_1) \cdots x^*(t - \tau_n)]$$
$$= \sum_{k=0}^{n} \binom{n}{k} \xi_{k,n}(\tau_1, \ldots, \tau_n) \tag{7.133}$$

where

$$\xi_{k,n}(\tau_1, \ldots, \tau_n) = E[x(t - \tau_1) \cdots x(t - \tau_k)\varepsilon(t - \tau_{k+1}) \cdots \varepsilon(t - \tau_n)] \tag{7.134}$$

First, let us study the second-order autocorrelation function of the error signal:

$$\phi_{\varepsilon\varepsilon}(\tau) = \lim_{T \to \infty} \frac{1}{2T} \int_{-T}^{T} \varepsilon(t) \dot{\varepsilon}(t-\tau) \, dt \qquad (7.135)$$

With the help of Eq. (7.132) we derive the values of $\phi_{\varepsilon\varepsilon}(\tau)$ (see Fig. 7.27):

$$\phi_{\varepsilon\varepsilon}(\tau) = \begin{cases} \dfrac{m_2 T_r}{\Delta t} \left\{ \exp\left(\dfrac{-|\tau|}{T_r}\right) - \exp\left(\dfrac{-\Delta t}{T_r}\right) \right. \\ \qquad \left. \times \left[\exp\left(\dfrac{-(\Delta t - |\tau|)}{T_r}\right) + \sinh\left(\dfrac{|\tau|}{T_r}\right) \right] \right\} & \text{for } 0 \leqslant |\tau| \leqslant \Delta t \\[6pt] -\dfrac{m_2 T_r}{2\Delta t} \exp\left[\dfrac{-(|\tau| - \Delta t)}{T_r}\right] \\ \qquad \times \left[1 - \exp\left(\dfrac{-2(2\Delta t - |\tau|)}{T_r}\right) \right] & \text{for } \Delta t \leqslant |\tau| \leqslant 2\Delta t \\[6pt] \approx 0 & \text{for } |\tau| > 2\Delta t \end{cases}$$

$$(7.136)$$

Notice that

$$-\frac{m_2 T_r}{2\Delta t} < \phi_{\varepsilon\varepsilon}(\tau) < \frac{m_2 T_r}{\Delta t} \qquad \text{for any } \tau \qquad (7.137)$$

Consequently, the values of this autocorrelation function become negligible if the response time T_r of the transducer is chosen much smaller than the step length Δt.

Similarly, we derive the expressions for the crosscorrelation function:

$$\psi_{x\varepsilon}(\tau) = \lim_{T \to \infty} \frac{1}{2T} \int_{-T}^{T} x(t) \varepsilon(t-\tau) \, dt \qquad (7.138)$$

using Eq. (7.132) (see Fig. 7.28), in terms of the second moment of the CSRS m_2, the step length Δt, and the transducer response time T_r:

$$\psi_{x\varepsilon}(\tau) = \begin{cases} \dfrac{m_2 T_r}{\Delta t} \left\{ 1 - \exp\left[\dfrac{-(\Delta t - \tau)}{T_r}\right] \right\} & \text{for } 0 \leqslant \tau \leqslant \Delta t \\[6pt] \dfrac{m_2 T_r}{\Delta t} \left[2 \exp\left(\dfrac{\tau}{T_r}\right) - 1 - \exp\left(\dfrac{-\Delta t}{T_r}\right) \right] & \text{for } -\Delta t \leqslant \tau \leqslant 0 \\[6pt] \dfrac{m_2 T_r}{\Delta t} \left\{ \exp\left(\dfrac{-\Delta t}{T_r}\right) - \exp\left[\dfrac{(\tau + \Delta t)}{T_r}\right] \right\} & \text{for } -2\Delta t \leqslant \tau \leqslant -\Delta t \\[6pt] \approx 0 & \text{for } \tau < -2\Delta t \text{ and } \tau > \Delta t \end{cases}$$

$$(7.139)$$

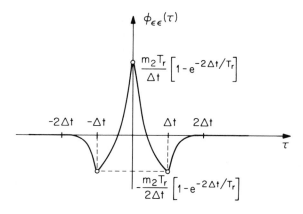

Fig. 7.27. Second-order autocorrelation function of the error signal.

We note again that

$$-\frac{m_2 T_r}{\Delta t} < \psi_{x\varepsilon}(\tau) < \frac{m_2 T_r}{\Delta t} \qquad \text{for any } \tau \qquad (7.140)$$

which implies that the values of this crosscorrelation become negligible, if T_r is chosen to be much smaller than Δt.

From the study of the autocorrelation and crosscorrelation properties of $\varepsilon(t)$ and $x(t)$, we deduce that the functions $\xi_{k,n}(\tau_1, \ldots, \tau_n)$ of Eq. (7.133) do not deviate significantly from quasiwhiteness, since their nonzero values remain concentrated within diagonal strips with width of the order of magnitude of Δt (see Figs. 7.27 and 7.28). In addition to that, it became evident from expressions (7.137) and (7.140) that the values of the functions $\xi_{k,n}(\tau_1, \ldots, \tau_n)$, for $k < n$, are much smaller than the values of the functions $\xi_{n,n}(\tau_1, \ldots, \tau_n)$, if T_r is chosen to be much smaller than Δt.

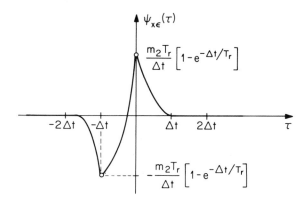

Fig. 7.28 Crosscorrelation function of the ideal stimulus and the error signal.

Thus, if we choose T_r to be much smaller than Δt, then the functions $\xi_{k,n}(\tau_1, \ldots, \tau_n)$, for $k < n$, become practically negligible compared to $\xi_{n,n}(\tau_1, \ldots, \tau_n)$. Consequently, Eq. (7.133) reduces approximately to

$$\phi_n^*(\tau_1, \ldots, \tau_n) \cong \xi_{n,n}(\tau_1, \ldots, \tau_n) = \phi_n(\tau_1, \ldots, \tau_n) \qquad (7.141)$$

Notice that even if the functions $\xi_{k,n}$ (for $k < n$) are not negligible the quasiwhiteness of $x^*(t)$ is not seriously affected. The only thing that is affected in this case is the value of the autocorrelation function at the full-diagonal strips. For this reason, special care must be taken in order to use the correct normalizing factors, since they are crucially dependent on the values of the autocorrelation functions at the full-diagonal strips.

In the case of an irreversible transition the differential equation that describes the operation of the transducer is not the same for upward and downward transitions. This complicates the analytical derivations, and we will confine ourselves to some qualitative remarks: (1) The significant values of the autocorrelation functions of the error signal will be concentrated within diagonal strips of width of the order of magnitude of Δt. The same is true for the crosscorrelation functions of the CSRS and the error signal. (2) The values of these autocorrelation and crosscorrelation functions can become practically negligible, if both the response times (of upward and downward transitions) are chosen to be much smaller than Δt.

The validity of these two remarks assures the preservation of the quasiwhiteness of $x^*(t)$ to a certain degree, but to a definitely lower degree than in the reversible transition case.

Notice, that, in the case of irreversible transitions, the expected value of the error signal (as well as all its odd-order moments) is not zero, while in the case of reversible transitions it is zero (along with all its odd-order moments). This is a clear indication of the fact that the case of irreversible transitions is disadvantageous, because it causes more significant deviations from the quasiwhiteness than the case of reversible transitions. Therefore, it is highly advisable to have a transducer with reversible transitions.

7.3.6. Computational Errors

There are three main sources of computational error in connection with the crosscorrelation technique. These sources are as follows:

    (1) discrete representation of continuous data
    (2) discrete integration in computing the crosscorrelations
    (3) numerical round-off errors

From these categories of computational errors, we discuss the first two as having some effect of practical interest. The effect of the last category is, for all practical purposes, negligible, if a contemporary digital computer is used to process the data.

(1) Discrete Representation of Continuous Data

If the input and output signals are continuous in time, their handling as data sets within a digital computer requires digitization, with which the continuous signal becomes a string of numbers. Thus, a continuous signal has to be sampled, at some proper sampling rate, and be represented thereafter within the digital computer as a discrete time series. This operation of "discretization" involves several pitfalls, which have received considerable attention in the literature (cf. Rabiner and Rader, 1972).

The most important of these pitfalls is the "aliasing problem" (cf. Sec. 2.9). This problem is the natural consequence of the simple mathematical fact that there is an infinite number of sinusoidal curves (of different frequencies) that pass through a set of equidistant points of a line, when the fundamental distance between any two points is finite (Fig. 7.29). The frequencies of these sinusoidal curves are integral multiples of a fundamental frequency called the Nyquist frequency

$$f_0 = 1/2d \tag{7.142}$$

If a finite interval d is chosen to sample a continuous signal, the power of the signal at the frequencies higher than the Nyquist frequency will be folded back upon the power of the symmetric (with respect to the Nyquist frequency) frequencies of the power spectrum (Fig. 7.30).

This very well known fact constitutes the main pitfall of discretizing a continuous signal. Obviously, if the sampling rate $f_s = 1/d$ is chosen to be greater than twice the bandwidth B of the signal, then the aliasing effect is

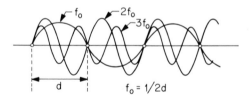

Fig. 7.29. Illustration of the aliasing problem.

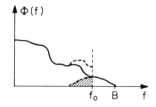

Fig. 7.30. Power spectrum folding due to aliasing.

eliminated. Thus, in practice we must always choose

$$f_s \geq 2B \qquad (7.143)$$

After sampling, the original continuous signal cannot be completely recovered (in general) but only approximated through some interpolation scheme. It is evident that in the case of a CSRS full and complete recovery of the original continuous signal from the discrete data set is possible. This is due to the special stairlike form of the CSRS. Nevertheless, the aliasing problem can be severe, even in the case of a CSRS, if the sampling rate is not sufficiently high.

(2) Discrete Integration Error

The computation of a crosscorrelation for the estimation of a kernel involves time integration of the product of the output signal with the proper number of time-shifted versions of the input signal:

$$\hat{\psi}_n(\sigma_1, \ldots, \sigma_n) = \frac{1}{T} \int_0^T y(t) x(t-\sigma_1) \cdots x(t-\sigma_n)\, dt \qquad (7.144)$$

where T is the record length.

Since the input and output signals are available within the computer only as discrete data sets, integration can never be completely accurate. However, almost any specified degree of accuracy can be achieved by using proper numerical interpolation–integration procedures. A prerequisite, of course, for this is that the discrete representation of the continuous signals is essentially free of the aliasing effect, and that the accuracy capacity (or word length) of the digital computer conforms with the desired degree of overall accuracy.

In practical applications of the crosscorrelation technique the computational burden is, by the method itself, very heavy, requiring that the numerical procedures that are used be kept as simple and efficient as possible. Thus, in the trade-off between computational accuracy and overall efficiency of the method, the balancing point is usually found on the side of simple numerical procedures with reasonable (but not the best possible) computational accuracy.

The simplest integration procedure for the computation of the crosscorrelation with discrete input and output data sets $\{y_i\}$ and $\{x_i\}$ is to compute the summation (consider the first-order case as an example):

$$\hat{\psi}_1(kDt) = \frac{1}{N} \sum_{i=1}^{N} y_i x_{i-k} \qquad (7.145)$$

where Dt is the sampling interval.

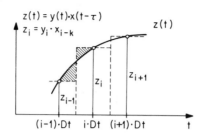

Fig. 7.31. Illustration of the deviation between continuous integration and discrete summation.

We now evaluate the difference of the integrals between $(i-1)Dt$ and iDt, obtained by analytical and numerical methods (Fig. 7.31). The integral obtained by simple numerical summation is

$$I_i = (z_{i-1} + z_i)Dt/2 \tag{7.146}$$

The integral obtained analytically is

$$J_i = \int_{(i-1)Dt}^{iDt} z(t)\, dt$$

$$= \int_{(i-1)Dt}^{(i-1/2)Dt} z_I(t)\, dt + \int_{(i-1/2)Dt}^{iDt} z_{II}(t)\, dt = L_1 + L_2 \tag{7.147}$$

where $z_I(t)$ and $z_{II}(t)$ are two Taylor expansions of $z(t)$ about z_{i-1} and z_i, respectively:

$$z_I(t) = z_{i-1} + z_{i-1}^{(1)}(z - z_{i-1}) + \frac{z_{i-1}^{(2)}}{2}(z - z_{i-1})^2 + \frac{z_{i-1}^{(3)}}{3!}(z - z_{i-1})^3 + \cdots \tag{7.148}$$

$$z_{II}(t) = z_i + z_i^{(1)}(z - z_i) + \frac{z_i^{(2)}}{2}(z - z_i)^2 + \frac{z_i^{(3)}}{3!}(z - z_i)^3 + \cdots \tag{7.149}$$

thus,

$$L_1 = \sum_{n=0}^{\infty} \frac{z_{i-1}^{(n)}}{(n+1)!}\left(\frac{Dt}{2}\right)^{n+1} \tag{7.150}$$

$$L_2 = \sum_{n=0}^{\infty} (-1)^n \frac{z_i^{(n)}}{(n+1)!}\left(\frac{Dt}{2}\right)^{n+1} \tag{7.151}$$

Consequently, the difference between the numerical and the analytical outcome of the ith integral portion is

$$D_i = J_i - I_i$$

$$= \sum_{n=1}^{\infty} \frac{[z_{i-1}^{(n)} + (-1)^n z_i^{(n)}]}{(n+1)!} \left(\frac{Dt}{2}\right)^{n+1} \qquad (7.152)$$

Now, consider the total difference between the two integrals when there are $N = T/Dt$ samples in the data set:

$$D = \sum_{i=1}^{N} D_i$$

$$\cong \sum_{m=1}^{\infty} \sum_{i=1}^{N} \frac{2z_i^{(2m)}}{(2m+1)!} \left(\frac{Dt}{2}\right)^{2m+1} \qquad (7.153)$$

and

$$z_i^{(2m)} = \sum_{j=0}^{2m} \binom{2m}{j} y_i^{(j)} x_{i-k}^{(2m-j)} \qquad (7.154)$$

Clearly, the exact value of $z_i^{(2m)}$ (and consequently the value of D) depends on the relative values of the derivatives of $y(t)$ and $x(t-\tau)$ at the sampling points, and the only general statement that can be made is that the difference D decreases very fast as Dt decreases.

If $x(t)$ is band-limited Gaussian white noise then the values of its derivatives at the sampling points are usually significant and, of course, depend mainly on the bandwidth of the signal. On the other hand, the values of the derivatives of $y(t)$ depend on the bandwidths of both the input $x(t)$ and the system under test.

Notice that if $x(t)$ is a CSRS all its derivatives at the sampling points are zero! Consequently, the expression (7.154) for $z_i^{(2m)}$ is dramatically simplified:

$$z_i^{(2m)} = y_i^{(2m)} x_{i-k} \qquad (7.155)$$

and, in most cases, it is expected to be much smaller than in the case of Gaussian white noise.

Since the sampling interval Dt is always fairly small (for aliasing reasons) and because the number of samples N is inversely proportional to Dt (for a constant record length) and the values of $z_i^{(2)}$ at closely neighboring points are only slightly different, in most of the cases, the difference D (and consequently the computational error) is approximately proportional to the square of the sampling interval:

$$D \cong \sum_{i=1}^{N} \frac{z_i^{(2)}}{24} Dt^3 \cong Dt^2 \left(Dt \sum_{i=1}^{N} \frac{z_i^{(2)}}{24}\right) \cong Dt^2(\text{const}) \qquad (7.156)$$

In conclusion, the basic factor affecting the numerical integration error is the sampling interval. For sufficiently small sampling interval, this error usually becomes negligible for all practical purposes.

7.3.7. General Error Management

In the previous sections we studied the several kinds of estimation error using CSRS for nonlinear system identification with the crosscorrelation technique. In this section, we will discuss the optimum strategy that ought to be followed in practical applications to achieve the highest possible accuracy in kernel estimates. We diagnosed the following errors:

(1) the deconvolution error (θ error)
(2) the statistical fluctuation error (ε error)
(3) the approximate orthogonality error due to the finite stimulus bandwidth (ξ error)
(4) the approximate orthogonality error due to the finite record length (ζ error)
(5) the erroneous power level error (π error)
(6) the finite transition time error
(7) the continuous signal discretization error
(8) the discrete integration numerical error

From these categories of error, some can be neglected as insignificant in practical applications, some can be corrected, and the rest, which cannot be either corrected or neglected, can be optimized with respect to the controllable test parameters.

Evidently, some errors can be neglected only if the controllable test parameters attain values within a proper range. More specifically we have the following:

(a) The discrete integration error can be neglected if the specified sampling interval Dt is sufficiently small.

(b) The discretization error can be neglected if Dt is smaller than $1/2B$, where B is the bandwidth of the input signal.

(c) The finite transition time error is similar to the erroneous power level error. This error can be corrected to a great extent (provided that the transitions are reversible) by computing the actual power levels corresponding to the imperfect experimental stimulus signal.

(d) The erroneous power level error, in those cases where it occurs, can be largely corrected by employing a final scaling procedure.

(e) The approximate orthogonality error due to finite record length can usually be neglected if the record length is reasonably long.

(f) The approximate orthogonality error due to the finite stimulus bandwidth can be either corrected, on the basis of the analysis made previously, or neglected, if the step length Δt is sufficiently small.

(g) The statistical fluctuation error (ε error) as well as the deconvolution error (θ error) can neither be neglected (in most cases) nor satisfactorily corrected. The θ error can be somewhat corrected by estimating the even-order derivatives of the kernels from the original kernel estimates. However, a short preliminary study of the numerical problems involved pointed to the limited efficiency of this correctional procedure. The ε error can be corrected somewhat by averaging several sample kernel estimates, but again the efficiency of this procedure is low.

Optimization of the controllable test parameters Δt and T, which influence the ε and θ errors, becomes the principal concern of error management in the case of the CSRS.

7.3.8. Minimization of the Deconvolution and Statistical Fluctuation Errors—The Fundamental Error Equation

As discussed before, the θ error is deterministic in nature and is due to the finite stimulus bandwidth. It amounts to some loss of high frequencies in the kernel estimates.

An explicit expression of this error for the nth-order kernel estimate is (the initial region is omitted)

$$\theta_n(\sigma_1, \ldots, \sigma_n) = \Delta t^2 D_{h_n}(\Delta t, \sigma_1, \ldots, \sigma_n) \tag{7.157}$$

where

$$D_{h_n}(\Delta t, \sigma_1, \ldots, \sigma_n) = \sum_{m=1}^{\infty} \frac{\Delta t^{2m-2}}{2m!} \sum_{j_1,\ldots,j_m=1}^{n} C_m(j_1, \ldots, j_m) \frac{\partial^{2m} h_n(\sigma_1, \ldots, \sigma_n)}{\partial \sigma_{j_1}^2 \cdots \partial \sigma_{j_m}^2} \tag{7.158}$$

Clearly, D_{h_n} depends very little on Δt, since Δt attains in practice fairly small values, and consequently

$$D_{h_n}(\sigma_1, \ldots, \sigma_n) \cong \frac{1}{12} \sum_{j_1=1}^{n} \frac{\partial^2 h_n(\sigma_1, \ldots, \sigma_n)}{\partial \sigma_{j_1}^2} \tag{7.159}$$

Thus, the θ_n error depends, in first approximation, on Δt^2 and the second partial derivatives of the kernel h_n.

On the other hand, as discussed before, the ε error is random in nature and is due to the finite record length. It amounts to random deviations of the kernel estimates, according to a Gaussian probability law. The first two moments of the Gaussian distribution of these deviations at the nodal points of the nth-order kernel are

$$E[\varepsilon_n(\sigma_1, \ldots, \sigma_n)] = 0 \tag{7.160}$$

$$\text{Var}\,[\varepsilon_n(\sigma_1, \ldots, \sigma_n)] = q_n^2(\sigma_1, \ldots, \sigma_n) = \frac{1}{T \Delta t^{n-1}} C_{h_n}^2(\Delta t, \sigma_1, \ldots, \sigma_n) \tag{7.161}$$

Again, it must be emphasized that $C_{h_n}^2$ depends very slightly on Δt, for Δt in the range of values of practical interest ($\Delta t \ll \mu_n$).

Summing up these two errors in practical applications of the CSRS:

$$\delta_n(\sigma_1, \ldots, \sigma_n) = \theta_n(\sigma_1, \ldots, \sigma_n) + \varepsilon_n(\sigma_1, \ldots, \sigma_n) \qquad (7.162)$$

Clearly, the total error δ_n is a Gaussian random variable with

$$E[\![\delta_n(\sigma_1, \ldots, \sigma_n)]\!] = \theta_n(\sigma_1, \ldots, \sigma_n) \qquad (7.163)$$

$$\mathrm{Var}\,[\![\delta_n(\sigma_1, \ldots, \sigma_n)]\!] = q_n^2(\sigma_1, \ldots, \sigma_n) \qquad (7.164)$$

Consequently, the mean-square error of the nth-order kernel estimate is

$$
\begin{aligned}
Q_n &= \int_0^{\mu_n} \cdots \int_0^{\mu_n} E[\![\delta_n^2(\sigma_1, \ldots, \sigma_n)]\!]\, d\sigma_1 \cdots d\sigma_n \\
&= \int_0^{\mu_n} \cdots \int_0^{\mu_n} \theta_n^2(\sigma_1, \ldots, \sigma_n)\, d\sigma_1 \cdots d\sigma_n \\
&\quad + \int_0^{\mu_n} \cdots \int_0^{\mu_n} q_n^2(\sigma_1, \ldots, \sigma_n)\, d\sigma_1 \cdots d\sigma_n \\
&= \Delta t^4 \int_0^{\mu_n} \cdots \int_0^{\mu_n} D_{h_n}^2(\Delta t, \sigma_1, \ldots, \sigma_n)\, d\sigma_1 \cdots d\sigma_n \\
&\quad + \frac{1}{T\Delta t^{n-1}} \int_0^{\mu_n} \cdots \int_0^{\mu_n} C_{h_n}^2(\Delta t, \sigma_1, \ldots, \sigma_n)\, d\sigma_1 \cdots d\sigma_n \\
&= A_n(\Delta t)\Delta t^4 + \frac{B_n(\Delta t)}{T\Delta t^{n-1}} \qquad (7.165)
\end{aligned}
$$

In applications, Δt is always much smaller than the kernel memory, and for this range of values A_n and B_n become approximately independent of Δt. Thus

$$Q_n \cong A_n \Delta t^4 + \frac{B_n}{T\Delta t^{n-1}} \qquad (7.166)$$

This equation will be called the "fundamental error equation" (FEE), and it constitutes the principal instrument of the optimization procedure for Δt and T. Notice that A_n and B_n depend on the specific kernel.

The function Q_n described by the FEE always has a single minimum for A_n and B_n positive (which is actually the case) and for a given T (Fig. 7.32). This single minimum is the optimum test position, corresponding to the optimum Δt (for a given T).

The value of the optimum Δt can be easily determined analytically from FEE:

$$(\Delta t_{opt})_n = \left[\frac{(n-1)B_n}{4TA_n}\right]^{1/(n+3)} \qquad (7.167)$$

and the resulting optimum MSE is

$$(Q_{opt})_n = \frac{(n+3)}{(n-1)} A_n^{(n-1)/(n+3)} \left[\frac{(n-1)B_n}{4T} \right]^{4/(n+3)} \tag{7.168}$$

Of course, these expressions are accurate only if the optimum Δt is in the neighborhood of very small Δt, where A_n and B_n can be considered approximately independent of Δt. Otherwise, the optimum Δt results as the solution in Δt of the equation

$$\Delta t^{n+4} \frac{dA_n}{d\Delta t} + \frac{\Delta t}{T} \frac{dB_n}{d\Delta t} + 4\Delta t^{n+3} A_n - \frac{(n-1)}{T} B_n = 0 \qquad (\Delta t \neq 0) \tag{7.169}$$

It is evident from Eqs. (7.167) and (7.168) that the optimum Δt and the corresponding Q_n are monotonically decreasing as T increases (Fig. 7.33). The continuous curve in Fig. 7.33 is the locus of the points $[(\Delta t_{opt})_n, (Q_{opt})_n]$. It is likely that the optimum Δt increases with higher-order kernels.

In the first-order kernel case, the optimum Δt, as determined by Eq. (7.167) is zero, which, of course, is not a realistic value. Therefore Δt is determined in the first-order case by signal-to-noise ratio considerations.

The power level of any CSRS diminishes as Δt goes to zero; therefore in cases where seriously contaminating external noise is present, the optimum Δt is determined as the minimum Δt for which the stimulus power level assures an acceptable signal-to-noise ratio in the response of the system.

Thus, we see that in some cases factors relating to characteristics of the experiment also participate in the determination of the optimum test parameters. One of the most important of these factors is external noise,

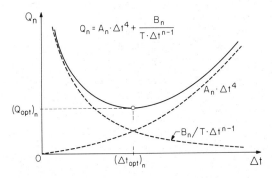

Fig. 7.32. Graphic representation of the fundamental error equation (FEE). [From Marmarelis, V.Z. (1977). *Biol. Cyb.* **27**, 49–56 by permission].

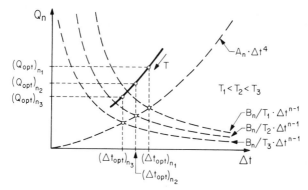

Fig. 7.33. Dependence of the optimum test position on the record length T (drawing for $n = 5$).

and in many applications it is a serious source of error in kernel estimation. The effect of external noise will be discussed in the following section.

We illustrate the form of the FEE in the case of identification of a computer-simulated nonlinear system. Consider a cascade system consisting of a linear subsystem followed by a second-degree polynomial zero-memory nonlinearity. Our intention is to compute the mean-square error of the CSRS kernel estimate as a function of the test parameters Δt and T, and verify the analytical relation described by the FEE.

In this example, the system has up to second-order nonlinearities. Therefore, the MSE of the zero-, first-, and second-order kernel estimates must be used to determine the optimum test parameters. In fact, the optimization procedure takes, in practice, the form of determining the optimum Δt for a given T.

There are two distinct ways this can be done. First, one can determine the optimum Δt by using the total estimation error for all the kernels. The second is to determine a different optimum Δt for each individual kernel estimate by using only the corresponding estimation error. It must be emphasized that in the second case (where we use stimuli with different Δt to estimate each one of the kernels) the operational ranges of the several stimuli must be adjusted in such a way that the power levels of all these stimuli are the same, so that they can be used compatibly in the same model.

In Fig. 7.34, we show the results obtained by computer simulation of this system, using ternary equirandom CSRS stimuli with several different record lengths ($T = 500$, 1000, and 2000 sec) and step lengths ($\Delta t = 0.15$, 0.30, 0.45, and 0.60 sec). The FEE curves for the zero-, first-, and second-order kernel estimates are shown along with the curve corresponding to the total estimation error. The total estimation error is computed as the

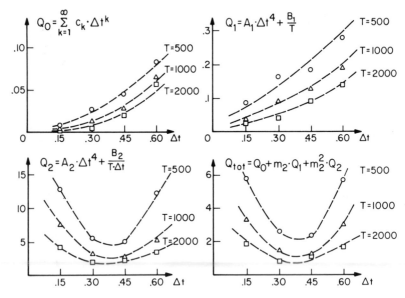

Fig. 7.34. Illustration of FEE curves.

weighted sum of the errors corresponding to the individual kernels:

$$Q_{tot} = Q_0 + m_2 Q_1 + m_2^2 Q_2 \tag{7.170}$$

where m_2 is the second moment of the CSRS stimulus.

The data points corresponding to record lengths of 500 sec are computed as averages from eight independent kernel estimates. The data points corresponding to record lengths of 1000 and 2000 sec are computed as averages from six and four independent kernel estimates, respectively. This is justified on the basis of the fact that the statistical variation of the kernel estimates decreases as the corresponding stimulus record length increases.

7.4. Errors Due to the Presence of Contaminating Noise

Biological signals are plagued with a high noise content. The presence of such noise affects the estimation of the system kernels. We consider the case of such additive noise (at the input, output, or internally) as shown in Fig. 7.35. In practice, of course, the several noise sources coexist. To simplify the present analysis, we examine the effect of each one separately, assuming at each stage that the other error sources do not exist.

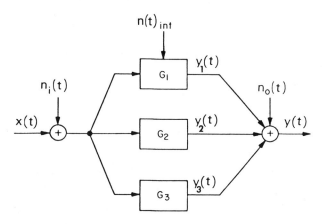

Fig. 7.35. System with input, output, and internal noise.

7.4.1. Noise at the Output

Consider the case of noise $\varepsilon(t)$ which is added to the output. We assume $x(t)$ is ideal Gaussian white noise with $\phi_{xx}(\tau) = P\delta(\tau)$. To estimate $h_1(\tau)$ we need to estimate $\phi_{yx}(\tau)$:

$$\hat{\phi}_{yx}(\tau) = E[x(t-\tau)[y_1(t) + y_2(t) + y_3(t) + \varepsilon(t)]] \tag{7.171}$$

where y_1, y_2, y_3 are the outputs of the linear, quadratic, and cubic terms, due to G_1, G_2, G_3, respectively, as shown in Fig. 7.35 (cf. Sec. 4.2.2).

Terms $y_2(t)$, $y_3(t)$ are, by construction, orthogonal to any functional of the first degree, such as $x(t-\tau)$, and thus Eq. (7.171) becomes

$$\hat{\phi}_{yx}(\tau) = E\left[x(t-\tau)\int_0^\infty h_1(\lambda)x(t-\lambda)\,d\lambda\right] + \phi_{x\varepsilon}(\tau)$$

$$= \int_0^\infty h_1(\lambda)\phi_{xx}(\tau-\lambda)\,d\lambda + \phi_{x\varepsilon}(\tau)$$

$$= Ph_1(\tau) + \phi_{x\varepsilon}(\tau) \tag{7.172}$$

and

$$\hat{h}_1(\tau) = h_1(\tau) + (1/P)\phi_{x\varepsilon}(\tau) \tag{7.173}$$

Thus, the error term due to the presence of corrupting noise is

$$\text{error} = (1/P)\phi_{x\varepsilon}(\tau) \tag{7.174}$$

i.e., proportional to $\phi_{x\varepsilon}(\tau)$ and, as expected, inversely proportional to the power level P of the stimulus signal. If $x(t)$ and $\varepsilon(t)$ are independent, then

$$\phi_{x\varepsilon}(\tau) = E[x(t-\tau)]E[\varepsilon(t)] = 0 \tag{7.175}$$

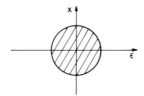

Fig. 7.36. Joint probability density of $x(t)$ and $\epsilon(t)$.

and the kernel estimate is unaffected by the presence of noise. Actually, the requirement of independence of $x(t)$ and $\varepsilon(t)$ is too strong since $\phi_{x\varepsilon}(\tau)$ will be zero (or very small) even in many cases where $x(t)$ and $\varepsilon(t)$ are dependent. For example, consider x and ε to have joint probability density distribution that is uniform over a circle with center at $x = 0$, $\varepsilon = 0$ (Fig. 7.36). Then, x and ε are dependent but uncorrelated, i.e., $\phi_{x\varepsilon}(\tau) = 0$. It is easily seen that the same result holds for dependent x and ε satisfying certain simple conditions.

What is the effect of record length R on this noise-induced error? Assuming that $\varepsilon(t)$ is a Gaussian process, the variance of the error term is given by

$$\text{Var}\left[\frac{1}{P}\hat{\phi}_{x\varepsilon}(\tau)\right] = \frac{1}{P^2}E[[\hat{\phi}_{x\varepsilon}(\tau) - \phi_{x\varepsilon}(\tau)]^2]$$

$$\cong \frac{1}{P^2}\frac{1}{R}\int_{-\infty}^{\infty}[\phi_{xx}(\lambda)\phi_{\varepsilon\varepsilon}(\lambda) + \phi_{x\varepsilon}(\tau + \lambda)\phi_{x\varepsilon}(\tau - \lambda)]\,d\lambda$$

$$(7.176)$$

And if $x(t)$ and $\varepsilon(t)$ are independent or simply uncorrelated, then

$$\text{Var}\left[\frac{1}{P}\hat{\phi}_{x\varepsilon}(\tau)\right] \cong \frac{1}{P^2}\frac{1}{R}\int_{-\infty}^{\infty}\phi_{xx}(\lambda)\phi_{\varepsilon\varepsilon}(\lambda)\,d\lambda \qquad (7.177)$$

In either case, the rms error varies with $1/R^{1/2}$, i.e., inversely with the square root of the record length. Figure 7.37 shows kernel estimates of a linear system whose output is corrupted by broadband noise, for various record lengths R.

Next, we consider noise $\varepsilon(t)$ that has a power spectrum

$$\Phi_{\varepsilon\varepsilon}(\omega) = \begin{cases} P_{\varepsilon}, & |\omega| \leq \omega_{\varepsilon} \\ 0, & |\omega| > \omega_{\varepsilon} \end{cases} \qquad (7.178)$$

and that the band-limited Gaussian white-noise stimulus has a spectrum

$$\Phi_{xx}(\omega) = \begin{cases} P, & |\omega| \leq \omega_x \\ 0, & |\omega| > \omega_x \end{cases} \qquad (7.179)$$

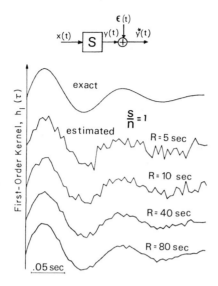

Fig. 7.37. First-order kernel estimates for various record lengths and output signal-to-noise ratio of 1.

Then it can be shown that, for uncorrelated $x(t)$ and $\varepsilon(t)$, Eq. (7.177) becomes approximately

$$\text{Var}\left[\!\!\left[\frac{1}{P}\hat{\phi}_{x\varepsilon}(\tau)\right]\!\!\right]\cong\frac{P_{\varepsilon}\min\{\omega_{\varepsilon},\,\omega_{x}\}}{\pi RP}\tag{7.180}$$

From this we see that the mean-square error is inversely proportional to the signal-to-noise ratio P/P_{ε}.

Similar expressions can be calculated if the noise has a different spectrum. For example, if the noise is low-pass filtered with power spectrum

$$\Phi_{\varepsilon\varepsilon}(\omega)=\frac{P_{\varepsilon}\alpha^{2}}{\alpha^{2}+\omega^{2}}\tag{7.181}$$

and therefore, autocorrelation

$$\phi_{\varepsilon\varepsilon}(\tau)=\frac{P_{\varepsilon}\alpha}{2}\,e^{-\alpha|\tau|}\tag{7.182}$$

we have

$$\text{Var}\left[\!\!\left[\frac{1}{P}\hat{\phi}_{x\varepsilon}(\tau)\right]\!\!\right]=\frac{1}{P^{2}}\frac{1}{R}2\int_{0}^{\infty}P\frac{\omega_{x}}{\pi}\frac{\sin\omega_{x}\lambda}{\omega_{x}\lambda}\frac{P_{\varepsilon}\alpha}{2}e^{-\alpha\lambda}\,d\lambda$$

$$=\frac{P_{\varepsilon}\alpha}{\pi PR}\tan^{-1}\left(\frac{\omega_{x}}{\alpha}\right)\tag{7.183}$$

again showing the dependence on the signal-to-noise ratio P/P_{ε}.

Figure 7.38 shows the first-order kernel estimates of a linear system, for several values of the signal-to-noise ratio and record length.

The derived expressions for the first-order kernel estimate can be extended to higher-order kernel cases. Thus, the nth-order kernel estimate is

$$\hat{h}_n(\tau_1, \ldots, \tau_n) = h_n(\tau_1, \ldots, \tau_n) + \frac{1}{n!P^n}\phi_{x\cdots x\varepsilon}(\tau_1, \ldots, \tau_n) \quad (7.184)$$

where $\phi_{x\cdots x\varepsilon}(\tau_1, \ldots, \tau_n)$ denotes the nth-order crosscorrelation between $x(t)$ and $\varepsilon(t)$. If signal $x(t)$ and noise $\varepsilon(t)$ are uncorrelated then the error becomes

$$\text{error} = \frac{1}{n!P^n}E[x(t-\tau_1)\cdots x(t-\tau_n)]E[\varepsilon(t)] \quad (7.185)$$

which is zero whenever $\varepsilon(t)$ has zero average or n is odd. Thus, we conclude that the determination of the system transfer characteristic by the white-noise method using crosscorrelation alleviates greatly the problem of response contamination by noise because of the smoothing effect (averaging) of the crosscorrelating procedure.

Figure 7.39 shows second-order (nonlinear) kernel estimates for a system whose output is contaminated by additive broadband noise. These estimates are shown for various record lengths R.

7.4.2. Internal Noise

A similar analysis can be made if noise internal to the system is present. For example, suppose noise contaminates the response after it passes through a linear filter with impulse response $g(\tau)$. Then

$$y(t) = \int_0^\infty h_1(\tau)x(t-\tau)\,d\tau + \int_0^\infty g(\tau)\varepsilon(t-\tau)\,d\tau$$

$$+ \iint_0^\infty h_2(\tau_1, \tau_2)x(t-\tau_1)x(t-\tau_2)\,d\tau_1\,d\tau_2 + \cdots \quad (7.186)$$

which means that the noise $\varepsilon(t)$ possibly follows a different course through the system than the input, in contaminating the output $y(t)$. We assume this to be a linear path. However, similar results are obtained if this path is nonlinear. We have

$$\hat{\phi}_{yx}(\tau) = E\left[x(t-\tau)\left[\int_0^\infty h_1(\lambda)x(t-\lambda)\,d\lambda + \int_0^\infty g(\lambda)\varepsilon(t-\lambda)\,d\lambda + \cdots\right]\right]$$

$$= Ph_1(\tau) + P\int_0^\infty g(\lambda)\phi_{x\varepsilon}(\tau-\lambda)\,d\lambda \quad (7.187)$$

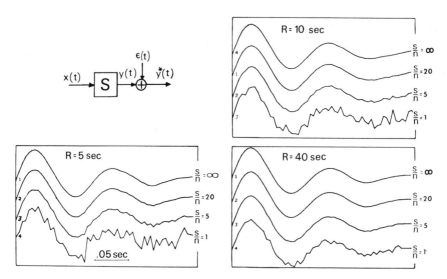

Fig. 7.38. First-order kernel estimates for various output signal-to-noise ratios and various record lengths.

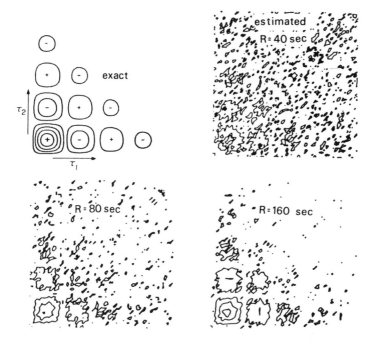

Fig. 7.39. Second-order kernel estimates for various record lengths and output signal-to-noise ratio of 1.

If $x(t)$ and $\varepsilon(t)$ are uncorrelated, then the error is zero. Otherwise, the error in the kernel estimate for any τ is given by

$$\text{error} = \frac{1}{P} \int_0^\infty g(\lambda)\phi_{x\varepsilon}(\tau - \lambda)\, d\lambda \tag{7.188}$$

In the case that the internal path followed by the noise $\varepsilon(t)$ is nonlinear with kernels $g_1(\tau)$ and $g_2(\tau_1, \tau_2)$ we find the error in the first-order kernel estimate is

$$\text{error} = \frac{1}{P} \int_0^\infty g_1(\lambda)\phi_{x\varepsilon}(\tau - \lambda)\, d\lambda$$

$$+ \frac{1}{P} \iint_0^\infty g_2(\lambda_1, \lambda_2)\phi_{x\varepsilon\varepsilon}(\tau - \lambda_1, \tau - \lambda_2)\, d\lambda_1\, d\lambda_2 \tag{7.189}$$

Assuming a linear path for the noise we obtain for the higher-order kernels

$$\hat{h}_n(\tau_1, \ldots, \tau_n) = h_n(\tau_1, \ldots, \tau_n) + \frac{1}{n!P^n} \int_0^\infty g(\lambda)\phi_{x\cdots x\varepsilon}(\tau_1 - \lambda, \ldots, \tau_n - \lambda)\, d\lambda \tag{7.190}$$

Therefore conclusions can be reached similar to those for the output noise case: The kernel estimates are unaffected by the presence of internal noise provided that $\phi_{x\cdots x\varepsilon}(\tau_1, \ldots, \tau_n)$ is zero, a condition easily satisfied in practice. For example, this condition is satisfied if $x(t)$ and $\varepsilon(t)$ are independent and n is odd or, in case of even n, if $E\{\varepsilon(t)\} = 0$. This again represents a great advantage in the study of internal-noise-plagued physiological systems.

7.4.3. Noise at the Input

The presence of noise at the input is, in general, the most disadvantageous situation of data contamination encountered in the white-noise method. Sources of noise at the input include extraneous factors that participate in the stimulation of the system, deviations of the actual test signal that is generated by the input transducer (e.g., truncation and skewness of the amplitude Gaussian distribution, spectrum distortion due to finite rise time of the transducer, etc.) and input measurement errors.

The several types of noise at the input can be classified into two categories. One category comprises the cases where the contaminating noise at the input goes through the system (see Fig. 7.40A). The other category comprises the case of measurement errors, in which the

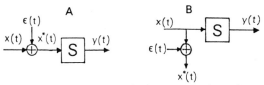

Fig. 7.40. Two cases of input contaminating noise.

contaminating noise does not go through the system (see Fig. 7.40B). We see below that the first category of contaminating noise is usually more hazardous.

To demonstrate the effect of input contaminating noise, consider a second-order nonlinear system described by the input–output relation:

$$y(t) = \int_0^\infty k_1(\tau)x(t-\tau)\,d\tau + \int\int_0^\infty k_2(\tau_1, \tau_2)x(t-\tau_1)x(t-\tau_2)\,d\tau_1\,d\tau_2 \quad (7.191)$$

The first-order kernel estimate in the case shown in Fig. 7.40A is

$$\hat{k}_1(\lambda) = \frac{1}{P}E[\![y(t)x(t-\lambda)]\!]$$

$$= k_1(\lambda) + \frac{1}{P}\int_0^\infty k_1(\tau)\phi_{x\varepsilon}(\lambda-\tau)\,d\tau$$

$$+ \frac{2}{P}\int\int_0^\infty k_2(\tau_1, \tau_2)\phi_{xx\varepsilon}(\lambda-\tau_1, \lambda-\tau_2)\,d\tau_1\,d\tau_2$$

$$+ \frac{1}{P}\int\int_0^\infty k_2(\tau_1, \tau_2)\phi_{x\varepsilon\varepsilon}(\lambda-\tau_1, \lambda-\tau_2)\,d\tau_1\,d\tau_2 \quad (7.192)$$

If $x(t)$ and $\varepsilon(t)$ are statistically independent and $\varepsilon(t)$ has a zero average, then all the error terms above vanish. Notice, however, that this is not true in the general case of a nonlinear system of order higher than 2. In that general case, the error terms that involve crosscorrelation functions of an even number of x's and ε's are preserved, despite the independence of $x(t)$ and $\varepsilon(t)$. Note that the number of error terms increases rapidly with the order of the computed kernel and with the order of nonlinearity of the system. This should be contrasted with the case of errors at the output that, as seen previously, do not increase with increasing order of the kernel or the order of nonlinearity. It should also be contrasted with "measurement" noise at the input, where the number of error terms increases only linearly with the number of nonlinear kernels present.

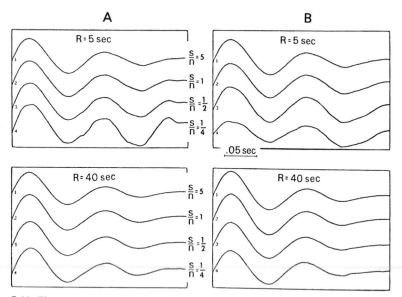

Fig. 7.41. First-order kernel estimates for various input signal-to-noise ratios and various record lengths for both cases A and B of Fig. 7.40.

The first-order kernel estimate in the case shown in Fig. 7.40B is

$$\hat{k}_1(\lambda) = \frac{1}{P} E[\![y(t)x^*(t-\lambda)]\!]$$

$$= k_1(\lambda) + \frac{1}{P} \int_0^\infty k_1(\tau)\phi_{x\varepsilon}(\lambda - \tau)\, d\tau$$

$$+ \frac{1}{P} \int\!\!\int_0^\infty k_2(\tau_1, \tau_2)\phi_{xx\varepsilon}(\lambda - \tau_1, \lambda - \tau_2)\, d\tau_1\, d\tau_2 \qquad (7.193)$$

Clearly, all the error terms vanish in this case (and for any system) provided that $x(t)$ and $\varepsilon(t)$ are statistically independent and $\varepsilon(t)$ has a zero average.

Comparison of Eqs. (7.192) and (7.193) demonstrates the relative severity of cases A and B of Fig. 7.40. Figure 7.41 shows first-order kernel estimates for various signal-to-noise ratios and record lengths in those two cases.

8

Tests and Analyses Preliminary to Identification Experiment

Introduction

Like most types of analysis, the application of the white-noise method for the characterization of a physiological system can become very difficult and involved if not preceded by considerable preliminary analysis of the system characteristics and the tools available for its study. In addition, the amount of difficulty depends on the nature of the system nonlinearities and the degree of accuracy which we require from the derived characterization (model). In certain cases the application of the method to a physiological system could produce poor results after long experimental procedures and digital computations. Therefore, it is desirable to develop preliminary criteria and simple experiments and tests that give an indication of how complex the system is and how successful the white-noise method will be in each particular case.

In developing these criteria and tests we shall take into account the characteristics of the system and the experimental limitations inherent in its study by stimulus–response experiments. This is especially important in the study of such physiological systems for which the measurement—and even the choice—of input and output is a difficult task (e.g., neural systems).

First, therefore, the inputs and outputs of a physiological system must be clearly defined and it must be shown that no other known inputs affect the system to a great extent. Of course, in practice, we know only a small number of the inputs to a system and we assume that all the other inputs have little effect on the response, justifiably clustering all the latter under the classification of "unwanted noise."

Second, the experimental conditions under which the system is stationary must be clearly established, since the method in its present form is applicable only to stationary systems.

Third, the nature of the contaminating noise must be determined in order to be able to smooth the stimulus–response data appropriately before processing them.

Fourth, we must choose the dynamic amplitude range of the white-noise signal to be used in the experiment. Often, physiological systems are sensitive over very large dynamic ranges of the stimulus amplitude (3–5 log units of sensitivity are rather common for sensory systems). Since stimuli produced in the laboratory have a much smaller dynamic range (usually at most 2 log units) the region of operation of the system must be carefully selected. More than one identifying experiment, covering different portions of the system operational range, are then necessary to identify the system completely.

Fifth, the memory of the system (settling time) must be measured from preliminary experiments. This information is needed in determining the length of the identifying experiment with regard to an acceptable statistical error and also in determining the time domain over which the kernels must be computed (recall that the computational burden depends drastically on the kernel memory). It should be noted that the memory is in general different for kernels of different order.

Sixth, the bandwidth of the system response must be determined approximately to determine the bandwidth of the stimulus white-noise signal. This, in turn, may place certain demands on the dynamic range of the stimulus signal from the experimental point of view (frequency response capability of the instruments producing the stimulus).

Seventh, the bandwidth of the white-noise input must be chosen. This choice depends on several factors. The white-noise bandwidth should cover the system bandwidth so that the system is exhaustively tested with all frequencies to which it responds. This provides a lower bound to the bandwidth of the white-noise stimulus. The upper bound is determined by statistical considerations, because if the white-noise bandwidth extends too far beyond the system bandwidth, the statistical error in estimating the kernels increases. This choice is also affected by sampling rate and computer storage considerations.

Eighth, the extent of the nonlinearity of the system must be determined. That is, how many and which of the kernels of the Wiener series must be computed. This also determines the degree of the computational complexity of the problem.

Finally, the length of the white-noise experiments should be determined. This depends on several factors such as the system memory, the system nonlinearity, the noise present in the system, experimental conditions, and computational considerations.

Once these parameters are set, the white-noise identification experiment can be performed and the stimulus–response data collected and preprocessed, in preparation for the estimation (computation) of the system kernels. This stage includes the recording of data through proper transductions (converting them from analog to digital forms to be processed by digital computers) and removing the drifts or otherwise reducing any other noise conditions that are present.

In this chapter we outline procedures and suggest methods for making all these decisions for the conduct of the white-noise experiment.

8.1. Determination of the System Input and Output and Region of Operation

Any physiological system, defined as an entity by the investigator, has a large number of inputs and outputs. In practice, however, it is not possible to monitor all these inputs and measure all the outputs. In the study of any system we do not need to know *all* the outputs but we do need to know *all* the inputs that contribute to the response of interest (measured response). However, the monitoring of all inputs is a difficult task in the case of physiological systems. Therefore, we usually monitor *some* of the inputs and assume that the effect of all other inputs on the measured response in question is negligible (and we call it contaminating "noise"). The so-called signal-to-noise ratio of a system is a measure of how important are the inputs that we are monitoring in comparison to the inputs that we neglect, in reference to the response that we are recording. For example, in recording the response of a neuron to a light stimulus we neglect inputs of temperature variation, pressure variation, inputs from endogenous sources, etc. Often, we can perform a preliminary test in determining the effect of the monitored inputs on the response as compared to the effect of the neglected inputs.

Next, we must decide on the dynamic amplitude range of the GWN stimulus. As this range is usually smaller than the total range over which the system responds (ranges of 3–5 log units in amplitude variation are quite common for sensory systems), the amplitude range of the stimulus must be chosen so that it covers the most "interesting" region of operation, often the range encountered in the natural environment of the system. In practice, the dynamic range of the instruments that produce the stimulus rarely exceeds two orders of magnitude. Therefore the choice of the stimulus range must be made very carefully to reveal the interesting properties of the system. Sometimes it will be necessary to perform more than a single white-noise experiment in order to cover the whole operational range of the system.

Let us take an example: The white-noise stimulus signal has a Gaussian distribution of amplitudes, such as that shown in Fig. 8.1. Figure 8.2 shows the response versus stimulus characteristic of a particular neuron. This kind of relationship is quite common for neurosensory systems (vision, audition, etc.). It is the well-known tanh–log relationship for stimulus and

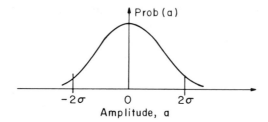

Fig. 8.1. Amplitude distribution of GWN.

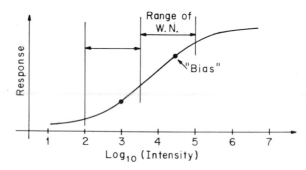

Fig. 8.2. Amplitude range in GWN experimental application.

response. Suppose that the amplitudes of the GWN stimulus signal cover part of this range. A bias point (the average of GWN) is chosen around which the white-noise modulation takes place. We expect that the derived characterization will be valid only within this range of amplitudes of the stimulus signal. However, if the system is analytic outside the stimulus amplitude range, then the characterization obtained can in principle be extended over the whole range of analyticity of the system. Nevertheless, this characterization in terms of estimated Wiener functionals will *not* be best (in the mean-square-error sense) outside the stimulus amplitude range, because the orthogonality of the estimated Wiener functionals holds strictly for that range (as reflected on the GWN power level).

The need for an orthogonal functional expansion becomes critical when we estimate (as is usually the case in practice) a truncated functional series (incomplete system model). Thus, it is advisable that we limit the validity of the estimated model to the stimulus amplitude range. If a functional description of the system outside the specified range is needed, then we have to either extend the amplitude range of the test stimulus or make a separate test with a stimulus amplitude range that is centered around a new bias and covers the adjacent region of interest (see Fig. 8.2). In this latter case, we must be aware of the fact that the set of kernels obtained is, in general, different and characteristic also of the new stimulus bias (cf. Sec. 4.1). This fact is mathematically demonstrated by Eqs. (4.24) and (4.25).

Another matter that needs clarification is related to the length of the white-noise experiment and the lowest frequency for which the system is tested. Of course, the white-noise experiment lasts only for a finite length of time. Therefore, conceivably, the lowest frequency for which we can measure the system response would be $1/T$. In practice, because of noise considerations, we cannot do so well and the lowest frequency that we can measure with accuracy has a period that is about $1/10$ of the total length of the experiment. This is due to the fact that for a limited-length white-noise experiment, the low frequencies are thinly represented. To this must be added uncertainties due to low-frequency nonstationarities (drift).

8.2. Examination of System Stationarity and Noise Conditions

The white-noise method, as presented in Chapter 4, is applicable to stationary systems. Thus, the stationarity of a system must be established before the white-noise method can be used for its identification and analysis.

8.2.1. System Stationarity

A system is stationary if its functional characteristics do not change with time. Since the input white-noise signal is a stationary random process, any system nonstationarities will be reflected as nonstationarities in the system response signal. Visual inspection of the response signal may often reveal the presence of nonstationarities (trends, etc). However, if visual inspection fails to be conclusive, a rigorous and systematic statistical test can be used to test the stability of several statistical measures of the response signal. This statistical test is known as the "run test" and was described in Sec. 5.5. An example of a nonstationary system taken from an actual neurophysiological experiment is given below. Figure 8.3 shows an experiment performed on a catfish retina horizontal cell. The input is light intensity and the output is the potential of the horizontal cell recorded intracellularly. The input and output records are segmented into overlapping segments and the mean and variance for each segment are computed. The results are plotted and shown in Fig. 8.3.

To analyze these data the trend was removed by fitting a least-squares parabola to the response data and subtracting it. Then the system kernels were computed. Notice, however, that the variance of the response also appears to be nonstationary. This signifies that the system dynamic gain is

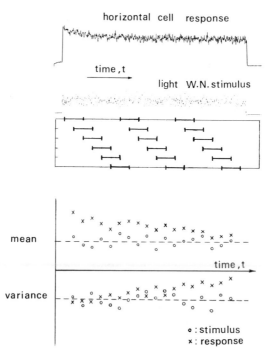

Fig. 8.3. Check on stationarity of the mean and variance of stimulus–response records from the catfish retina. The record is segmented into overlapping pieces and the statistics of each segment are computed.

also nonstationary. Therefore, if the kernels are computed using the entire length of this record, the resulting characterization will be an average characterization taking into account both the high and low gains of the system. These results may also be used as a guide to delete part of the stimulus–response record (e.g., the initial part, in which changes in both the mean and variance occur) and compute the kernels using only the remaining record.

8.2.2. Noise Conditions

The noise conditions in the system must also be examined. As shown in Chapter 7, the kernel estimates are little affected by such noise in most cases. However, if we measure some noise characteristics such as bandwidth and amplitude range, it is possible to improve even further the accuracy of the characterization of the system.

In practice, we usually assume that the noise is additive to the input or output of the system and therefore examine it by holding the system input

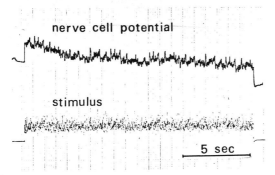

Fig. 8.4. Slow trend in intracellular response potential of a horizontal cell to stationary GWN stimulus.

at zero. Two important aspects of the noise are needed for the analysis: first, the bandwidth and autocorrelation function (power spectrum) of this noise, and second, whether the noise is independent of the white noise stimulus and/or response. The study of these aspects is not a simple task. The stimulus- and response-independent noise is usually ignored not because the noise level is low, but because the crosscorrelation approach to measuring the system kernels greatly alleviates this problem.

8.3. Removal of Drifts in the Response Data

Physiological response data often exhibit slow trends such as those shown in Fig. 8.4. These trends are usually unjustified by the low-frequency components in the stimulus data and therefore must be assumed to be caused by other mechanisms (such as light adaptation, breathing, etc.). Often, it is not easy to remove these components by high-pass filtering. Therefore, certain other drift-removal techniques are needed. It has been found useful to use a least-squares procedure in which the response data are fitted with a low-order polynomial that minimizes the mean-square error and that is subsequently subtracted from these data to produce data that have no mean or trend. This was done for the data of Fig. 8.5A. However, the type of trend shown in Fig. 8.5B is of higher frequency and is best removed by high-pass filtering. We examine both of these procedures here since both arise in applications of the white-noise method.

8.3.1. Trend Removal by Fitting Least-Squares Polynomials

This procedure is used if the period of the unwanted signal (trend) is comparable to or greater than the length of the response record. Therefore, the degree of the polynomial to be fitted is usually 1 (linear), 2

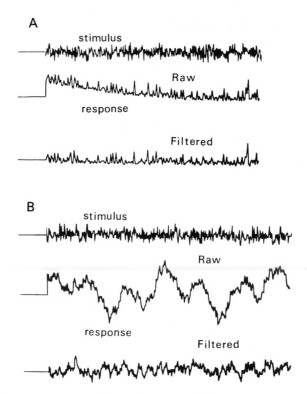

Fig. 8.5. (A) Parabolic type of drift in response data; (B) low-frequency noise in response data.

(parabolic), or 3 (cubic). In applications of the white-noise method to physiological systems a parabolic fit has been found suitable since trends are often of the type shown in Fig. 8.5A. The actual procedure of trend removal using a least-squares deviation criterion was illustrated in Sec. 2.8.

The removal of trends prior to the computation of the system kernels is important. If not done properly, it could result in large errors in the estimation of the system kernels, especially in the low-frequency region. In the above discussion of trend removal from the response the following assumption is implicit: The response is the sum of two components, one being the trend (perhaps the result of a nonstationarity) and the other being the "true" stimulus-dependent system response.

8.3.2. High-Pass Filtering of the Response

High-pass filtering of the response is advisable if the response record has trends of the form shown in Fig. 8.5B. Then, one of the high-pass filters discussed in Sec. 2.8 can be used. We should keep in mind, though, that the estimation of the kernels involves phase information of the response relative to the stimulus. Therefore, a proper digital filter must be used in processing the response, so that little or no phase shift is introduced.

For example, the "raw" response data shown in Fig. 8.5B are filtered by a digital high-pass filter to produce the "filtered" response record shown in the same figure. This filtered response is then used in computing the system kernels. In this particular case, the filter used is of the moving-average type. That is, the filtered record $y^*(t)$ is obtained from the raw data $y(t)$ by the following procedure:

1. Form the low-pass filtered signal samples

$$y_F(k\,\Delta t) = \sum_{i=-m}^{m} a_i y[(k+i)\Delta t] \tag{8.1}$$

i.e., by forming a weighted average of neighboring values of $y(t)$. By choosing these weights to be symmetrical for the past and future y values, no phase shift is introduced.

2. To get the high-pass filtered signal $y^*(t)$ we simply subtract:

$$y^*(t) = y(t) - y_F(t) \tag{8.2}$$

8.4. The Measurement of System Memory and Bandwidth

The extent to which the different kernels must be evaluated, that is the magnitude of $\tau_1, \tau_2, \ldots, \tau_n$ for $h_n(\tau_1, \tau_2, \ldots, \tau_n)$ to be nearly zero, depends only on the memory of the system (settling time). The memory, μ, of the system can be loosely defined as the time required for the effect of the stimulus on the response to become almost zero. That is, if the memory of the system is μ, the stimulus at time $t - \mu$ will have no (or negligible) effect at times $T \geq t$ and on. In general, however, the memory associated with the nth-order kernel may be different from the memory associated with any other kernel. Simple preliminary experiments can be performed to measure the memory of a specific kernel. For instance, in order to measure the second-order kernel memory, the system is stimulated by an impulse at time t and an impulse at time $t + \alpha$; the delay α is increased until the response of the system to the second impulse is identical to the response to the first impulse (Fig. 8.6).

The determined value of α constitutes an upper bound for the memory extent of all kernels of order higher than the first. The same procedure can be repeated with three impulses to obtain an upper bound for the memory extent of all kernels of order higher than the second. Comparing those two bounds we can determine the second-order kernel memory extent.

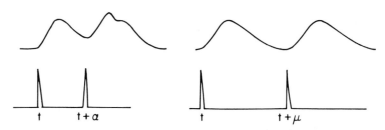

Fig. 8.6. Two-impulse experiment for the measurement of the second-order kernel memory.

These procedures are tedious and time consuming, and thus, in practice, we usually seek merely a single bound for the memory extent of all
kernels. This can be easily attained through the impulse response or the
autocorrelation function of the system response to white noise. Note that in
most cases the memory extent has an arbitrary (conventional) character
since it is determined on the basis of a criterion (convention) that is chosen
by the investigator according to the effect of the estimated kernel upon the
model-predicted response. For this reason the term "effective memory
extent" is appropriate.

To illustrate the concept of the effective memory extent consider the
system shown in Fig. 8.7, consisting of a cascade combination of linear and
nonlinear subsystems. We wish to estimate the system kernels and examine
the extent to which they need to be computed (i.e., determine the effective
memory extent of these kernels). We have

$$v(t) = \frac{1}{\alpha} \int_0^\infty e^{-\nu/\alpha} x(t-\nu) \, d\nu \tag{8.3}$$

$$w(t) = v(t) + cv^2(t) \tag{8.4}$$

$$y(t) = \frac{1}{\beta} \int_0^\infty e^{-\mu/\beta} w(t-\mu) \, d\mu \tag{8.5}$$

After some manipulation of these relations we find that the system
(note that the system is of second order) kernels are given by

$$h_1(\tau) = \frac{1}{\alpha - \beta} (e^{-\tau/\alpha} - e^{-\tau/\beta}) \tag{8.6}$$

$$h_2(\tau_1, \tau_2) = \frac{c}{\alpha(\alpha - 2\beta)} (e^{-(\tau_1+\tau_2)/\alpha} - e^{-|\tau_2-\tau_1|/\alpha - \min\{\tau_1, \tau_2\}/\beta} \tag{8.7}$$

It is easily seen that the decay rate of the first-order kernel is dominated by
α or β, whichever is greater, although, the decay rate of the second-order
kernel is dominated by α since it enters both terms. Notice the big increase

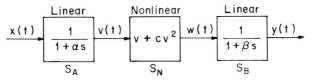

Fig. 8.7. Cascade nonlinear system.

of the values of $h_2(\tau_1, \tau_2)$ as α decreases towards zero. The system configuration of Fig. 8.7 is quite general and we may even think of S_A and S_B as general linear systems.

If $\alpha \gg \beta$ then the effective memory extent of h_1 is determined by the term $e^{-\tau/\alpha}$ and of h_2 by $e^{-(\tau_1+\tau_2)/\alpha}$. We usually compute $h_1(\tau)$ up to a maximum τ of 4α or 5α. Now we consider $h_2(\tau_1, \tau_2)$ and the extent to which each of τ_1 and τ_2 needs to be computed. We note that at any point (τ_1, τ_2) this kernel has decayed as $e^{-(\tau_1+\tau_2)/\alpha}$. Therefore it decays faster than $e^{-\tau/\alpha}$, i.e., h_1, for similar values of τ and τ_1, τ_2. Consequently, the effective memory extent seems to be smaller for h_2 than for h_1 (if the criterion for the memory extent is a measure of the overall kernel magnitude). Therefore, in this case—i.e., $\alpha \gg \beta$—we usually compute h_2 for τ_1, τ_2 up to about 3α. Of course, the h_2 kernel decays fastest along the diagonal $\tau_1 = \tau_2$ (decay constant of $\alpha/2$) and it has a decay rate equal to that of h_1 along the $\tau_1 = 0$ or $\tau_2 = 0$ line (decay constant of α). It should be noticed, however, that in the case of $\beta \gg \alpha$, the effective memory extent of the nonlinear kernel $h_2(\tau_1, \tau_2)$ is determined by the second exponent, the decay rate of which is not faster than the decay rate of h_1—$\exp(-\tau/\beta)$ in this case—but about the same (for similar values of τ and τ_1, τ_2).

In computing the error that results from using a finite effective memory, the integral of the truncated kernel may be the deciding factor, as it is the one that usually enters in the system response calculation. In four time constants, we have for $h_1(\alpha \gg \beta)$, that the area of this truncated kernel is

$$\int_0^{4\alpha} e^{-\tau/\alpha}\, d\tau = \alpha(1 - e^{-4}) = 0.98\alpha \tag{8.8}$$

i.e., 98% of the total area. Because of geometry, to include 98% of the h_2 *volume* we must go up to 4.5 time constants, i.e., max $\{\tau_1\}$, max $\{\tau_2\} = 4.5\alpha$. However, in practice, the deciding factor of the extent to which the kernel is computed is the question *How big* can τ_1, τ_2 be and still be able to estimate $h_2(\tau_1, \tau_2)$ reliably given the noise conditions, length of record, stimulus bandwidth, and system characteristics? Thus, the *amplitude* attenuation of the h_2 kernel becomes, in practice, a more realistic criterion.

In any case, the question of amplitude or integral criterion depends on the type of stimulus that we want to use the model for. For example, if the stimulus is a delta function (impulse), then the response is

$$y(t) = h_1(t) + h_2(t, t) \tag{8.9}$$

Clearly, in this case, it is the amplitude of the kernels that matters and not their integral. The converse is true if the stimulus is a unit step function. The response in that case is

$$y(t) = \int_0^t h_1(\tau) \, d\tau + \int_0^t \int_0^t h_2(\tau_1, \tau_2) \, d\tau_1 \, d\tau_2 \tag{8.10}$$

and the integral of the kernels becomes of importance.

Related to the system memory is the *system bandwidth*. This is a measure of the frequency range within which the system responds significantly. The bandwidth of the system should be estimated by preliminary tests in order to determine the bandwidth of the white-noise stimulus signal to be used for the experiment. This can be done, in a simple and approximate way, by testing the system with sine waves or pulses or, better yet, with broadband white-noise signal. The question may arise: Why not take the system with as large a white-noise bandwidth as possible? It was shown in Sec. 7.1 that the statistical variance of the kernel estimates increases if the white-noise bandwidth extends much beyond the system bandwidth. Of course, on the other hand the white-noise bandwidth should not be too narrow, because then the high-frequency behavior of the system is not identified. A related consideration entering in this picture is that of the sampling *rate* of the input–output records as related to the white-noise bandwidth and aliasing. In turn, the sampling rate has to take into account the computing power available (memory storage, computing speed, etc.).

In a system of more than one input, it is conceivable that the response bandwidth for each input could be quite different. It is also conceivable that these bandwidths are affected by the presence (or not) of the other inputs.

8.5. Measurement of Extent of System Nonlinearity

The next concern in designing a white-noise experiment deals with the question of how many kernels are needed to represent the system accurately. The exact mathematical answer to this question is rather difficult. However, this question in practice can be answered in a simple, approximate, and useful way.

We note from the Volterra series that the nth-order term of the series would produce the nth-order harmonic in addition to several lower harmonics—if a sine wave stimulus were used. This suggests a simple way of determining approximately which kernels are important in a given system by analyzing the harmonic content of the response to sine wave stimuli. In the case of a system with more than one input the possible sums and differences of the frequencies of the inputs must be taken into account. The procedure is straightforward, as in the one-input case. It should be noted, however, that this practical way of measuring the extent of nonlinearity is an approximate one; it provides only a rough index of the size of the kernels of the Volterra series. It should also be noticed that the results depend crucially on the specific frequency of the sinusoidal stimulus. It is possible that certain types of kernels may give misleading indications of their magnitude following this procedure. To illustrate the nature of this index of kernel magnitude we present the following analysis. Consider a second-order nonlinear system described by

$$y(t) = \int_0^\infty h_1(\tau)x(t-\tau)\,d\tau + \int_0^\infty \int_0^\infty h_2(\tau_1, \tau_2)x(t-\tau_1)x(t-\tau_2)\,d\tau_1\,d\tau_2$$

$$(8.11)$$

A stimulus $x(t) = \cos \omega t$ is applied to the system input. The first integral term will give rise to response at frequency ω and the second integral term will produce a harmonic of frequency 2ω plus a constant. Let us examine the size of this second harmonic. We have

$$\int_0^\infty\!\!\int h_2(\tau_1, \tau_2)\cos\left[\omega(t-\tau_1)\right]\cos\left[\omega(t-\tau_2)\right]\,d\tau_1\,d\tau_2$$

$$=\frac{1}{2}\int_0^\infty\!\!\int h_2(\tau_1, \tau_2)\{\cos\left[\omega(2t-\tau_1-\tau_2)\right]+\cos\left[\omega(\tau_1-\tau_2)\right]\}\,d\tau_1\,d\tau_2$$

$$=\frac{1}{2}\int_0^\infty\!\!\int h_2(\tau_1, \tau_2)\cos\left[2\omega t-\omega(\tau_1+\tau_2)\right]\,d\tau_1\,d\tau_2+\text{const} \qquad (8.12)$$

Thus, the second harmonic will be

$$A(\omega)\cos 2\omega t + B(\omega)\sin 2\omega t$$

$$=\frac{1}{2}\int_0^\infty\!\!\int h_2(\tau_1, \tau_2)\sin\left[\omega(\tau_1+\tau_2)\right]\,d\tau_1\,d\tau_2\cos 2\omega t$$

$$+\frac{1}{2}\int_0^\infty\!\!\int h_2(\tau_1, \tau_2)\cos\left[\omega(\tau_1+\tau_2)\right]\,d\tau_1\,d\tau_2\sin 2\omega t \qquad (8.13)$$

Consequently, Fourier analysis of $y(t)$ will give for the amplitude of the second harmonic

$$F_2(\omega) = [A^2(\omega) + B^2(\omega)]^{1/2} \tag{8.14}$$

Let us see how $A(\omega)$ and $B(\omega)$ are related to $h_2(\tau_1, \tau_2)$. We have

$$A(\omega) = \frac{1}{2} \int\!\!\int_0^\infty h_2(\tau_1, \tau_2) \sin\left[\omega(\tau_1 + \tau_2)\right] d\tau_1 \, d\tau_2$$

$$= \frac{1}{2} \int_0^\infty g_2(\sigma) \sin \omega\sigma \, d\sigma \tag{8.15}$$

where

$$g_2(\sigma) = \int_0^\infty h_2(\tau_1, \sigma - \tau_1) \, d\tau_1 \tag{8.16}$$

Similarly,

$$B(\omega) = \frac{1}{2} \int_0^\infty g_2(\sigma) \cos \omega\sigma \, d\sigma \tag{8.17}$$

Therefore, we see that $F_2(\omega)$ is actually the magnitude of the Fourier transform of the function $g_2(\sigma)$ at the frequency ω; and $g_2(\sigma)$ is nothing else but the accumulated (integrated) values of $h_2(\tau_1, \tau_2)$ over the lines $\tau_1 + \tau_2 = \sigma$, as shown in Fig. 8.8.

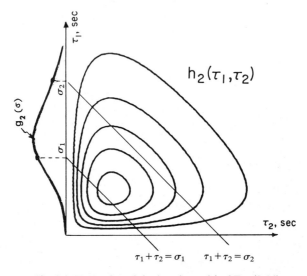

Fig. 8.8. Evaluation of the function $g_2(\sigma)$ of Eq. (8.16).

From this analysis it becomes obvious that $g_2(\sigma)$ is a *rough* index of the magnitude of $h_2(\tau_1, \tau_2)$. Alternate negative and positive values of $h_2(\tau_1, \tau_2)$ on the line of integration $\tau_1 + \tau_2 = \sigma$ would cancel out and the resulting value of $g_2(\sigma)$ could be a misleading description of $h_2(\tau_1, \tau_2)$. However, greatly misleading results would be obtained if this cancellation occurred for all σ—an unlikely situation in most cases.

Examples of Certain Physiological Systems. We present here examples from actual physiological applications—i.e., how the extent of nonlinearity is assessed and the decision on the number of kernels to be estimated is made. These are systems with distinctly different nonlinearities.

In the first example, the system under study is a retinal neuron chain (in catfish) whose input is light intensity, uniformly distributed in space and modulated by a GWN signal. The output is the resulting potential of the horizontal cell recorded intracellularly. Several sine wave stimuli of different frequencies are presented and the corresponding response is recorded. We show these in Fig. 8.9(A). The responses exhibit a distinct asymmetric characteristic of slow-on fast-off changes. These are a good example of unidirectional rate sensitivity. Let α denote the fraction of the response cycle during which there is increase within the cycle (therefore $1 - \alpha$ is the portion of the cycle during which the response decreases). Fourier analysis of these responses shows that the normalized harmonic content is given by

$$A_n = (1/n^2) \sin n\pi\alpha \qquad (8.18)$$

where A_n is the normalized coefficient of the nth harmonic. The following are the amplitude values for the first five harmonics with the amplitude of the fundamental frequency normalized to unity and $\alpha = \frac{3}{4}$:

n	1	2	3	4	5
A_n	1	0.35	0.11	0	0.04

If $\alpha = \frac{2}{3}$ then $A_3 = 0$. From the results of the experiments α appears to be between $\frac{2}{3}$ and $\frac{3}{4}$. Therefore, from this preliminary analysis we note that we only need to compute up to the third-order kernel in order to get a satisfactory model (in fact, the h_3 kernel would be very small or nearly zero if $\alpha = \frac{2}{3}$).

In the second example, again from retinal experiments, the stimulus is modulated light intensity and the response is the recorded electroretinogram (ERG). Figure 8.9(B) shows some typical response waveforms. It is obvious that the system is nonlinear since the response to sine wave stimulation is quite distorted; specifically, it exhibits a strong second harmonic distortion, which is most pronounced when the stimulus is in the range of 5–12 Hz. This distortion is substantially smaller for the lower

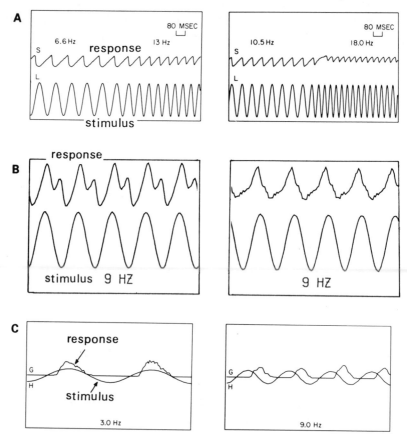

Fig. 8.9. Sinusoidal responses of system (A) light → horizontal cell, (B) light → ERG, and (C) horizontal cell → ganglion cell.

amplitudes of stimulation (right frame of Fig. 8.9(B)]. Fourier analysis of this waveform gives the following normalized results:

n	1	2	3	4	5
A_n	1	0.6	0.1	0.02	0.01

We conclude that we only need to compute the linear and second-order nonlinear kernels, h_1 and h_2, in order to obtain an accurate characterization of this system.

A third example is also taken from experiments on the catfish retina. The system input in this case is current injected intracellularly into a horizontal cell and the output is the response of a ganglion cell recorded extracellularly. It is noted from Fig. 8.9(C) that the response is half-wave rectified for most of these frequencies. Harmonic analysis of these responses reveals the harmonic content shown below:

n	1	2	3	4	5
A_n	1	0.22	0.10	0.05	0.002

We note that most of the signal energy, in fact 90% of it, is in the first two harmonics. Thus, we only need to compute h_1 and h_2 in order to obtain an accurate description of the system dynamics.

The final example is taken from the visual nervous system of the fly, from an experiment with two inputs and one output. The system has two inputs, each one a source of light modulated by independent GWN signals. The response is the spike frequency recorded from a motion-sensitive ganglion cell in the fly optic lobe. It is suggested that the two lights, which are placed along the axis of motion detection, simulate motion in one direction or the other, depending on the phase difference of their signals. To estimate the kernels that are important in this system, we excite each one of the two light sources by sine wave stimuli of the same or different frequencies and we record the response, on which we then perform harmonic analysis. Since in this case we can have products of sine waves of different frequencies, the response may contain components that are found at frequencies formed by adding and subtracting the stimuli frequencies. The experimental results are shown in Fig. 8.10. Notice the presence of a strong second harmonic.

8.6. Recording and Digitalization of Stimulus–Response Data

Figure 8.11 outlines the procedures involved in recording the stimulus–response data. The stimulus and response signals are physical quantities that are translated through proper transducers into electrical signals representing these quantities.

For example, consider the eye movement system for which the input is the motion of a visual target and the output is the motion of the eyes trying to track this target. One transducer is needed that translates the motion of the visual target into an electrical signal, and another is needed to translate the motion of the eye into an electrical signal such as shown in Fig. 8.11.

We wish ideally to have this translation of the physical quantity into electrical signal to be accomplished without any distortion or dependence on frequency, that is, as in Fig. 8.11, we wish $x^*(t) = Cx(t)$, where C is a constant, and similarly for $y(t)$ and $y^*(t)$. In practice, we usually assume this. However, the transducer does introduce some distortion depending on amplitude and frequency characteristics of the physical quantity that is being measured. For the proper application of the white-noise method we are, of course, interested in knowing these alterations and distortions introduced by the transducers measuring the stimulus and response signals.

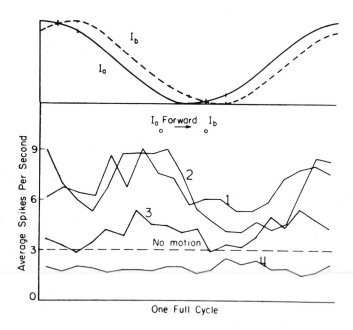

Fig. 8.10. Experimental results from the visual nervous system of the fly, Phaenicia. A two-input, one-output system. Two spots of light (*a* and *b*) are placed along the axis of motion detection and modulated by sine waves having a phase difference of 45°. Curve 1: forward motion, stimulus frequency 0.5 Hz. Curve 2: forward, 1 Hz. Curve 3: forward, 0.2 Hz. Curve 4: reverse, 1 Hz. Forward motion is simulated when the signal at *a* (I_a) is leading in phase (and reverse when it is lagging).

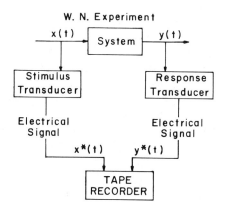

Fig. 8.11. Outline for recording the data on tape.

If they can be determined, then it is often possible to obtain $x(t)$ from a measurement of $x^*(t)$ and therefore to correct for the estimated system kernels at the end of the processing or even before we start processing the data.

The electrical signals produced by the transducers are usually recorded on tape before being transmitted to a digital computer. Sometimes, of course, they could be directly digitalized and transmitted to the computer. Here, an additional transduction of the stimulus–response signals takes place. In the most common form the data are frequency modulated for tape recording. The various errors that occur during tape recording and/or playback are outside the scope of this book, and details can be found in G. L. Davies, 1961. For our purposes here we will note that we are interested in stimulus–response data that are *synchronized*. Therefore, we must take care to minimize any error introduced by the tape recorder that will affect this synchronization. The most disturbing such error is attributable to the variations in the angle at which the tape passes over the recording head. This will clearly affect the analysis of the data (stimulus and response signals recorded on different channels) used in computing the kernels (crosscorrelations). Such problems can be minimized if the data are recorded on adjacent heads. In addition, a clock pulse may be used on the two channels for synchronization purposes. It should also be noted that, in most tape recorders, both the record and playback tracks are divided into two heads. For example, the odd-numbered tracks are on one head and the even-numbered tracks are on the other head. Therefore, to have close synchronization, it is important to record the stimulus and the response data on the same head. Finally, the errors due to the difference in channels depend on the speed of recording and playback, and, in general, greater speed would tend to minimize most of these errors.

After the data have been recorded on tape, they are digitalized and sent to the computer, as shown in Fig. 8.12.

The choice of the sampling interval Δt depends on several considerations: (1) the bandwidth of the white-noise stimulus signal, (2) the highest frequency in the response that is detectable above the noise level, (3) the memory of the system, (4) the computing capacity available, and (5) the highest-order kernel that we are interested in computing.

For example, assume that we want to compute kernels h_1 and h_2. It is usually impractical to compute the $h_2(\tau_1, \tau_2)$ kernels for more than about 100 values (lags) of the arguments τ_1, τ_2. Therefore, if the memory of the system is μ, then the sampling interval Δt should be chosen such that $\mu/\Delta t$ is approximately equal to 100. However, it is possible, in some cases, to digitalize the data at a fine sampling interval and compute the kernels at points that are further apart than this interval Δt—i.e., at points that are integral multiples of Δt.

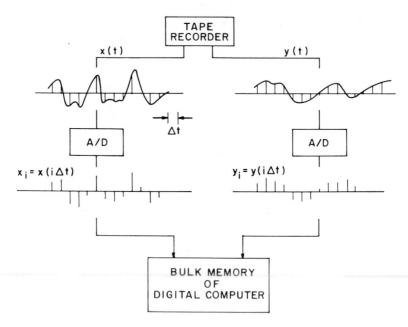

Fig. 8.12. Digitalization and transmission of stimulus–response data.

Usually, since the bandwidth of the GWN stimulus is normally higher than the bandwidth of the system, the GWN bandwidth becomes the determining factor of the *sampling rate*. That is, the highest frequency f_m in the white-noise stimulus is chosen and then the sampling interval is adjusted according to the Nyquist folding frequency to be $\Delta t = 1/2f_m$. Of course, if Δt is too small, the resulting samples are very close together and, consequently, highly correlated in the output. This will tend to increase the computational burden considerably. Therefore, an *optimum value* of Δt must be chosen such that the high-frequency behavior is adequately represented and at the same time the computational burden is not increased impractically.

If frequencies higher than f_m exist in the recorded data, because of "noise," for example, then it is desirable to low-pass-filter the records before sampling in order to avoid aliasing.

8.6.1. Effect of Aliasing on Kernel Estimation

Assume that we are studying a linear system and that we are trying to estimate its impulse response $h_1(\tau)$ using the following relationship:

$$|H_1(f)|^2 = \Phi_{yy}(f)/\Phi_{xx}(f) \qquad (8.19)$$

where $H_1(f)$ is the Fourier transform of $h_1(\tau)$ and $\Phi_{xx}(f)$, $\Phi_{yy}(f)$ are the power spectra of the stimulus and the response. Suppose the stimulus used has the power spectrum shown in Fig. 2.17, but has been sampled at a rather low rate $1/\Delta t$, which produces a cutoff frequency f_c (as shown in that figure), below the highest frequency present in the stimulus. Then, as discussed in Sec. 2.9, the power spectrum of this stimulus signal, when computed, will be aliased in the range of frequencies from $f_c - f_w$ to f_c. Therefore, in trying to estimate the magnitude of $H_1(f)$ from Eq. (8.19), $\Phi_{yy}(f)$ will be divided by a number greater than the actual spectrum of x in that range. Therefore, the estimate of the transfer function will tend to be lower than its true value, in this high-frequency range, because of aliasing.

An analogous effect takes place in the time domain when crosscorrelations are computed. That is, if the stimulus signal has high frequencies that have not been accounted for by a suitably high sampling rate, they appear as lower frequencies in the crosscorrelation estimates.

It is, therefore, imperative that the sampling interval Δt be chosen sufficiently small so that it is good enough in describing all the frequencies up to the highest frequency existent in the data. For example, if the highest frequency present in the data is 50 Hz, then Δt should be less than 0.01 sec. In practice, it is advisable to use a Δt that is one-half of this value. If the choice of Δt, following these considerations, leads to too many samples and therefore computational difficulties, it may be advisable to filter the data prior to sampling them so that any frequencies above the maximum frequency of interest are no longer present, and the estimates of the kernels are not aliased by the higher frequencies in the stimulus. In fact, this method seems to be preferable since it alleviates both the aliasing problem and the computational problem. Notice that this applies in the case of a linear system where each frequency f of the input produces the same frequency f in the output, and therefore simultaneous low-pass filtering of the input and output records leaves the input–output data relation unaffected. However, in the case of a nonlinear system, each harmonic f of the input produces several harmonics f, $2f$, $3f$, etc. (depending on the order of nonlinearity of the system) in the output, and therefore simultaneous low-pass filtering of the input and output records could alter the input–output data relation.

8.6.2. Effect of Digitalization on Kernel Estimation

There is one final matter to be considered in the process of analog-to-digital conversion of the data. This is the matter of *digitalization* of signals, that is, assigning a digital number to each sample value. Obviously, this is directly related to the number of *binary* digits that the analog-to-digital converter produces. The question of interest that arises *in practice* concerns the effect of digitalization on the statistical properties of a random signal.

To study this, consider a random signal $x(t)$ with continuous amplitude probability density function $p(x)$, which is digitalized at equidistant discrete values $k\Delta x (k = 0, \pm 1, \pm 2, \ldots)$. The amplitude probability density function of the digitalized signal $x_D(t)$ is

$$p_D(x_D) = \sum_{n=-\infty}^{\infty} c_n \delta(x_D - n\Delta x) \qquad (8.20)$$

where

$$c_n = \int_{n\Delta x - \Delta x/2}^{n\Delta x + \Delta x/2} p(x)\, dx \qquad (8.21)$$

Therefore, the deviation in the mth-order statistical moment caused by digitalization is

$$\varepsilon_m = \sum_{n=-\infty}^{\infty} \int_{n\Delta x - \Delta x/2}^{n\Delta x + \Delta x/2} p(x)[x^m - (n\Delta x)^m]\, dx \qquad (8.22)$$

If the probability density function $p(x)$ is symmetric around zero, then it is easily seen that the deviation of any odd-order statistical moment is zero. The deviation of any even-order statistical moment, in first approximation, is

$$\varepsilon_m \cong \sum_{n=-\infty}^{\infty} m(n\Delta x)^{m-1} \int_{n\Delta x - \Delta x/2}^{n\Delta x + \Delta x/2} p(x)(x - n\Delta x)\, dx \qquad (8.23)$$

and obviously depends strongly on the magnitude of Δx. Similar expressions can be derived in the study of the joint statistical properties of two or more digitalized random signals.

The error introduced by the digitalization process is usually small compared to other errors encountered in the study of physiological systems by the white-noise method (cf. Chapter 7). This is especially true if the number of binary digits employed by the analog-to-digital converter is more than 8.

8.7. Choice of GWN Bandwidth and Record Length

The white-noise theory has been formulated for an input that is ideal Gaussian white noise, i.e., it has a flat power spectrum over all frequencies and a Gaussian amplitude distribution. In practice, of course, white-noise sources exhibit a flat power spectrum only over a finite range of frequencies with cutoff at high frequencies. The low-frequency cutoff is usually determined by the length of the record. It was found that if the bandwidth of the

white noise extends too much beyond the system bandwidth, at the high-frequency end, then statistical estimation errors increase in the computation of the kernels (cf. Chapter 7). However, the input noise bandwidth should cover the system bandwidth completely so that the system is tested with all frequencies to which it responds appreciably.

Naturally, the response of any physical system attenuates for high enough frequencies. Therefore, the range of *frequencies of interest* is determined by the highest frequency for which the system response is distinguishable from the noise level. Since this level of noise is usually quite high for physiological systems, the response is usually not detectable below 20–30 db. This is the highest frequency of interest in the system response. At this point it is of interest to consider the linear (h_1) and nonlinear (h_2) kernels and the responses they produce. The linear kernel produces a response of the same frequency as the stimulus, and therefore this argument is directly applicable to it. However, the nonlinear kernel h_2 gives rise to a *second-harmonic* response, which represents power at a *higher* frequency, and its detectability at that range must be considered. In this latter respect, it should be noted that as the signal-to-noise ratio decreases, the *non*linearity of the response appears to decrease from the *measurement* point of view. That is, noise has a linearizing effect, as demonstrated in Sec. 3.6.

To illustrate the effect of the limited bandwidth of the white-noise stimulus on the system kernel estimates, let us consider the following nonlinear (second-order, i.e., $h_k = 0$ for $k \geq 3$) system, where $x(t)$ is the input and $y(t)$ is the output:

$$y(t) = \int_0^\infty h_1(\tau)x(t-\tau)\,d\tau + \int\int_0^\infty h_2(\tau_1, \tau_2)x(t-\tau_1)x(t-\tau_2)\,d\tau_1\,d\tau_2$$

$$\tag{8.24}$$

Suppose the system is tested with band-limited Gaussian white noise $x(t)$ and the response $y(t)$ is obtained. From these input–output data the kernels h_1, h_2 are estimated through crosscorrelation.

Consider the estimation of h_1:

$$\hat{h}_1(\lambda) = \frac{1}{P}\int_0^{\mu_1} h_1(\tau)\hat{\phi}_{xx}(\lambda - \tau)\,d\tau$$

$$+ \frac{1}{P}\int\int_0^{\mu_2} h_2(\tau_1, \tau_2)\hat{\phi}_{xxx}(\lambda - \tau_1, \lambda - \tau_2)\,d\tau_1\,d\tau_2$$

$$= \hat{A}_1(\lambda) + \hat{A}_2(\lambda) \tag{8.25}$$

where P is the power level of GWN, μ_1 and μ_2 are the effective memory

extent of h_1 and h_2, respectively, and

$$\hat{\phi}_{xx}(\lambda - \tau) = \frac{1}{R} \int_0^R x(t-\tau)x(t-\lambda)\,dt \tag{8.26}$$

$$\hat{\phi}_{xxx}(\lambda - \tau_1, \lambda - \tau_2) = \frac{1}{R} \int_0^R x(t-\tau_1)x(t-\tau_2)x(t-\lambda)\,dt \tag{8.27}$$

where R is the record length of stimulus–response data.

The estimate $\hat{h}_1(\sigma)$ is a biased estimate of $h_1(\sigma)$ because of the limited bandwidth of $x(t)$ (cf. Sec. 7.1). The variance of this estimate is determined by the variance of the autocorrelation estimates $\hat{\phi}_{xx}$ and $\hat{\phi}_{xxx}$. Notice that $\hat{\phi}_{xx}$ and $\hat{\phi}_{xxx}$ are uncorrelated and consequently

$$\mathrm{Var}\,[\![\hat{h}_1(\sigma)]\!] = \mathrm{Var}\,[\![\hat{A}_1(\sigma)]\!] + \mathrm{Var}\,[\![\hat{A}_2(\sigma)]\!] \tag{8.28}$$

In Sec. 7.1 we studied the variance of $\hat{A}_1(\sigma)$ and we demonstrated its dependence on both the record length and the bandwidth of the GWN stimulus. The dependence of the variance of $\hat{A}_2(\sigma)$ on those two stimulus parameters can be similarly demonstrated. Thus, it is evident that the GWN stimulus bandwidth affects both the bias and the variance of the kernel estimates. In general, the bias increases and the variance decreases as the stimulus bandwidth decreases. Therefore, an optimum bandwidth can be found for which the total estimation error is minimized, although analytically this is a complicated task (cf. Sec. 7.1) and trial-and-error procedures are recommended in practice. Note that this is a relative disadvantage of GWN as compared to CSRS (cf. Sec. 7.3).

Clearly, the variance of the kernel estimates depends on the record length of the stimulus–response data. As shown in Sec. 7.1, to a first approximation the variance is inversely proportional to the record length, for all orders of kernel estimates. Thus, the limit on the record length is usually posed by computational considerations or by the experimental lifetime of the physiological preparation. In the unusual case where our computational capacity is unlimited and the physiological preparation remains stable over very long periods, the statistical error of the kernel estimates becomes the determining factor of the record length. It must be emphasized that, in all cases, the optimum stimulus bandwidth depends on the record length chosen.

8.8. Optimal Choice of CSRS Step and Record Length

The optimal determination of the record and step length of a CSRS stimulus is based upon the fundamental error equation (cf. Sec. 7.3):

$$Q_n = A_n \Delta t^4 + \frac{B_n}{T \Delta t^{n-1}} \tag{8.29}$$

where Q_n is the combined deconvolution and statistical fluctuation mean-square error of the nth-order kernel estimate, Δt is the CSRS step length, T is the CSRS record length, A_n and B_n are positive constants characteristic of the specific kernel (cf. V. Z. Marmarelis, 1976, 1977). Obviously, for a given value of T, there is always an optimum value of Δt for which Q_n reaches a minimum.

Thus, first we determine the record length T. In this process, we distinguish two main cases:

Case I. The experimentation time is limited by the nature of the specific system under study or by the specific experimental procedure, but computational capacity is practically unlimited. For example, the limited physical endurance of a nerve cell being probed by a measurement electrode puts a strict limitation on the experimentation time and, consequently, on the length of the input–output data records.

In this case, the record length is chosen to be the maximum experimentation time for which reliable data can be obtained. The determination of the optimum Δt then follows from the fundamental error equation (8.29).

Of course, the determination of an optimum Δt in the nth-order kernel case requires some knowledge of the values of A_n and B_n. These two constants depend on the specific nth-order kernel. We assume that for all practical purposes A_n and B_n are independent of Δt, in the range of Δt of practical interest. There are several ways to estimate A_n and B_n using the basic facts discussed in Sec. 7.3. In any case, we will have to utilize the different nature of the deconvolution and statistical fluctuation errors (deterministic and random, respectively) in order to distinctly estimate A_n and B_n. We outline below one such procedure.

We perform k preliminary tests with independent CSRS stimuli of the same T_1 and Δt_1. Of course, Δt_1 attains a value from the range of practical interest, as determined by the system bandwidth. The record length T_1 of these preliminary tests can be short, so that the experimental and computational burden is light. Actually, it is usually practicable to obtain these k independent short records as segments of a single longer record.

In any case, from each one of these k preliminary tests we estimate the nth-order kernel by crosscorrelation. According to Sec. 7.3 we have

$$\hat{h}_n(\sigma_1, \ldots, \sigma_n) = h_n(\sigma_1, \ldots, \sigma_n) + \theta_n(\sigma_1, \ldots, \sigma_n) + \varepsilon_n(\sigma_1, \ldots, \sigma_n)$$

$$(8.30)$$

where

$$\theta_n(\sigma_1, \ldots, \sigma_n) = \Delta t^2 D_{h_n}(\sigma_1, \ldots, \sigma_n) \tag{8.31}$$

and, $\varepsilon_n(\sigma_1, \ldots, \sigma_n)$ is a Gaussian random variable with

$$E[\![\varepsilon_n(\sigma_1, \ldots, \sigma_n)]\!] = 0 \tag{8.32}$$

$$\text{Var}\,[\![\varepsilon_n(\sigma_1,\ldots,\sigma_n)]\!] = q_n^2(\sigma_1,\ldots,\sigma_n) = \frac{1}{T\Delta t^{n-1}}C_{h_n}^2(\sigma_1,\ldots,\sigma_n) \qquad (8.33)$$

From the k kernel estimates $\{\hat{h}_{n_i}\}$, we can estimate, for each point $(\sigma_1,\ldots,\sigma_n)$, the mean and the variance of the random variable $\hat{h}_n(\sigma_1,\ldots,\sigma_n)$:

$$\hat{m}_{h_n}(\sigma_1,\ldots,\sigma_n) = \frac{1}{k}\sum_{i=1}^{k}\hat{h}_{n_i}(\sigma_1,\ldots,\sigma_n) \qquad (8.34)$$

$$\hat{v}_{h_n}(\sigma_1,\ldots,\sigma_n) = \frac{1}{k-1}\sum_{i=1}^{k}[\hat{h}_{n_i}(\sigma_1,\ldots,\sigma_n) - \hat{m}_{h_n}(\sigma_1,\ldots,\sigma_n)]^2 \qquad (8.35)$$

Clearly,

$$m_{h_n}(\sigma_1,\ldots,\sigma_n) = h_n(\sigma_1,\ldots,\sigma_n) + \theta_n(\sigma_1,\ldots,\sigma_n) \qquad (8.36)$$

$$v_{h_n}(\sigma_1,\ldots,\sigma_n) = q_n^2(\sigma_1,\ldots,\sigma_n) \qquad (8.37)$$

Estimation of B_n is now straightforward since

$$\hat{C}_{h_n}^2(\sigma_1,\ldots,\sigma_n) = T_1\Delta t_1^{n-1}\hat{v}_{h_n}(\sigma_1,\ldots,\sigma_n) \qquad (8.38)$$

and from that

$$\hat{B}_n = \int_0^{\mu_n}\cdots\int_0^{\mu_n}\hat{C}_{h_n}^2(\sigma_1,\ldots,\sigma_n)\,d\sigma_1\cdots d\sigma_n \qquad (8.39)$$

For the estimation of A_n, we need another set of k preliminary tests with different step length Δt_2. From this second set, we obtain another estimate $\hat{m}_{h_n}^*$ of the mean of the nth-order kernel estimates. Subtracting these two estimates of the mean, we obtain an estimate of A_n, since

$$\hat{D}_{h_n}(\sigma_1,\ldots,\sigma_n) = \frac{\hat{m}_{h_n}(\sigma_1,\ldots,\sigma_n) - \hat{m}_{h_n}^*(\sigma_1,\ldots,\sigma_n)}{\Delta t_1^2 - \Delta t_2^2} \qquad (8.40)$$

and from that

$$\hat{A}_n = \int_0^{\mu_n}\cdots\int_0^{\mu_n}\hat{D}_{h_n}^2(\sigma_1,\ldots,\sigma_n)\,d\sigma_1\cdots d\sigma_n \qquad (8.41)$$

Now that the basic parameters A_n and B_n have been estimated, the fundamental error equation can be used to determine the optimum step length for the estimation of the nth-order kernel of the system at hand. This actual determination can be done either graphically (see Fig. 8.13) or analytically as

$$(\Delta t_{\text{opt}})_n = \left[\frac{(n-1)B_n}{4TA_n}\right]^{1/(n+3)} \qquad (8.42)$$

We discuss the graphical determination of $(\Delta t_{\text{opt}})_n$ later in this section.

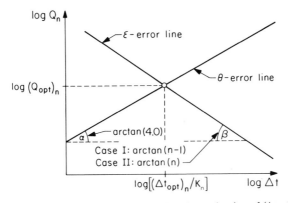

Fig. 8.13. Illustration of graphical determination of $(\Delta t_{\text{opt}})_n$.

Case II. The experimentation time is not limited and our principal practical restriction now becomes the computational burden. In this case, of concern is the number N of data points in the record, and it must be chosen to conform to some maximum computational restriction. Note that

$$T = \alpha N \Delta t \tag{8.43}$$

where N is the number of samples in the record and α the inverse of the number of samples per stimulus step. The optimization procedure for Δt is now performed based on the modified fundamental error equation:

$$Q_n = A_n \Delta t^4 + \frac{B_n}{\alpha N \Delta t^n} \tag{8.44}$$

The steps for the estimation of A_n and B_n are similar to those in case I, with some small modifications in the formulas resulting from the substitution of T with $(\alpha N \Delta t)$.

After A_n and B_n have been estimated, the optimum value of Δt is determined either graphically (see Fig. 8.13) or analytically as

$$(\Delta t_{\text{opt}})_n = \left[\frac{n}{4\alpha N} \frac{B_n}{A_n} \right]^{1/(n+4)} \tag{8.45}$$

Notice that in the expression above, α is another determinable parameter. For a given N, α determines the number of steps in the stimulus signal. Clearly, α can only attain values in the range between 0 and 1. In most cases α is chosen to be $\frac{1}{2}$ (i.e., two sampling points per stimulus step), the case where the sampling rate is equal to the Nyquist frequency of the stimulus.

However, α can also be used to achieve the optimum solution which exhausts the remaining margins of computational capacity or experimentation time, since it is a regulating parameter between the number of samples and the number of stimulus steps (and consequently the record length). In other words, the optimum choice of α, which exhausts the possible margins of both the "quantities in scarcity" (namely, computational capacity and experimentation time), is

$$(\alpha_{opt})_n = \frac{T_{max}}{N_{max}(\Delta t_{opt})_n} \tag{8.46}$$

where T_{max} and N_{max} are determined by the practical limitations as discussed in cases I and II.

If $(\alpha_{opt})_n$ as computed from Eq. (8.46) is bigger than 1, then the optimum feasible choice is 1. Of course in this case we encounter significant aliasing problems.

It must be noted that in most applications we know which of the principal practical limitations (experimentation time or the computational burden) dominates but are unable to determine $(\alpha_{opt})_n$ through Eq. (8.46). Thus, we usually choose the value of α in a more or less arbitrary fashion from a reasonable range of values (usually from $\frac{1}{4}$ to $\frac{1}{2}$).

The graphical determination of $(\Delta t_{opt})_n$ is much simplified if logarithmic paper is used (Fig. 8.13). The optimum position is determined from the Δt value corresponding to the cross section of the ε-error and θ-error lines by properly scaling it with $K_n = [4/(n-1)]^{1/(n+3)}$ (in Case I).

The ε-error line is described in the previously discussed two cases by the following equations:*

$$\text{Case I:} \qquad \log Q_n = \log B_n - \log T - (n-1)\log \Delta t \tag{8.47}$$

$$\text{Case II:} \qquad \log Q_n = \log B_n - \log (\alpha N) - n \log \Delta t \tag{8.48}$$

The θ-error line is described by the same equation in both cases I and II:

$$\log Q_n = \log A_n + 4 \log \Delta t \tag{8.49}$$

This graphical representation is very illustrative. First, it illustrates clearly how $(\Delta t_{opt})_n$ decreases when T increases. Second, it shows nicely the dependence of $(\Delta t_{opt})_n$ on the order n. Third, it illustrates the role of A_n and B_n, and, consequently, the effect of small estimation errors of $\hat{A}_n$ and $\hat{B}_n$ upon the determination of $(\Delta t_{opt})_n$.

Suppose, for example, that we have an estimation error δ of $\log A_n$ in case I; then, as shown geometrically in Fig. 8.14, the resulting error in the

---

*Where, as here, the base of the logarithm is not given, the expressions given are valid for any base.

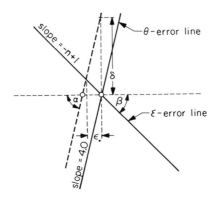

Fig. 8.14. Illustration of sensitivity of determined $(\Delta t_{opt})_n$.

determination of $\log (\Delta t_{opt})_n$ is $\varepsilon_* = \delta/(n+3)$ and is in the opposite direction (increase–decrease).

Similarly, if an estimation error δ occurs with $\log B_n$, then it can be shown easily that the resulting error in the determination of $\log(\Delta t_{opt})_n$ is again $\varepsilon_* = \delta/(n+3)$ but in the same direction as δ.

Therefore, the sensitivity of the determined $(\Delta t_{opt})_n$ is lower in the higher-order kernel cases, and the resulting deviation is, in any case, smaller than the estimation error of $\log \hat{A}_n$ or $\log \hat{B}_n$ that causes it.

9

Peeking into the Black Box

Introduction

Thus far we have approached the problem of analysis of a physiological system from the point of view of *identifying* its stimulus–response relationship and describing quantitatively its dynamics. That is, our objective has been the determination of the system functional F, where $y(t) = F[x(t)]$ and $x(t)$, $y(t)$ are the stimulus and response, respectively. The identification problem was posed as follows: Given a system $y(t) = F[x(t)]$, choose a set of stimuli $\{x_i(t)\}$ such that the stimulus–response pairs $\{x_i(t), y_i(t)\}$ allow you to determine F as completely and accurately as possible, under given experimental conditions.

We have argued—and, we hope, shown—that a quasiwhite stimulus is indeed the most desirable stimulus with regard to both *completeness* and *accuracy* of the identification, for the kind of nonlinear systems that appear functionally to us as "black boxes," as most physiological systems do.

Following the determination of F, the next question concerns the *structure* of the system. That is, how is F realized by the different interacting components of the system? How do changes in the characteristics of a particular component affect the system function F? Paradoxically, subanalysis of the system structure often becomes possible if the system is nonlinear, while it is nearly impossible if the system is linear. This is due to the fact that nonlinear operators, unlike linear ones, do not commute, in general. For example, as shown in Fig. 9.1, if systems U and/or W are nonlinear, it may be possible to determine whether U precedes or follows W, while this is not possible if U and W are linear. We show how below.

9.1. Analysis of Cascades in Physiological Systems

This process is directly applicable to signal processing by neuron chains, a processing taking place by a concatenation of a finite number of discrete elements (neurons or neural aggregates). Let us take a simple example to illustrate the plausibility of the above remarks before we describe the process in detail. Consider the systems shown in Fig. 9.1. We have *a priori* information (or we hypothesize) that the system consists of

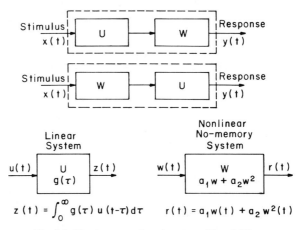

Fig. 9.1. The two cascades of systems U and W.

two subsystems connected in series: a linear system and a nonlinear zero-memory (no-memory) system. We wish to determine the sequence of these two subsystems, i.e., whether the configuration is U–W or W–U, a matter of some interest in connection with the internal structure of the overall system. In this example, the nonlinearity is, for a limited range and for a suitable choice of α_1, α_2, a half-wave rectifier. We have the following:

If U–W is the Sequence

$$r(t) = \alpha_1 w(t) + \alpha_2 w^2(t)$$

$$= \int_0^\infty \alpha_1 g(\tau) x(t-\tau)\, d\tau + \int\!\!\int_0^\infty \alpha_2 g(\tau_1) g(\tau_2) x(t-\tau_1) x(t-\tau_2)\, d\tau_1\, d\tau_2 \tag{9.1}$$

then, the linear and (second-order) nonlinear kernels would be related by

$$h_1(\tau) = \alpha_1 g(\tau) \tag{9.2}$$

$$h_2(\tau_1, \tau_2) = \alpha_2 g(\tau_1) g(\tau_2) = (\alpha_2/\alpha_1^2) h_1(\tau_1) h_1(\tau_2) \tag{9.3}$$

If W–U is the Sequence

$$r(t) = \int_0^\infty g(\tau)[\alpha_1 x(t-\tau) + \alpha_2 x^2(t-\tau)]\, d\tau$$

$$= \int_0^\infty \alpha_1 g(\tau) x(t-\tau)\, d\tau$$

$$+ \int\!\!\int_0^\infty \alpha_2 g(\tau_1) \delta(\tau_1 - \tau_2) x(t-\tau_1) x(t-\tau_2)\, d\tau_1\, d\tau_2 \tag{9.4}$$

then the linear and (second-order) nonlinear kernels in this case are related by

$$h_1(\tau) = \alpha_1 g(\tau) \tag{9.5}$$

$$h_2(\tau_1, \tau_2) = \alpha_2 g(\tau_1)\delta(\tau_1 - \tau_2) = (\alpha_2/\alpha_1)h_1(\tau_1)\delta(\tau_1 - \tau_2) \tag{9.6}$$

Note that in both cases ($U-W$ or $W-U$) the linear kernel is the same. Thus, from Eqs. (9.3) and (9.6) we see that by looking at the second-order system kernels we can decide whether $U-W$ or $W-U$ is the actual sequence of the input–output transformation. These techniques have been applied to the analysis of certain retinal neuron chains [cf. P. Z. Marmarelis and Naka, 1973a–c].

Recently, Korenberg (1973a,b) suggested an elegant method for identifying each component in cascades such as the one shown in Fig. 9.2 consisting of a linear, a no-memory (static) nonlinear, and another linear element. This is accomplished by a single Gaussian white-noise experiment, unlike methods previously proposed for the identification of such cascades, which involved repeated experiments using special test inputs (Spekreijse, 1969).

In addition to being more general and experimentally more convenient, the method proposed by Korenberg yields an exact description of the nonlinearity and a complete identification of *each* linear system component.

If the static nonlinearity can be described by a polynomial

$$z(t) = \sum_{m=0}^{M} \alpha_m v^m(t) \tag{9.7}$$

to an arbitrary degree of accuracy for large enough M, then we have

$$z(t) = \alpha_0 + \int_0^\infty \alpha_1 g(\tau)x(t - \tau)\,d\tau + \cdots$$

$$+ \int_0^\infty \cdots \int_0^\infty \alpha_M g(\tau_1)\cdots g(\tau_M)x(t - \tau_1)\cdots x(t - \tau_M)\,d\tau_1 \cdots d\tau_M$$

$$\tag{9.8}$$

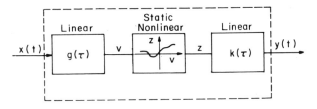

Fig. 9.2. A three-subsystem cascade: linear → zero-memory nonlinear → linear.

and, of course,

$$y(t) = \int_0^\infty k(\lambda)z(t-\lambda)\,d\lambda \qquad (9.9)$$

Then

$$y(t) = \alpha_0 \int_0^\infty k(\lambda)\,d\lambda + \alpha_1 \int_0^\infty \int_0^\infty k(\lambda)g(\tau)x(t-\lambda-\tau)\,d\lambda\,d\tau + \cdots$$

$$+ \alpha_M \int_0^\infty \cdots \int_0^\infty k(\lambda)g(\tau_1)\cdots g(\tau_M)x(t-\lambda-\tau_1)\cdots$$

$$\times x(t-\lambda-\tau_M)\,d\tau_1 \cdots d\tau_M\,d\lambda \qquad (9.10)$$

We recall that for $x(t)$ being a zero-mean Gaussian white-noise signal we have

$$E[x(t-\tau_1)\cdots x(t-\tau_n)]$$

$$= \begin{cases} 0 & \text{if } n \text{ is odd} \\ P^m \sum\prod \delta(\tau_i - \tau_j) & \text{if } n \text{ is even (where } m = n/2) \end{cases} \qquad (9.11)$$

where P is the power level of the GWN and, as in Chapter 2 (Sec. 2.5.1), $\sum\prod$ is the sum of products of $\delta(\tau_i - \tau_j)$ over all distinct ways of partitioning $\tau_1, \ldots, \tau_n$ into pairs. The number of terms in this sum is $(2m)!/m!2^m$.

Taking the first-order crosscorrelation

$$\phi_{yx}(\sigma) = E[y(t)x(t-\sigma)] = A_1 \int_0^\infty k(\nu)g(\sigma-\nu)\,d\nu \qquad (9.12)$$

where

$$A_1 = \sum_{m=1}^{[M/2]} \frac{(2m)!}{m!2^m}\alpha_{2m-1}P^m\left[\int_0^\infty g^2(\tau)\,d\tau\right]^{m-1} \qquad (9.13)$$

and $[M/2]$ denotes the largest integer which is less than or equal to $M/2$. It should be noted that if the nonlinearity is even (implying that all α_{2m-1} are zero), then A_1 is zero. This case is treated later. From Eq. (9.12), taking the Fourier transform, we have

$$\Phi_{yx}(\omega) = A_1 K(\omega)G(\omega) \qquad (9.14)$$

Similarly, it can be shown (cf. Korenberg, 1973) that

$$\phi_{yxx}(\sigma_1, \sigma_2) = A_2 \int_0^\infty k(\nu)g(\sigma_1-\nu)g(\sigma_2-\nu)\,d\nu + A_3\delta(\sigma_1-\sigma_2) \qquad (9.15)$$

where

$$A_2 = \sum_{m=1}^{[M/2]} \frac{m(2m)!}{m!2^{m-1}} P^m \alpha_{2m} \left[\int_0^\infty g^2(\nu)\, d\nu \right]^{m-1} \tag{9.16}$$

$$A_3 = \sum_{m=0}^{[M/2]} \frac{(2m)!}{m!2^m} P^m \alpha_{2m} \left[\int_0^\infty k(\nu)\, d\nu \right] \left[\int_0^\infty g^2(\nu)\, d\nu \right]^m \tag{9.17}$$

It is easily seen that

$$y_a = E[y(t)] = A_3 \tag{9.18}$$

which is consistent with the use of the response residual in the crosscorrelation technique (cf. Sec. 4.3). We can simplify matters if the mean of the response is subtracted before the second-order crosscorrelation is computed. Thus, the A_3 term in Eq. (9.15) is eliminated. Taking the two-dimensional Fourier transform of Eq. (9.15), we have

$$\Phi_{yxx}(\omega_1, \omega_2) = A_2 K(\omega_1 + \omega_2) G(\omega_1) G(\omega_2) \tag{9.19}$$

From Eqs. (9.14) and (9.19) we have

$$\frac{G(\omega_1)G(\omega_2)}{G(\omega_1 + \omega_2)} = \frac{A_1}{A_2} \frac{\Phi_{yxx}(\omega_1, \omega_2)}{\Phi_{yx}(\omega_1 + \omega_2)} \tag{9.20}$$

We wish now to find $G(\omega)$ and $K(\omega)$ explicitly. To this end, let $\omega_1 = -\omega/2$, $\omega_2 = \omega$. Then from Eq. (9.20) we have

$$\frac{G(-\omega/2)G(\omega)}{G(\omega/2)} = \frac{A_1}{A_2} \frac{\Phi_{yxx}(-\omega/2, \omega)}{\Phi_{yx}(\omega/2)} \tag{9.21}$$

Then, since $|G(\omega/2)| = |G(-\omega/2)|$, we have

$$|G(\omega)| = \left| \frac{A_1}{A_2} \right| \frac{|\Phi_{yxx}(-\omega/2, \omega)|}{|\Phi_{yx}(\omega/2)|} \tag{9.22}$$

and then from Eq. (9.14)

$$|K(\omega)| = \frac{|A_2|}{A_1^2} \frac{|\Phi_{yx}(\omega)| \, |\Phi_{yx}(\omega/2)|}{|\Phi_{yxx}(-\omega/2, \omega)|} \tag{9.23}$$

Therefore, since $\Phi_{yx}(\ )$ and $\Phi_{yxx}(\ )$ are measurable from the stimulus–response data, then $G(\omega)$ and $K(\omega)$ are determinable up to a scaling constant by use of Eqs. (9.22) and (9.23). Note that, for a minimum-phase linear system, the gain function suffices to determine the transfer function.

Figure 9.3 shows an example of identification of the linear component dynamics in a cascade system. The various quantities of interest (spectra) that participate in Eqs. (9.22) and (9.23) are shown along with the final answer for the linear component transfer functions $G(f)$ and $K(f)$ (gain

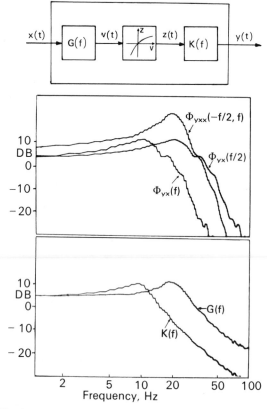

Fig. 9.3. Identification and decomposition of a three-subsystem cascade from the cross-spectra.

plots). They both appear to be underdamped second-order systems with bandwidths of about 30 and 15 Hz, respectively. This analysis was done by simulating the original "black box" system on a digital computer. The results are indeed very close to the originally specified transfer functions for $G(f)$ and $K(f)$.

Similarly we can find the phase of $G(\omega)$ and $K(\omega)$. Letting $\omega_1 = -\Delta\omega$ and $\omega_2 = N\Delta\omega$, where N is a positive integer, we have from Eq. (9.20)

$$G(N\Delta\omega) = \frac{A_1}{A_2} \frac{G((N-1)\Delta\omega)}{G(-\Delta\omega)} \frac{\Phi_{yxx}(-\Delta\omega, N\Delta\omega)}{\Phi_{yx}((N-1)\Delta\omega)} \qquad (9.24)$$

However, assuming absence of power terms, we may set the phase of $G(-\Delta\omega)$, $\theta[G(-\Delta\omega)]$, equal to zero. Thus from Eq. (9.24) we have

$$\theta[G(N\Delta\omega)] = \theta[G((N-1)\Delta\omega)] + \theta\left[\frac{\Phi_{yxx}(-\Delta\omega, N\Delta\omega)}{\Phi_{yx}((N-1)\Delta\omega)}\right], \quad N \geq 2 \quad (9.25)$$

Thus we obtain a recursive formula for calculating the phase $\theta[G(N\Delta\omega)]$ in terms of the previous value $\theta[G((N-1)\Delta\omega)]$. From Eq. (9.25) an explicit solution (in a discrete form) may be obtained for the phase of $G(\omega)$:

$$\theta[G(N\Delta\omega)] = \sum_{i=2}^{N} \theta\left[\frac{\Phi_{yxx}(-\Delta\omega, i\Delta\omega)}{\Phi_{yx}((i-1)\Delta\omega)}\right], \qquad N \geqslant 2 \qquad (9.26)$$

Combining Eqs. (9.14) and (9.26), we find an expression for $K(\omega)$:

$$\theta[K(N\Delta\omega)] = \theta[\Phi_{yx}(N\Delta\omega)] - \sum_{i=2}^{N} \theta\left[\frac{\Phi_{yxx}(-\Delta\omega, i\Delta\omega)}{\Phi_{yx}((i-1)\Delta\omega)}\right], \qquad N \geqslant 2 \qquad (9.27)$$

$$\theta[K(\Delta\omega)] = \theta[\Phi_{yx}(\Delta\omega)] \qquad (9.28)$$

Thus, both the magnitude and the phase of $G(\omega)$ and $K(\omega)$ can be found as a function of frequency in a discrete form with resolution $\Delta\omega$. The magnitude is determinable up to a multiplying constant. Therefore in Fig. 9.3, the input $v(t)$ and output $z(t)$ of the nonlinearity can be determined—multiplied by an unknown constant. We have

$$V(\omega) = C_1 G(\omega)X(\omega) \qquad (9.29)$$

$$Z(\omega) = C_2 Y(\omega)/K(\omega) \qquad (9.30)$$

from which $v(t)$ and $z(t)$ can be found. Then the nonlinearity can be found as follows: We pick the coefficients $\{\alpha_m\}$ and C_1, C_2 so as to minimize the mean-square error between $z(t)$ and $\sum_{m=0}^{M} \alpha_m v^m(t)$, where we choose M large enough to achieve as small a mean-square error as desired.

One case that needs caution was mentioned earlier: If the static nonlinearity is an even function, then all α_{2m-1} in Eq. (9.13) are zero and consequently $\phi_{yx}(\sigma)$ is zero. However, the analysis can still be performed if we find the crosscorrelation

$$\phi_{yxx}(\sigma, \alpha) = E[\![y(t)x(t-\sigma)x(t-\alpha)]\!] \qquad (9.31)$$

for a fixed α. Then, we notice that $\phi_{yxx}(\sigma, \alpha) \neq 0$. Alternatively, in this case Eq. (9.14) may be replaced by a different equation of $G(\omega)$, $K(\omega)$:

$$G(0)G(\omega_1)K(\omega_1) = (1/A_2)\Phi_{yxx}(\omega_1, 0) \qquad (9.32)$$

which is derived from Eq. (9.19) by setting $\omega_2 = 0$.

Similarly, if the nonlinearity is odd, then all α_{2m} are zero and consequently $\phi_{yxx}(\sigma_1, \sigma_2) = 0$. Again, the analysis may proceed by finding the crosscorrelation

$$\phi_{yxxx}(\sigma_1, \sigma_2, \alpha) = E[\![y(t)x(t-\sigma_1)x(t-\sigma_2)x(t-\alpha)]\!] \qquad (9.33)$$

for a fixed α. Then $\phi_{yxxx}(\sigma_1, \sigma_2, \alpha) \neq 0$.

In studying a physiological system, however, we will often not know *a priori* if indeed the system can be represented by such a cascade combination. We may wish to investigate this possibility using Eq. (9.20). We have

$$G(0) = \frac{A_1}{A_2} \frac{\Phi_{yxx}(\omega, 0)}{\Phi_{yx}(\omega)} \qquad (9.34)$$

and, therefore, a necessary condition is

$$\Phi_{yxx}(\omega, 0) = C\Phi_{yx}(\omega) \qquad (9.35)$$

where C is a constant. If this system can be represented by such a cascade combination, then this condition between the cross-spectra must be satisfied.

Two special cases of interest are those of Fig. 9.1; the case of a linear system followed by a static nonlinearity [i.e., $K(\omega) = 1$] and the case of a static nonlinearity followed by a linear system [i.e., $G(\omega) = 1$].

9.1.1. Linear System Followed by Zero-Memory Nonlinearity

In this case $K(\omega) = 1$ and Eq. (9.19) yields

$$H_2(\omega_1, \omega_2) = (A_2/2P^2)G(\omega_1)G(\omega_2) \qquad (9.36)$$

or in the time domain:

$$h_2(\tau_1, \tau_2) = (A_2/2P^2)g(\tau_1)g(\tau_2) \qquad (9.37)$$

where $h_2(\tau_1, \tau_2)$ is the second-order Wiener kernel of the cascade system, estimated by the use of a Gaussian white-noise stimulus with power level P (recall the dependence of Wiener kernels on the power level of the white-noise stimulus).

From Eq. (9.14) we also have that

$$H_1(\omega) = (A_1/P)G(\omega) \qquad (9.38)$$

or in the time domain

$$h_1(\tau) = (A_1/P)g(\tau) \qquad (9.39)$$

where $h_1(\tau)$ is the first-order Wiener kernel of the cascade system for the same power level.

Thus, the first- and second-order Wiener kernels of the cascade system are related as

$$H_2(\omega_1, \omega_2) = (A_2/2A_1^2)H_1(\omega_1)H_1(\omega_2) \qquad (9.40)$$

and, alternatively,

$$\Phi_{yxx}(\omega_1, \omega_2) = (A_2/A_1^2)\Phi_{yx}(\omega_1)\Phi_{yx}(\omega_2) \qquad (9.41)$$

in the frequency domain; or

$$h_2(\tau_1, \tau_2) = (A_2/2A_1^2)h_1(\tau_1)h_1(\tau_2) \qquad (9.42)$$

and, alternatively,

$$\phi_{yxx}(\tau_1, \tau_2) = (A_2/A_1^2)\phi_{yx}(\tau_1)\phi_{yx}(\tau_2) \qquad (9.43)$$

in the time domain.

9.1.2. Linear System Preceded by Zero-Memory Nonlinearity

In this case $G(\omega) = 1$ and Eq. (9.19) yields

$$H_2(\omega_1, \omega_2) = (A_2/2P^2)K(\omega_1 + \omega_2) \qquad (9.44)$$

or in the time domain

$$h_2(\tau_1, \tau_2) = (A_2/2P^2)k(\tau_1)\delta(\tau_1 - \tau_2) \qquad (9.45)$$

From Eq. (9.14) we also have

$$H_1(\omega) = (A_1/P)K(\omega) \qquad (9.46)$$

or in the time domain

$$h_1(\tau) = (A_1/P)k(\tau) \qquad (9.47)$$

There the relations between the first- and second-order Wiener kernels of this cascade system are

$$H_2(\omega_1, \omega_2) = (A_2/2A_1P)H_1(\omega_1 + \omega_2) \qquad (9.48)$$

and, alternatively,

$$\Phi_{yxx}(\omega_1, \omega_2) = (A_2/A_1)\Phi_{yx}(\omega_1 + \omega_2) \qquad (9.49)$$

in the frequency domain; or

$$h_2(\tau_1, \tau_2) = (A_2/2A_1P)h_1(\tau_1)\delta(\tau_1 - \tau_2) \qquad (9.50)$$

and, alternatively,

$$\phi_{yxx}(\tau_1, \tau_2) = (A_2/A_1)\phi_{yx}(\tau_1)\delta(\tau_1 - \tau_2) \qquad (9.51)$$

in the time domain.

Korenberg (1973*b*) has extended this type of analysis to cascades containing any finite number of linear systems alternating in sequence with static nonlinearities (as in Fig. 9.4).

9.1.3. Illustrative Applications to Physiological Systems

The cascade analysis described above is well suited to systems that have been identified by GWN stimulation and for which estimates of the

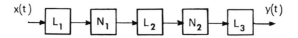

Fig. 9.4. Alternating linear and zero-memory nonlinear subsystems in cascade.

system Wiener kernels are available. In this light we may analyze certain neural chains whose kernels have been estimated (cf. P. Z. Marmarelis and Naka, 1973b). Figure 9.5 shows the kernels $h_1(\ )$ and $h_2(\ )$ for three such systems experimentally identified in the catfish retina, namely,

light → horizontal cell

horizontal cell → ganglion cell

light → ganglion cell

Obviously the third one is the cascade combination of the first two. Preliminary approximate analysis has indicated that the first system, light → horizontal cell, exhibits a "logarithmic compression" nonlinearity occurring near the beginning of the chain, while the second system exhibits primarily a rectifying nonlinearity occurring near the end of the chain.

Another application of cascade analysis was made on the photoreceptor of the fly *Calliphora erythrocephala* (cf. V. Z. Marmarelis, 1976; V. Z. Marmarelis and McCann, 1977). The first and second kernel estimates are shown in Fig. 9.6 and they exhibit approximately the relation described by Eq. (9.42). This is demonstrated better in Fig. 9.7, where a cross section of the second-order kernel estimate is compared to the first-order kernel; the form of the system kernels suggests that the physiological system under study can be formalized as a cascade of a linear subsystem followed by a saturating zero-memory nonlinearity. The characteristics of those two subsystems have been determined and are shown in Fig. 9.8.

It must be emphasized that under the cascade arrangement the physiological system under study has been completely identified, since the linear subsystem is completely describable by its impulse response, which in turn is identifiable through the first-order kernel estimate, and the zero-memory nonlinear subsystem is identified by relating a properly phase-shifted sinusoidal stimulus with the system response to that sinusoidal stimulus. Thus, this special cascade formalization of the system makes its complete identification a feasible and relatively simple task.

9.2. Zero-Memory Systems

In the analysis of physiological systems zero-memory nonlinear systems play a prominent role, as demonstrated by the examples given in

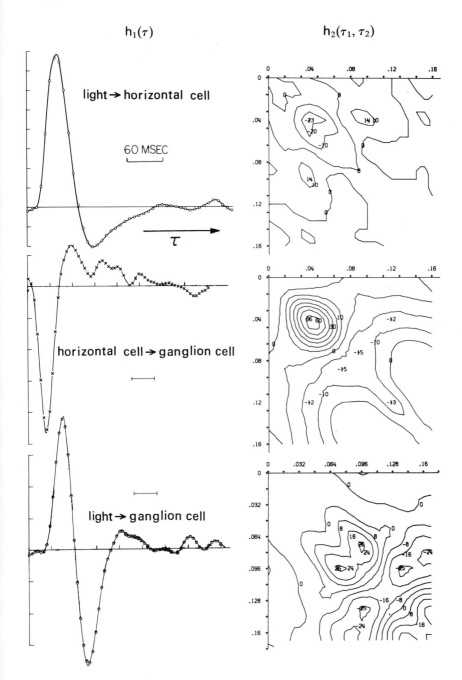

Fig. 9.5. First- and second-order kernels of three neuroretinal systems. The third one (light → ganglion cell) is a concatenation of the first two.

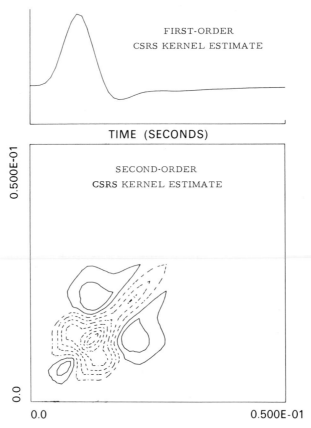

Fig. 9.6. First- and second-order kernel of the photoreceptor of *Calliphora erythrocephala*.

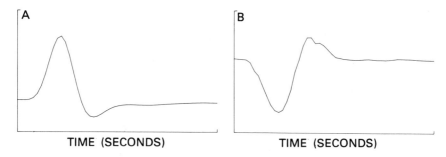

Fig. 9.7. Comparison of first-order kernel (A) and cross section of second-order kernel (B).

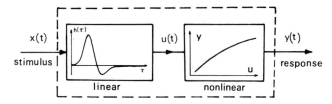

Fig. 9.8. The estimated cascade configuration of the photoreceptor light-potential transduction.

the previous section. Thus, some further study of zero-memory nonlinear systems is justified.

Consider the general case of a polynomial zero-memory nonlinearity:

$$y(t) = \sum_{m=0}^{n} a_m x^m(t) \tag{9.52}$$

Considering the uniqueness of representation in a Volterra series [Eq. (4.21)], it is easily seen that the Volterra kernels of this system are

$$k_m(\tau_1, \ldots, \tau_m) = a_m \delta(\tau_1) \cdots \delta(\tau_m) \tag{9.53}$$

and, in the Laplace domain

$$K_m(s_1, \ldots, s_m) = a_m \tag{9.54}$$

For example, consider the saturating nonlinearity shown in Fig. 9.9. Suppose we fit (in the least-squares sense) an nth-degree polynomial to this curve. The coefficients $\{a_0, \ldots, a_n\}$ of the polynomial determine the Volterra kernels of this approximation [cf. Eqs. (9.52) and (9.53)]. To determine the coefficients a_0, a_1, a_2, etc. we follow the standard mathematical procedure of expanding a function of x onto a basis $\{1, x, x^2, \ldots, x^n\}$, so that the mean-square error of the approximation is minimum, for a certain range of values of x. The resulting generalized Fourier coefficients

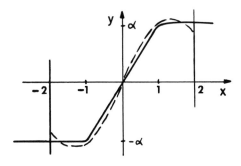

Fig. 9.9. Saturating zero-memory nonlinearity.

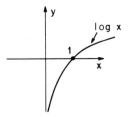

Fig. 9.10. Logarithmic zero-memory nonlinearity.

of a third-order polynomial expansion, for the saturating nonlinearity of Fig. 9.9, are found to be

$$a_0 = 0, \qquad a_1 = 1.28\alpha, \qquad a_2 = 0, \qquad a_3 = -0.23\alpha$$

for a range of x values from -2 to 2. Notice that $a_0 = 0$ and $a_2 = 0$ because the function $y(x)$, shown in Fig. 9.9, is an odd function of x and, therefore, all the even powers are absent from the expansion. The approximation $\tilde{y} = 1.28\alpha x - 0.23\alpha x^3$ of $y(x)$ is shown in Fig. 9.9 as a dashed line. By construction, this approximation is the best, in the mean-square-error sense, of all third-order polynomial approximations in the range $[-2, 2]$. However, the system described by $y(x)$ has an infinite number of Volterra kernels, and if, for example, we sought the best fifth-order polynomial approximation we would obtain different values for a_1 and a_3, since the basis $\{1, x, x^2, x^3, \ldots\}$ is not orthogonal.

Of course, an orthogonal basis of third polynomial order can be constructed for the interval $[-2, 2]$ through a Gram–Schmidt orthogonalization procedure. It is found to be $\{1, x, (x^2 - 4/3), (x^3 - 12x/5)\}$. The coefficients resulting from an expansion on this basis will now remain invariant in any extension of the basis to include higher-order polynomial terms. This expansion, in terms of *orthogonal* polynomials, compared to the expansion in terms of $\{1, x, x^2, \ldots\}$ demonstrates the difference between the expansions in terms of the Wiener functionals and expansions in terms of Volterra functionals. It should be noted, finally, that the two finite expansions given above could result in least-squares error approximations which, in general, would be different and would result in a different mean-square error (with the orthogonal expansion being expected to be more accurate).

Considering now the logarithmic transformation, commonly found in sensory systems (Fig. 9.10), we can determine the Volterra kernels of an expansion around 1, by considering simply the Taylor expansion of $y = \ln(x)$ around $x = 1$ (see Sec. 4.2):

$$\ln x = (x - 1) + \frac{(x - 1)^2}{2} + \frac{(x - 1)^3}{3} + \cdots + \frac{(x - 1)^m}{m} + \cdots \qquad (9.55)$$

Thus

$$k_0^1 = 0$$

$$k_1^1(\tau_1) = \delta(\tau_1)$$

$$k_2^1(\tau_1, \tau_2) = \tfrac{1}{2}\delta(\tau_1)\delta(\tau_2)$$

$$k_3^1(\tau_1, \tau_2, \tau_3) = \tfrac{1}{3}\delta(\tau_1)\delta(\tau_2)\delta(\tau_3)$$

$$\vdots$$

$$k_m^1(\tau_1, \ldots, \tau_m) = (1/m)\delta(\tau_1) \cdots \delta(\tau_m) \tag{9.56}$$

$$\vdots$$

Of course, if we only wanted to consider the first n kernels for the representation of the system, then we could obtain, for a certain range of x, the best—in the mean-square-error sense—approximation as previously for the saturating nonlinearity by using an orthogonal expansion basis.

Let us illustrate this difference by considering the case of a zero-memory nonlinear system $y = e^x$ (Fig. 9.11). The Taylor expansion around zero is

$$y = e^x$$

$$= 1 + x + \frac{x^2}{2!} + \frac{x^3}{3!} + \cdots + \frac{x^m}{m!} + \cdots \tag{9.57}$$

The best second-order polynomial approximation in the interval $[-1, 1]$ is found to be

$$\tilde{y} = 0.92 + 1.08x + 0.72x^2 \tag{9.58}$$

which deviates clearly from the Taylor approximation:

$$y^T = 1 + x + 0.50x^2 \tag{9.59}$$

So, practically if we want to confine ourselves to the first two kernels, Eq. (9.58) is a better approximation.

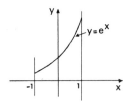

Fig. 9.11. Exponential zero-memory nonlinearity.

9.3. Combinations of Systems

The analysis of physiological systems is complicated by the fact that it is usually very difficult to measure the state variables (responses) from many points of a complex system such as, for example, a neural net. Fortunately, the white-noise approach and the accompanying representation of systems in terms of their kernels can greatly alleviate this problem.

Figure 9.12 shows some typical systems that are found in physiology. Consider the first one, a cascade combination of two subsystems, S_A and S_B. Suppose the experimental realities are such that we can only stimulate an input x and record the response at z and y. We apply, therefore, a GWN stimulus at x and from the recorded responses at z and y we can measure the kernels of subsystem S_A as well as those of the overall system x to y. The question arises: From these results, can we find a description in terms of kernels for subsystem S_B? This evidently is of utmost importance in the study of *complex* physiological systems. The answer to this question is yes. The same applies to the composite systems of cases B and C in Fig. 9.12. That is, knowing the overall system transfer characteristics, x to y, and those of one of the subsystems (S_A or S_B), we can find the characteristics of the other. The calculus of the input–output relations is simplified if we make use of the multidimensional Laplace transform of an nth-order kernel $g_n(\tau_1, \ldots, \tau_n)$:

$$G_n(s_1, \ldots, s_n) = \int_0^\infty \cdots \int_0^\infty g_n(\tau_1, \tau_2, \ldots, \tau_n) \exp(-s_1\tau_1 - s_2\tau_2 - \cdots$$

$$- s_n\tau_n)\, d\tau_1 \cdots d\tau_n \tag{9.60}$$

Let us consider now a few simple combinations of systems and derive expressions that will allow us to find the characteristics of their components

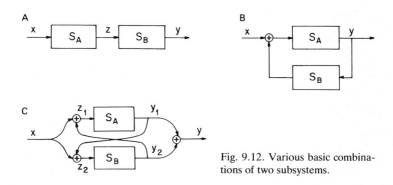

Fig. 9.12. Various basic combinations of two subsystems.

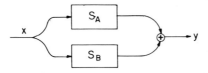

Fig. 9.13. Sum system.

from the knowledge of the overall characteristics and of some of the components. In each case, we call the overall system R and its kernels in the Laplace domain $R_1(s)$, $R_2(s_1, s_2)$, $R_3(s_1, s_2, s_3) \cdots$. To simplify matters we assume that the zero-order kernel is zero.

9.3.1. Identity System

This is, of course, an extremely simple case. It is the system

$$y(t) = x(t) \tag{9.61}$$

This system has only one kernel:

$$R_1(s) = 1 \tag{9.62}$$

9.3.2. Sum System

This is the configuration shown in Fig. 9.13. It is easily seen that, in this case,

$$R_n(s_1, \ldots, s_n) = A_n(s_1, \ldots, s_n) + B_n(s_1, \ldots, s_n) \tag{9.63}$$

That is, the kernels of the combination are simply the sum of the kernels of the components.

9.3.3. Cascade System

This system configuration is shown in Fig. 9.12A. Then, it can be shown (cf. Brilliant, 1958; Barrett, 1963) that

$$R_1(s) = B_1(s)A_1(s) \tag{9.64}$$

$$R_2(s_1, s_2) = B_1(s_1 + s_2)A_2(s_1, s_2) + B_2(s_1, s_2)A_1(s_1)A_1(s_2) \tag{9.65}$$

$$R_3(s_1, s_2, s_3) = B_1(s_1 + s_2 + s_3)A_3(s_1, s_2, s_3)$$
$$+ \tfrac{2}{3}[B_2(s_1, s_2 + s_3)A_1(s_1)A_2(s_2, s_3)$$
$$+ B_2(s_2, s_1 + s_3)A_1(s_2)A_2(s_1, s_3)$$
$$+ B_2(s_3, s_1 + s_2)A_2(s_1, s_2)A_1(s_3)]$$
$$+ B_3(s_1, s_2, s_3)A_1(s_1)A_1(s_2)A_1(s_3) \tag{9.66}$$

9.3.4. Feedback System

This is the system configuration shown in Fig. 9.12B. To find the kernels use the operator notation

$$y = R(x) \tag{9.67}$$

meaning y is the response, x is the stimulus, and system R operates on x to produce y. We have

$$R(x) = A[x + B(R(x))] \tag{9.68}$$

where

$$B[R(x)]$$

means the cascade combination of R followed by B to produce $B[R(x)]$. But, for a cascade we have formulas relating the kernels. Calling the combination

$$Q(x) = x + B[R(x)] = I(x) + B[R(x)] \tag{9.69}$$

where I is the identity operator, we find

$$Q_1(s) = 1 + B_1(s)R_1(s) \tag{9.70}$$

$$Q_2(s_1, s_2) = B_1(s_1 + s_2)R_2(s_1, s_2) + B_2(s_1, s_2)R_1(s_1)R_1(s_2) \tag{9.71}$$

Finally, combining Eqs. (9.68)–(9.71), we get the results

$$R_1(s) = \frac{A_1(s)}{1 - A_1(s)B_1(s)} \tag{9.72}$$

familiar from linear system theory, and

$$R_2(s_1, s_2) = [A_1(s_1)A_1(s_2)B_2(s_1, s_2) + B_1(s_1 + s_2)A_2(s_1, s_2)]$$
$$\times \{[1 - A_1(s_1)B_1(s_1)]$$
$$\times [1 - A_1(s_2)B_1(s_2)][1 - A_1(s_1 + s_2)B_1(s_1 + s_2)]\}^{-1} \tag{9.73}$$

$R_3(s_1, s_2, s_3)$ becomes quite complicated to write down in terms of A_i, B_i, but it is of a form similar to R_2 and R_1. For simplicity of expressions, let us use H_1, H_2, and H_3 to denote the kernel transforms of the cascade system S_A followed by S_B, as given by Eqs. (9.64), (9.65), and (9.66), respectively. Then

$$R_3(s_1, s_2, s_3) = \tfrac{1}{3}\{[2H_2(s_1, s_2 + s_3)H_2(s_2, s_3) - H_3(s_1, s_2, s_3)][1 - H_1(s_2 + s_3)]^{-1}$$
$$+ [2H_2(s_2, s_3 + s_1)H_2(s_3, s_1) - H_3(s_1, s_2, s_3)]$$
$$\times [1 - H_1(s_3 + s_1)]^{-1} + [2H_2(s_3, s_1, s_2)H_2(s_1, s_2)$$
$$- H_3(s_1, s_2, s_3)][1 - H_1(s_1 + s_2)]^{-1}\}\{[1 - H_1(s_1)]$$
$$\times [1 - H_1(s_2)][1 - H_1(s_3)][1 - H_1(s_1 + s_2 + s_3)]\}^{-1} \tag{9.74}$$

Clearly, all systems that can be constructed by sum, cascade, and feedback combinations, as examined above, can be described and analyzed. Let us consider another type of system, which often occurs in physiological systems and which does not belong to any of these categories. This is the type of system shown in Fig. 9.12C, which involves mutual cross couplings as seen, for example, in systems with lateral inhibition.

We have (using operator notation)

$$y_1 = A(z_1) = A(x + y_2) = A[x + B(x + y_1)] \tag{9.75}$$

Let K be the system with input x and output y_1:

$$K(x) = A\{x + B[x + K(x)]\} \tag{9.76}$$

Now in terms of the transforms of kernels this is a linear equation in the transformed kernels of K and therefore it can be easily solved. For example, for the linear kernel

$$K_1(s) = A_1(s)\{1 + B_1(s)[1 + K_1(s)]\} \tag{9.77}$$

$$K_1(s) = \frac{A_1(s) + A_1(s)B_1(s)}{1 - A_1(s)B_1(s)} \tag{9.78}$$

This is analogous to the way that the kernels for the feedback combination were calculated. Similarly, let L be the system from x to y_2. Then, in operator notation

$$L(x) = B\{x + A[x + L(x)]\} \tag{9.79}$$

Thus, the original system becomes as shown in Fig. 9.14 and

$$R_n(s_1, \ldots, s_n) = K_n(s_1, \ldots, s_n) + L_n(s_1, \ldots, s_n) \tag{9.80}$$

For example, for the linear representation

$$R_1(s) = \frac{A_1(s) + B_1(s) + 2A_1(s)B_1(s)}{1 - A_1(s)B_1(s)} \tag{9.81}$$

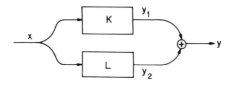

Fig. 9.14. Alternate configuration for system of Fig. 9.12C.

9.3.5. *Illustrative Applications to Physiological Systems*

The methods presented in the previous section can be readily applied to the analysis–synthesis problem of certain physiological systems. Several are presented in this section: (a) synthesis of a neuron model exhibiting self-inhibition, synaptic integration, threshold phenomena, etc.—this represents the first step to the systematic synthesis of neural networks; (b) a feedback system in the vertebrate retina; and (c) a cascade system in the retina.

Synthesis of a Neuron Model

A neuron model is shown in Fig. 9.15. This model accounts for most physiological phenomena present in the functioning of a neuron. The components are as follows:

T: We assume this to be a zero-memory half-wave rectifier. Then, when the input membrane potential exceeds a threshold value θ, an output is generated.

F_1:   A linear filter whose function is to inhibit the neuron immediately after it fires, thus producing the effect of absolute refractoriness. For simplicity, we could, for example, take $F_1(s) = A_1/(s + b_1)$.

F_2:   A linear filter simulating the integrating behavior of the membrane potential, e.g., $F_2(s) = A_2/(s + b_2)$.

F_3:   A linear filter that provides the neuron with long-term "refractoriness' after firing or with "facilitation," e.g., $F_3(s) = A_3/(s + b_3)$, where $A_3 > 0$ for facilitation and $A_3 < 0$ for refractoriness.

I_1, I_2:   Linear filters, one for each synapse, for the integration of the various incoming neural input pulses, e.g., $I_k(s) = D_k/(s + d_k)$. They can be excitatory ($D_k > 0$) or inhibitory ($D_k < 0$).

Now, we wish to find the kernels of the overall system. We start with the nonlinearity T. We approximate it in the interval $[-2\theta, 2\theta]$ by a quadratic (see Fig. 9.15):

$$T(x) \cong \alpha_1 x + \alpha_2 x^2 \tag{9.82}$$

where α_1, α_2 are the generalized Fourier coefficients of the expansion of $T(x)$ on the function basis $[x, x^2]$ (cf. Sec. 9.2).

In order to find the intermediate combination shown in Fig. 9.16A we apply the feedback formulas [Eqs. (9.72) and (9.73)] and, calling the

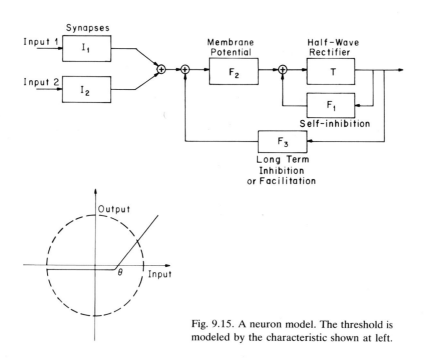

Fig. 9.15. A neuron model. The threshold is modeled by the characteristic shown at left.

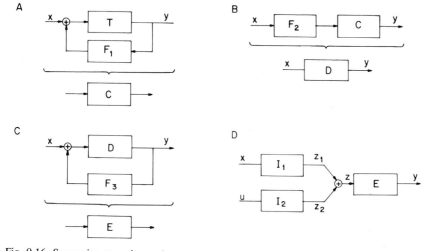

Fig. 9.16. Successive steps in a subsystem synthesis to derive intput–output expression for neuron model.

resultant system C, we have

$$C_1(s) = \frac{\alpha_1}{1 - \alpha_1 F_1(s)} \tag{9.83}$$

$$C_2(s_1, s_2) = \frac{\alpha_2}{[1 - \alpha_1 F_1(s_1)][1 - \alpha_1 F_1(s_2)][1 - \alpha_1 F_1(s_1 + s_2)]} \tag{9.84}$$

Next, we put F_2 in series with C (Fig. 9.16B), and using the cascade formulas [Eqs. (9.64) and (9.65)] we find for the combination (system D)

$$D_1(s) = \frac{\alpha_1 F_2(s)}{1 - \alpha_1 F_1(s)} \tag{9.85}$$

$$D_2(s_1, s_2) = \frac{\alpha_2 F_2(s_1) F_2(s_2)}{[1 - \alpha_1 F(s_1)][1 - \alpha_1 F_1(s_2)][1 - \alpha_1 F_1(s_1 + s_2)]} \tag{9.86}$$

Next, we put F_3 in feedback, as in Fig. 9.16C, and we obtain [cf. Eqs. (9.72) and (9.73)] for the overall system E:

$$E_1(s) = \frac{\alpha_1 F_2(s)}{[1 - \alpha_1 F_1(s) - \alpha_1 F_2(s) F_3(s)]} \tag{9.87}$$

$$E_2(s_1, s_2) = \alpha_2 F_2(s_1) F_2(s_2)\{[1 - \alpha_1 F_1(s_1) - \alpha_1 F_2(s_1) F_3(s_1)]$$
$$\times [1 - \alpha_1 F_1(s_2) - \alpha_1 F_2(s_2) F_3(s_2)][1 - \alpha_1 F_1(s_1 + s_2)$$
$$- \alpha_1 F_2(s_1 + s_2) F_3(s_1 + s_2)]\}^{-1} \tag{9.88}$$

Finally, we arrive at the final stage, in which we have to incorporate the filters of the two synapses. This is a case of a system with two inputs and one output (cf. Sec. 4.4). We have (see Fig. 9.16D)

$$Z_1(s) = I_x(s) X(s) \tag{9.89}$$

$$Z_2(s) = I_u(s) U(s) \tag{9.90}$$

Then

$$y(t) = \int_0^\infty e_1(\tau) z(t - \tau)\, d\tau + \int\int_0^\infty e_2(\tau_1, \tau_2) z(t - \tau_1) z(t - \tau_2)\, d\tau_1\, d\tau_2$$

$$= \int_0^\infty e_1(\tau)[z_1(t - \tau) + z_2(t - \tau)]\, d\tau$$

$$+ \int\int_0^\infty e_2(\tau_1, \tau_2)[z_1(t - \tau_1) + z_2(t - \tau_1)][z_1(t - \tau_2) + z_2(t - \tau_2)]\, d\tau_1\, d\tau_2$$

$$\tag{9.91}$$

from which we finally find the kernels of the overall two-input-one-output system:

First-order kernels:

$$H_{1x}(s) = I_x(s)E_1(s) \tag{9.92}$$

$$H_{1u}(s) = I_u(s)E_1(s) \tag{9.93}$$

Second-order self-kernels:

$$H_{2xx}(s_1, s_2) = I_x(s_1)I_x(s_2)E_2(s_1, s_2) \tag{9.94}$$

$$H_{2uu}(s_1, s_2) = I_u(s_1)I_u(s_2)E_2(s_1, s_2) \tag{9.95}$$

Second-order cross-kernel:

$$H_{2xu}(s_1, s_2) = 2I_x(s_1)I_u(s_2)E_2(s_1, s_2) \tag{9.96}$$

Application to Physiological Feedback and Cascade Systems

There is evidence that the system light → horizontal cell in the catfish retina has a feedback path from the horizontal cells back to the photoreceptors, which becomes active at high light levels and is inactive at low ones (cf. P. Z. Marmarelis and Naka, 1973*b,c*). Thus, this system can be studied under both open-loop and closed-loop conditions simply by varying the mean light level of stimulation. Experiments were performed at both low and high mean light levels (points B and A in Fig. 9.17). The kernels $h_1(\ )$ and $h_2(\ )$ for both cases are shown in Fig. 9.17. From these results we see that $h_2(\ )$ for the low light level is almost zero. Then, letting $F_1(s)$ be the Laplace transform of the first-order kernel at high light level, $F_2(s_1, s_2)$ be the Laplace transform of the second-order kernel at high light level, $G_1(s)$ be the Laplace transform of the first-order kernel at low light level, $L_1(s)$ be the Laplace transform of the first–order kernel of the feedback path, and $L_2(s_1, s_2)$ be the Laplace transform of the second-order kernel of the feedback path, we have from Eqs. (9.72) and (9.73) for a feedback nonlinear system that

$$F_1(s) = \frac{G_1(s)}{1 - G_1(s)L_1(s)} \tag{9.97}$$

$$F_2(s_1, s_2) = \frac{G_1(s_1)G_1(s_2)L_2(s_1, s_2)}{[1 - G_1(s_1)L_1(s_1)][1 - G_1(s_2)L_1(s_2)][1 - G_1(s_1+s_2)L_1(s_1+s_2)]} \tag{9.98}$$

Since $F_1(s)$, $F_2(s_1, s_2)$, $G_1(s)$ are known (measured experimentally) we can find the nonlinear dynamics of the feedback path from these two equations by solving for $L_1(s)$ and $L_2(s_1, s_2)$.

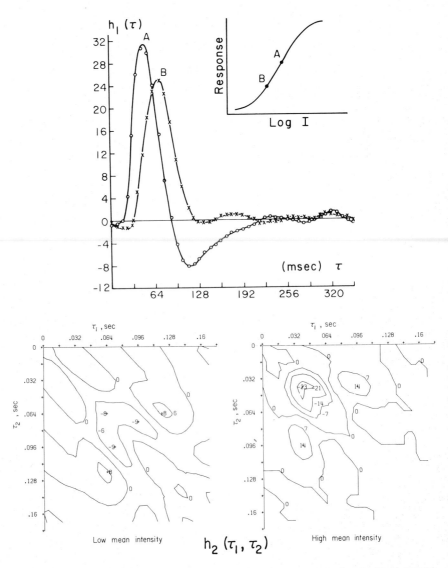

Fig. 9.17. First- and second-order kernels of system light → horizontal cell under low and high mean light levels. [From Marmarelis, P.Z., and K.-I. Naka (1973). *J. Neurophysiol.*, **36**, 605–648, by permission.]

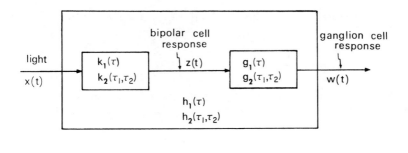

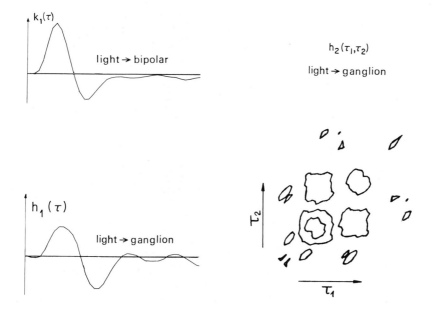

Fig. 9.18. Kernels for the cascade light → bipolar cell → ganglion cell. The second-order kernel of subsystem light → bipolar cell is negligible.

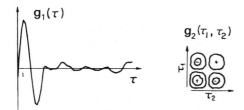

Fig. 9.19. First- and second-order kernels for subsystem bipolar cell → ganglion cell.

We turn now our attention to another physiological system. Using the analysis of Sec. 9.3 for general nonlinear systems in cascade, we can analyze the cascade of systems light→bipolar cell and bipolar cell→ ganglion cell. The data we have are for the system light→bipolar cell and the overall system light→ganglion cell. We seek to find the (nonlinear, dynamic) characteristics of the system bipolar cell→ganglion cell.

Figure 9.18 shows the kernels obtained experimentally. The system light→bipolar cell is nearly linear, and we thus have taken its second-order kernel to be zero. Using Eqs. (9.64) and (9.65) for a cascade combination we can find the desired kernels for the system bipolar cell→ganglion cell. The results are shown in Fig. 9.19. We note that this system seems to act as a differentiator (bandpass filter) followed by a rectifier.

10

Applications of the White-Noise Method to Neural Systems

Introduction

In the previous chapters we covered the theoretical foundation of the white-noise method and the practical considerations of its actual use in physiological system identification and analysis. In this chapter we present some representative applications of the white-noise method to neural system identification and analysis. These applications are chosen because they include rather interesting cases of physiological system identification (e.g., one or two inputs, continuous or discrete input or output, etc.) and illustrate the various techniques and strategies of the white-noise method (e.g., choice of quasiwhite stimulus, representation of discrete data etc.).

10.1. Practical Considerations in Application of the White-Noise Method to Neural Systems

In identifying neural systems through white-noise stimulation, several considerations come into play in practice. These must be carefully assessed in each case. For this purpose the following comments are made.

10.1.1. Dynamic Range of Stimulus

Neural systems, especially sensory ones, respond to stimuli covering a very wide dynamic range: 4–6 log units for sensory neural systems are quite common. It is technically impossible (unless very expensive and sophisticated means are employed) to produce quasiwhite noise signals that will cover such large dynamic ranges with typical laboratory equipment. Therefore, in practice, we can identify a system only over a portion of its total dynamic range with a single white-noise experiment.

Accordingly, a particular system can be analyzed over its total range with white-noise stimuli employed at several stimulus average levels that cover its total operating region. Although this approach burdens us with long identifying experiments (several separate experiments have to be conducted to cover the total dynamic range of the system), it has the advantage that the resolution of the derived characterization for a given stimulus average level is better than in the case where one tries to cover the total system range with a single experiment.

10.1.2. Stationarity of System Response

The method requires that the system under study be stationary. This is a difficult condition to meet in practice rigorously, especially in the case of intracellular recording from smaller neurons. Usually, the cell response is stationary only over a limited period of time. The identification task must then be carried out over this short time as efficiently as possible. The white-noise approach fulfills this requirement in that it allows the system to be tested with a great variety of stimulus waveforms in a short period of time. The resulting system characterization in terms of kernels is a statistical average characterization in the sense that it describes the "average" dynamic nonlinear characteristics of the system. Such an averaging approach results, in many cases, in noise-free estimates provided the biological noise present satisfies certain weak requirements. In comparison with the traditional approach of using sinusoidal or pulse inputs, the white-noise approach has, therefore, three great advantages: (a) It allows a complete and systematic description of the system nonlinearities; (b) it provides system characterizations that are in many cases free of the contaminating noise; and (c) given the limited life of the preparation (with respect to the stationarity of the system) it provides a testing signal that has a very high "information content," meaning that the system is tested at a high rate with many different waveforms. The last point is extremely important in the case of nonlinear biological systems. It is made stronger in the extension of the method to multi-input systems, because the orthogonality of the functional terms in the series and the independence of the white-noise signals exciting each input incorporates the results that would be obtained by performing several single-input experiments and, in addition, together with a description of the interaction between the several inputs. Thus, the information gained per unit time of experiment is increased more than linearly with the number of inputs.

10.1.3. Lower-Frequency Limitations

Since the signal-to-noise ratio for neural systems is usually low, and since these systems tend to be nonstationary over long periods of experimentation, the period of lowest frequency component of the white-noise signal for which the system can be reliably tested is about 1/10 to 1/20 of the total record length of the identifying experiment. Moreover, the computation time needed to obtain the nonlinear kernels increases rapidly with increasing length of the stimulus–response record for a given sampling rate (determined by the highest frequency present). These considerations determine the limits of the frequency range over which the system can be identified with reasonable accuracy within the usual experimental time.

10.1.4. Intracellular Recording

There are two significant advantages in applying the white-noise method to intracellular response recording from smaller neurons (such as bipolar, amacrine, or ganglion cells), where it is difficult to record reliably for a long time: (a) The white-noise test utilizes the whole recording time to obtain a great variety of stimulus–response data, as compared with a brief pulse test given once every few seconds or sinusoidal stimulation, which tends to be rather repetitious and redundant; and (b) many types of noise, such as electrode noise or interference noise, can be eliminated through the crosscorrelation procedure of the method.

10.1.5. Modeling of Neural Systems

Identification through white-noise analysis is a "black-box" modeling approach in the sense that it defines the transfer characteristics of a given neural system without specifying the internal structure of this system. However, as we develop the ability to record from more points in the neuronal network, these "black boxes" will be broken up into smaller "black-box" subsystems whose organization will reflect intimately the morphological and physiological structure of the system (cf. Naka *et al.*, 1975).

This is the black-box approach to modeling by which large systems are analyzed (modeled) in terms of their component systems. It should be stressed that there is no stimulus–response experiment that would reveal the "internal structure" of a system without making certain assumptions about alternative structural configurations. That is, a stimulus–response experiment could conceivably, in certain cases, distinguish between two possible structural configurations, but cannot determine uniquely the system structure without any *a priori* information. In both cases (i.e., whether assumptions are made or not) the white-noise approach has advantages over the traditional approaches since it nearly maximizes the rate of information gathering about the system behavior and results in a complete quantitative description.

Finally, it should be pointed out that the traditional pulse-stimulus testing of neural systems is less "natural" than the stimulus conditions involved in the white-noise experiment. Fluctuation of stimulus intensity around a certain average level is probably what most neural systems encounter in their natural environment.

10.2. Identification of One-Input Neural Systems Using GWN Stimulus

10.2.1. System with Continuous Input and Continuous Output: Light → Horizontal Cell

In this application the stimulus is a light covering the entire receptive field and projected uniformly in space upon the retina; it is modulated in time by a GWN signal. The average light intensity of the GWN stimulus is such as to "bias" the system near the middle of its operational range. The bandwidth of the GWN stimulus is 50 Hz and its dynamic range is about 1.6 log units. This means that

$$\log_{10}\left(\frac{I_{av}+3\sigma}{I_{av}-3\sigma}\right) = 1.6 \tag{10.1}$$

where I_{av} is the average light intensity and σ is the standard deviation of the amplitude at the Gaussian distribution of the stimulus signal. Clearly, this dynamic range of the stimulus covers only part of the total operational range of this sensory system. Typically, this system has a dynamic range of operation that spans 4–6 log units. Therefore, in order to characterize it completely, several GWN experiments are necessary, each covering a different portion of its operational range.

Following procedures discussed in Sec. 8.4 it was found that the system has a bandwidth that varies from about 6 Hz at low mean intensity levels to about 13 Hz at high mean intensity levels; accordingly, a GWN stimulus bandwidth of 50 Hz was chosen for the experiments. The number of kernels to be evaluated was estimated from the horizontal cell responses to sine wave stimuli, following Fourier analysis (cf. Sec. 8.5). Following procedures described in Chapter 8, we estimated the memory of the system (settling time) at about 150 msec and the length of the required GWN stimulus–response record, in order to obtain a statistical error of less than 5% in the estimation of the kernel values, to be about 1 min.

Figure 10.1 shows the estimated first-order kernel $h_1(\tau)$. From $h_1(\tau)$ we deduce that the system has a latency of about 15 msec and it is slightly underdamped. The same figure shows a contour map of the second-order kernel $h_2(\tau_1, \tau_2)$. This is interpreted to signify the deviations from linearity due to temporal interaction between different portions of the input. The set $\{h_1(\tau), h_2(\tau_1, \tau_2)\}$ is equivalent to the second-order nonlinear dynamic characterization (model) of the system under study.

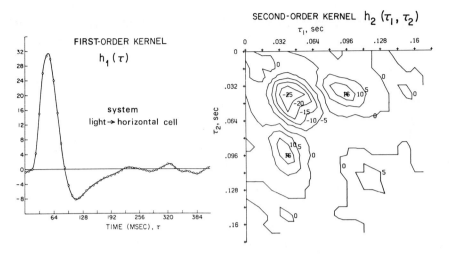

Fig. 10.1. First- and second-order kernels for the system light → horizontal cell.

Given this characterization, the question arises: How good is it? How does one measure "goodness" of a nonlinear model for which the principle of superposition does not apply?

According to the Wiener theory (Wiener, 1942), the criterion of "goodness" of a nonlinear model is how well it performs when tested with a Gaussian white-noise input. Such an input tests a system with a great variety of stimuli (waveforms) and therefore it is general and stringent as a test of "goodness" of a given model. In fact, Wiener showed that two systems are equivalent if and only if they respond identically to a Gaussian white-noise input. Therefore, "goodness" of the model can be measured by calculating its response to GWN and comparing it to the experimental response of the system under study when it is excited by the same stimulus. Such a comparison can be made by measuring the agreement in waveshape of the responses of the two systems (model and physical) to GWN, e.g., in terms of the mean-square deviation. Other criteria of "goodness" of the model consist of comparing the model and physical system responses, to such specialized inputs as pulses and sine waves, comparing, for example, their output frequency spectra.

Figure 10.2 shows samples of horizontal cell responses to GWN and model responses to this same input for the first- (linear) and second-order (nonlinear) models. We note that the linear model description—resulting from $h_1(\tau)$—is quite good in duplicating the horizontal cell response. This indicates that, for this limited dynamic range of input, the system is almost linear. There are, however, some small improvements resulting from the addition of the nonlinear term (represented by h_2).

The mean-square error for the linear and nonlinear models is computed as follows. The zeroth-order model $\{h_0\}$ is a constant equal to the average value of the response over the entire record. The mean-square-error for this model is computed and normalized to 100 (arbitrary) units. The error is measured over the entire length of the GWN record. The mean-square error for the linear (h_1) model is 26 units and the error for the nonlinear (h_1, h_2) model is 16 units. There is, therefore, substantial improvement by adding the second-order nonlinear term. The improvement is mainly due to correcting rise and fall times of the response and peak-to-valley relationships. This will become clear when we examine sine wave responses for these models (Fig. 10.3).

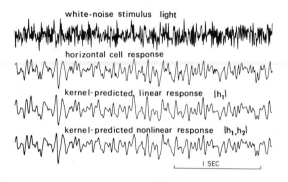

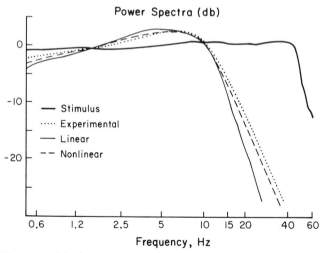

Fig. 10.2. Response of horizontal cell to white-noise stimulus and corresponding kernel-predicted responses (linear and nonlinear). The power spectra of these signals are also shown.

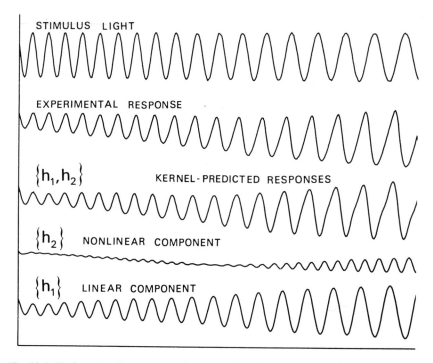

Fig. 10.3. Horizontal cell response to sine wave stimuli and corresponding kernel-predicted responses to this same stimulus.

Figure 10.2 also shows the power spectra of the GWN stimulus, the experimentally obtained horizontal cell response, and the corresponding linear and nonlinear model responses. It is seen that the system has a bandwidth of around 10 Hz. Note how the nonlinear model improves significantly the performance, over that of the linear model, in the high-frequency region. This is intuitively expected, since a nonlinearity introduces harmonics that show up in the higher frequencies.

Although the nonlinearity in the light → horizontal cell system is small, it can, under some conditions, be very conspicuous. One such case can be found with sine wave stimuli in the range of 4–18 Hz. A response with a slow-rising and fast-falling waveform is then evoked. The linear model (h_1 alone), of course, fails to describe any nonlinear phenomena, but the additon of the response due to h_2 can reproduce these nonlinearities with reasonable accuracy (Fig. 10.3). Figure 10.3 shows a sinusoidal stimulus and the experimental and model (both linear and nonlinear) responses for a range of frequencies. Note that the model reproduces well the asymmetric rising and falling phases of the response as well as the upward drift of the mean level of the response with an increase in frequency. The inflection point in the rising phase of the model response indicates the second harmonic introduced by the response component due to the nonlinear kernel (h_2).

10.2.2. System with Continuous Input and Discrete Output: Horizontal Cell → Ganglion Cell

Figure 10.4 shows a schematic diagram of the neuron chain horizontal cell → bipolar cell → ganglion cell that forms part of the catfish retinal network. The stimulus is extrinsic electrical current injected into the

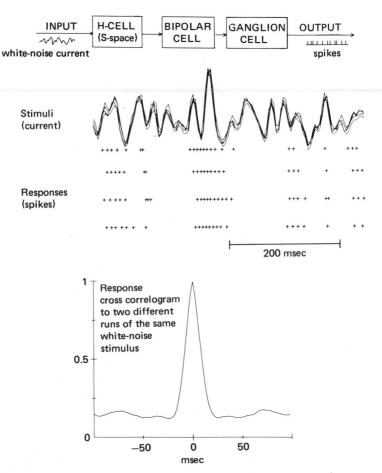

Fig. 10.4. Schematic diagram of catfish retinal neural chain and its reponse to identical GWN stimuli. The crosscorrelogram between two of these responses is also shown. [From Marmarelis, P.Z., and K.-I. Naka (1973) , *J. Neurophysiol.*, **36**, 605–648.]

horizontal cell (at a location approximately 0.3 mm away from the spike-recording site) and the response is the spike train (point process) from the ganglion cell. We wish to obtain a nonlinear dynamic characterization of this system.

The discrete output data are treated as continuous using the following procedure. A GWN stimulus (32 sec long) is repeated ten times and the evoked ganglion responses (spikes) are superposed and histogrammed in time, resulting in continuous-response waveform that signifies the instantaneous spike frequency of the ganglion discharge. The GWN stimulus bandwidth in this case extends from 0 to about 30 Hz. Figure 10.4 shows a short portion of the identical white-noise stimuli (superposed) and the corresponding evoked spike responses for four such runs (the occurrence of each spike is marked in time by a cross mark). The crosscorrelogram (Figure 10.4) between two of these records measures the signal-to-noise ratio in the system, as indicated by the peak-to-background ratio of the correlogram.

Figure 10.5 shows the first-order and the second-order kernels of this system. The first-order kernel, h_1, is a sharp positive wave followed by a smaller negative undershoot. This indicates that a hyperpolarizing (in the figure hyperpolarization of the horizontal cell is plotted as an upward deflection) impulse of the horizontal cell potential produces an initial excitation of the ganglion response (on-discharge) followed by a depression.

In the plot of the second-order kernel we notice two distinct areas: a small area of high positivity (for $\tau_1 = 16$–40 msec, $\tau_2 = 16$–40 msec), and a larger area of low negativity. This indicates that, if for example two impulses are given within an interval of 24 msec, the evoked response 20 msec after the occurrence of the second impulse will be enhanced more than indicated by linear superposition (due to h_1), while if the two impulses are approximately 32 msec apart, the ganglion discharge 32 msec after the occurrence of the second impulse will be depressed (i.e., less than that expected from linear superposition).

To assess the goodness of this characterization, Fig. 10.6 shows a portion of the white-noise stimulus, the evoked (experimental) ganglion response, and the corresponding responses to this same stimulus as they are predicted by the estimated kernels. As indicated in the figure, the first-order (linear) characterization performed poorly (MSE of 43%), while addition of the second-order (nonlinear) term improved markedly the model performance (MSE of 20%), indicating a strong second-order nonlinearity in the system. The improvement resulted in a sharpening of the peaks and rectification of the negative deflection seen in the first-order model response. The same figure also shows the power spectra for the stimulus, the experimental response, the linear and the nonlinear

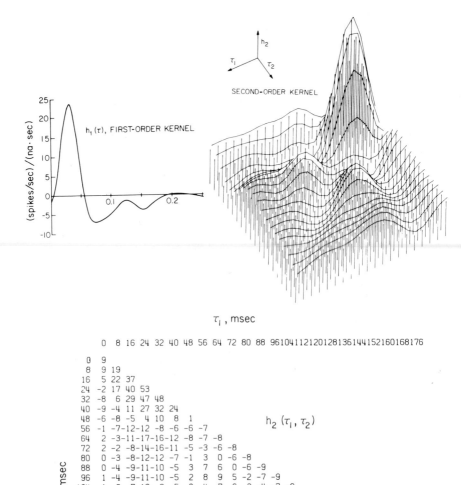

Fig. 10.5. First- and second-order kernels for the system horizontal cell → ganglion cell.

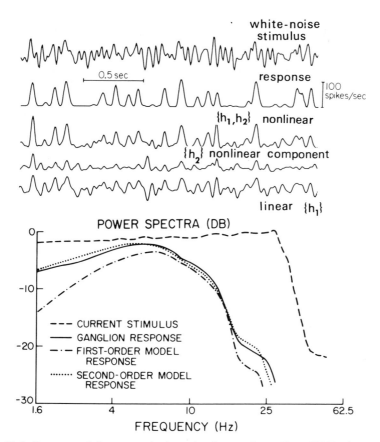

Fig. 10.6. Response of the system horizontal cell→ganglion cell to GWN stimulus and corresponding kernel-predicted responses. The power spectra of these signals are also shown.

(second-order) model responses. Notice how the incorporation of the nonlinear term improves both the low- and high-frequency characterization; specifically, notice the secondary peak around 20 Hz introduced by h_2.

Figure 10.7 shows the response to an impulse predicted by the linear model for this neural system as well as the experimentally obtained response of the system to an (hyperpolarizing) impulse-current stimulus. Agreement is good between experimental responses and kernel-predicted responses in terms of rise–fall times, but it is bad regarding the absence of spike discharge for the negative portion of h_1. If the nonlinear part of the model response (h_2) is added—the total model response to an impulse $\delta(t)$ is $h_1(t) + h_2(t, t)$—then the agreement between model and experiment improves somewhat. This improvement consists mainly of a sharpening in the rise and fall times and a reduction of the negative undershoot. This is expected because the

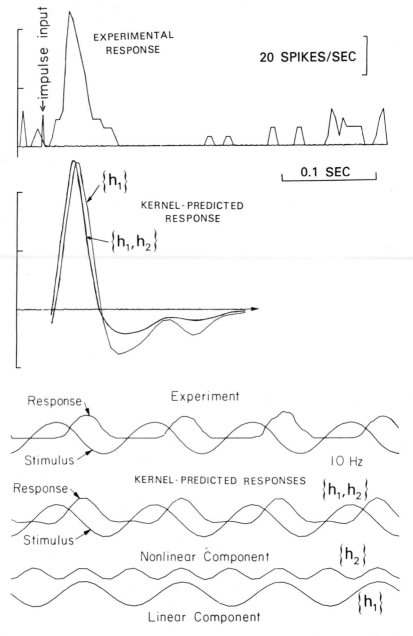

Fig. 10.7. System response to impulse and sine wave compared to responses predicted by estimated kernels of Fig. 10.5 for the horizontal cell → ganglion cell system.

nonlinear term (h_2) primarily describes a rectification process (taking place in the neural chain), which is not very evident in the case of an impulse stimulus, but is revealed by sinusoidal stimulation. Figure 10.7 shows model and experimental stimulus–response waveforms for a sinusoidal input of 10 Hz. The agreement, including the rectifying nonlinearity, is remarkably good. In this figure, it is interesting to notice how the nonlinear component, a sine wave of twice the frequency, introduces half-wave rectification.

10.3. Identification of Two-Input Neural Systems Using GWN Stimulus

As discussed in Chapter 4, physiological systems must often be studied in configurations entailing more than one input and output. We present here examples of two-input analysis. The first example is taken from applications on the vertebrate retina in which both the stimulus and response are continuous signals. The second example is from applications on an invertebrate retina in which the stimulus is continuous and the response is a discrete spike train.

10.3.1. System with Continuous Inputs and Continuous Output: Spot and Annulus Light → Horizontal Cell

The common form of "receptive field" for a neuron in the vertebrate retina is a geometric area consisting of two distinct components, a spot (receptive-field center), and a concentric annulus (receptive-field surround), as determined by the distinct type of response they elicit from the retinal neurons when each is stimulated. Thus a natural way to study these systems is to consider them as two-input one-output systems and employ two photic stimuli: a small spot of light (in this case, 0.3 mm in diameter) and a concentric annulus of light (in this case, with inner diameter of 0.3 mm and an outer diameter of 5 mm), each modulated by statistically independent GWN signals. These two stimuli were designed to cover the two distinct components of the receptive field: center and surround. The GWN stimuli used (light intensities modulated in GWN fashion) in the identifying experiment had a flat power spectrum up to 55 Hz and a dynamic amplitude range of 1.6 log units.

In the previous sections we described results of white-noise analysis of the catfish retinal neuron systems in which a single stimulus was used, such as a spot or annular GWN light stimulus. It was assumed that these two modes of stimulation (spot or annulus) evoked responses by activating distinct neural pathways in this retina. The two-input white noise experiments described in this section permit the study of the interaction between

Table 10.1. Notation for Kernels of Two-Input System

h_0	Zero-order kernel, a constant (one- or two-input experiment)
$h_{1s/a}(\tau)$	First-order self-kernel for spot input (two-input experiment)
$h_{1a/s}(\tau)$	First-order self-kernel for annulus input (two-input experiment)
$h_{2ss}(\tau_1, \tau_2)$	Second-order self-kernel for spot input (two-input experiment)
$h_{2aa}(\tau_1, \tau_2)$	Second-order self-kernel for annulus input (two-input experiment)
$h_{2as}(\tau_1, \tau_2)$	Second-order cross-kernel between spot and annulus inputs
$h_{1s}(\tau)$	First-order kernel for spot input (one-input experiment)
$h_{1a}(\tau)$	First-order kernel for annulus input (one-input experiment)

these pathways subserving the center and surround mechanisms of the receptive field; in addition they permit the study of the role and contribution of each mechanism separately, in the presence of the other. As discussed in Sec. 4.4, the response arising from the simultaneous stimulation of the two inputs can be separated into the components evoked by each input stimulus separately, as well as the component due to the interaction of the two inputs. The former are described completely by the self-kernels of each input while the latter is given by the cross-kernel (or interaction kernel). Thus, the self-kernels of input "spot" characterize the response of the system to the "spot" input, considering the other input (i.e., the annulus) as having a constant value equal to its average. We denote the kernels as shown in Table 10.1.

Figure 10.8 shows the first-order kernels for the light $\rightarrow$ horizontal cell system obtained through GWN stimulation for the following three cases: a one-input spot stimulus; a one-input annular stimulus; and a two-input stimulus composed of a spot and an annulus independently modulated by GWN signals. Hyperpolarization of the cell has been plotted upwards. We note that the annular self-kernel $h_{1a/s}$ is very similar to h_{1a}. However, $h_{1s/a}$ is larger and faster than h_{1s}; i.e., the mechanism responsible for generation of the horizontal cell response to a light spot becomes faster and its gain increases in the presence of a constant annular input. On the other hand, presence of the spot input does not affect the annular response to any appreciable extent.

Figure 10.8 shows portions of the two GWN input signals (one for spot and the other for annulus) and the resulting horizontal cell response obtained experimentally together with the corresponding model response to these same inputs. The model response was computed from the kernel estimates of $h_{1s/a}$, $h_{1a/s}$, h_{2aa}, h_{2ss}, h_{2as}. Agreement between the system response and the model prediction is extremely good (MSE is 5%). The first-order contribution brings the error down to 12%, suggesting that the system is fairly linear.

An experiment similar to the one described above for the horizontal cell response was performed on a bipolar cell in the catfish retina (cf. P. Z.

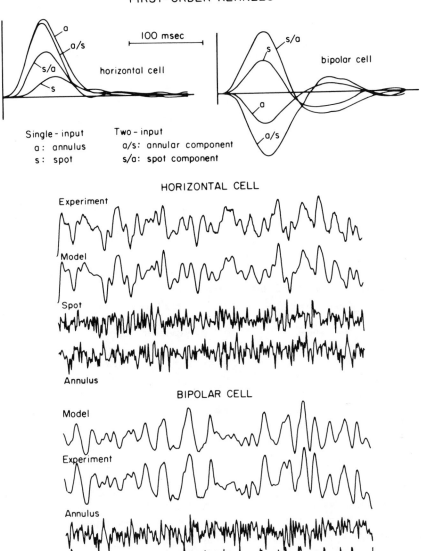

Fig. 10.8. First-order kernels and experimental and model responses of the two-input system (spot–annulus) for the horizontal and the bipolar cell.

*Table 10.2. Percentage MSE of Responses Predicted
by Several Models of a Two-Input System*

Response due to	Mean-square error
$\{h_0\}$	100
$\{h_{1s/a}, h_{1a/s}\}$	18
$\{h_{1s/a}, h_{1a/s}, h_{2aa}, h_{2ss}\}$	12
$\{h_{1s/a}, h_{1a/s}, h_{2aa}, h_{2ss}, h_{2as}\}$	6

Marmarelis and Naka, 1974d). The linear kernels (for one-input and two-input GWN stimuli) are shown in Fig. 10.8. Notice how the presence of the "other" input enhances the response to a spot or annulus in both cases. Responses to GWN stimuli, both experimental and kernel-predicted are shown in Fig. 10.8. The agreement in waveform is very good. The reduction in MSE is as shown in Table 10.2. We conclude that this system, under the indicated stimulating conditions, is fairly linear.

10.3.2. System with Continuous Inputs and Discrete Output: Two Spot Light → Horizontal Motion Detection Fiber

The system under study involves motion detecting neurons which are part of the visual nervous system of insects. It has been found that these neurons respond maximally when motion takes place within their receptive field in a preferred direction. The mechanisms underlying this basic sensory process have been under extensive investigation (cf. McCann, 1966, 1969; Poggio, 1973; Reichardt, 1961, 1970; Reichardt and Poggio, 1975, 1976; Poggio and Reichardt, 1973a,b, 1976).

The compound eye of insects consists of a matrix of "smaller eyes" called ommatidia, each with its own optical system (lens, etc.). Each ommatidium contains a small number of retinula cells, each of which has a distinct optical axis. They are arranged in a fairly regular array, as shown in Fig. 10.9. Motion-sensitive neurons, located in the optic lobe of the insect brain, respond maximally to motions along two coordinate directions— approximately horizontally and vertically, as shown in Fig. 10.9. For each direction there is a pair of neurons, each tuned to respond maximally to one of the two vector senses of this direction; e.g., for the horizontal direction, there is one fiber responding maximally to motions from left to right and one responding to motions in the opposite sense, i.e., from right to left. The functional properties (dynamics) of each fiber type are approximately the same. Our objective is to identify this neural system.

A two-input experiment was performed (cf. P. Z. Marmarelis and McCann, 1973) in which the stimulus consisted of two spots of light placed with the line connecting them aligned with the axis of motion detection (Fig. 10.9) and properly spaced for maximum motion-induced response from the neuron. The two lights (light a and light b) were modulated by two independent GWN sources. The power spectrum of this stimulus was flat from zero up to about 80 Hz. The spike-train response of the horizontal motion detection cell was measured by an extracellular electrode. The following procedure was followed in order to convert the output spike records into continuous functions of time: The GWN stimulus record was formed by several sequences (6–12) of identical (40-sec duration) GWN records. The neuron spike responses to these runs of identical stimuli were superimposed and histogrammed in time to produce a continuous function, which denotes the spike frequency as a function of time.

From this two-input, one-output experiment five characterizing kernels are obtained: $\{h_{1a}(\tau), h_{1b}(\tau), h_{2aa}(\tau_1, \tau_2), h_{2bb}(\tau_1, \tau_2), h_{2ab}(\tau_1, \tau_2)\}$. The set $\{h_{1a}(\tau), h_{2aa}(\tau_1, \tau_2)\}$—the self-kernels due to input a—describe the contribution of this input to the total system response. Similarly for set $\{h_{1b}(\tau), h_{2bb}(\tau_1, \tau_2)\}$. Kernel $h_{2ab}(\tau_1, \tau_2)$ is the cross-kernel (or interaction kernel) and denotes the nonlinear interaction of the two inputs as it affects the system response (Fig. 10.10) assuming a second-order system.

Figure 10.11 shows the two first-order kernels h_{1a} and h_{1b}, which are quite different. Kernel $h_{1b}(\tau)$ is positive while $h_{1a}(\tau)$ is somewhat negative; this is a manifestation of selectivity. If an impulse is given at input b, a positive response (increase from the mean response level) will be evoked, while an impulse given at input a will elicit a negative reaction (decrease of the mean response). In interpreting these results it should be noted that the two signals at a and b have a certain mean level (dc value) and are measured with respect to this level taken as reference (zero level).

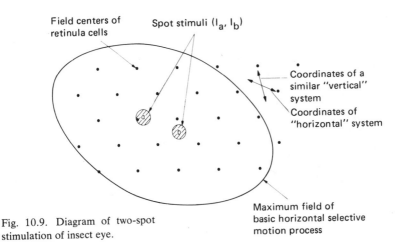

Fig. 10.9. Diagram of two-spot stimulation of insect eye.

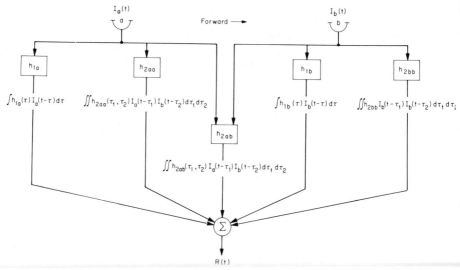

Fig. 10.10. Diagram of second-order two-input system functional relation between stimulus and response. [From Marmarelis, P. Z., and G. D. McCann (1973). *Biol. Cyb.* (formerly *Kybernetik*), **12**, 74–89, by permission.]

Figure 10.11 also shows the two self-kernels h_{2aa} and h_{2bb} as square arrays of numbers. Similar comments apply to them: self-kernel h_{2aa} is very small (nearly null) while self-kernel h_{2bb} has significant values. This is again a manifestation of selectivity. The contribution of these self-kernels to the system response can be seen in Fig. 10.12. It should be noted that while the self-kernels describe the contribution of each input separately, their effect is dependent upon the fact that there is a nonzero, steady (dc) signal at the other input.

Figure 10.11 also shows the interaction kernel $h_{2ab}(\tau_1, \tau_2)$. It is here that selectivity in motion detection is clearly exhibited. In the region $\tau_1 > \tau_2$ there is a large positive peak (forward motion) while in the region $\tau_2 > \tau_1$ there is a large negative peak (reverse motion). As described earlier, this kernel denotes quantitatively the contribution to the response that is due to the nonlinear dynamic interaction between the input signal at a and the input signal at b. From this kernel we see that a pulse at a followed by a pulse at b (i.e., $\tau_1 > \tau_2$) will elicit a large positive response, while a pulse at b followed by a pulse at a (i.e., $\tau_2 > \tau_1$) will produce a negative response. These expectations are indicated by h_{2ab}, which also clearly shows the temporal extent of such "cross-talk" (about 60 msec) as well as what the time course of the elicited response would be. In essence, h_{2ab} is a concise nonlinear dynamic description of the selective part of the response of the neuron evoked by the two spot stimuli.

A portion of the GWN stimuli as well as the corresponding experimental and kernel-predicted responses are shown in Fig. 10.12. The kernel

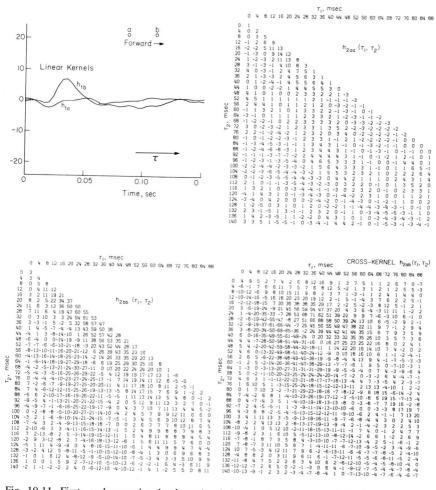

Fig. 10.11. First- and second-order kernels of the two-input system of Fig. 10.9. [From Marmarelis, P. Z., and G. D. McCann (1973). *Biol. Cyb.* (formerly *Kybernetik*), **12**, 74–89, by permission.]

responses have been partitioned into the different components that they represent. The mean-square-error reduction, where the error for the $\{h_0\}$ model (i.e., a constant equal to the average response) is 100 units, is as shown in Table 10.3. It is noted that the system is strongly nonlinear (the linear model produces only a 3% reduction of the error) and that the nonlinear dynamic cross talk (between a and b) term is very large (31% error reduction from the self-kernel model). The same figure also shows the response power spectra for both experimental and kernel-predicted responses as well as the spectra of the two GWN stimuli. The system has a

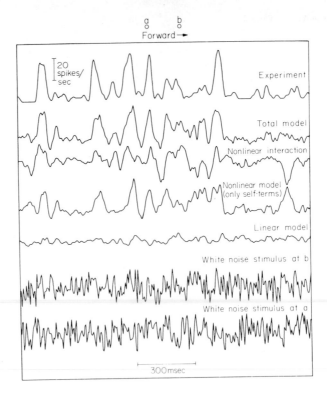

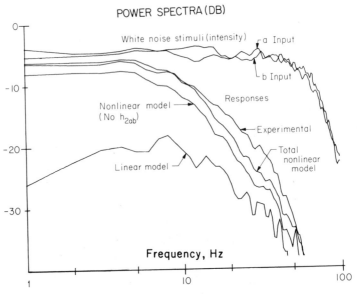

Fig. 10.12. Experimental and model-predicted responses of the two-input system of Fig. 10.9, and the respective power spectra of the signals. [From Marmarelis, P. Z., and G. D. McCann (1973). *Biol. Cyb.* (formerly *Kybernetik*), **12**, 74–89, by permission.]

Table 10.3. Percentage MSE of Responses Predicted by Several Models of a Two-Input System

Model	Kernel composition	Error
Constant	$\{h_0\}$	100
Linear	$\{h_{1a}, h_{1b}\}$	97
Self-, nonlinear	$\{h_{1a}, h_{1b}, h_{2aa}, h_{2bb}\}$	69
Total, nonlinear	$\{h_{1a}, h_{1b}, h_{2aa}, h_{2bb}, h_{2ab}\}$	38

corner frequency of about 5 Hz and rolls off at very high frequencies at a rate of 24 db/octave. It should be noted that the model performance at high frequencies (above 20 Hz approximately) deviates somewhat from the experimental response. This is due to "smoothing" of the response function and the fact that the characterization has been computed only up to second order (producing only up to the second harmonic). In this respect, it should be noted that the addition of the second-order nonlinearity improves the high-frequency model performance.

Thus, the characterization in terms of the set of kernels describes the system behavior fairly accurately in the case of GWN inputs. Typical experiments employing sequences of step stimuli at a and b that approximate forward and reverse motion are illustrated in Fig. 10.13. The kernel-predicted response to such forward and reverse sequences is compared to actual responses in Fig. 10.13. These tests were made using a preparation different from the one used for the kernel calculations. The agreement for this type of experiment is good.

10.4. Identification of One-Input Neural System Using Pseudorandom Binary Stimulus*

As an illustration of the use of pseudorandom signals in physiological system identification, we summarize here the work done by O'Leary *et al.* (1974), who used pseudorandom binary stimuli in a series of experiments aimed at the characterization of responses of afferent fibers in the semicircular canal. These responses are evoked by angular motion (cf. O'Leary *et al.*, 1974). Classically, the semicircular canal is considered to be a sensor of angular head motion during animal navigation. However, the transduction and encoding of specific head trajectories by the receptor hair cells is not

---

*Initial material provided by D. O'Leary.

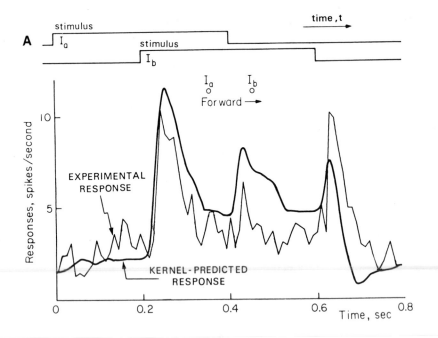

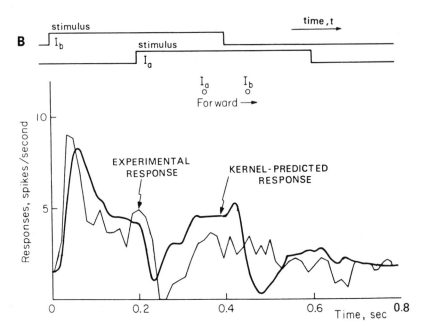

Fig. 10.13. Experimental and model-predicted responses to pulse stimuli for the system of Fig. 10.9. (A) Forward movement; (B) backward movement.

well understood. In addition, the correlation between the dynamic characteristics of these receptors and their local anatomical innervation, although of great importance, was described only recently (O'Leary *et al.*, 1974). To achieve this latter objective an experimentally efficient procedure was needed to accurately identify the dynamic characteristics of the various afferent bundles of fibers under the experimental difficulties present in such an undertaking. To this end, a pseudorandom binary stimulus provides significant advantages over the use of conventional deterministic stimuli such as sinusoidal and constant acceleration. These include the accurate determination of the small-signal linear characteristics of the system over wide bandwidths and in a fraction of the time required for conventional techniques. In addition, other noise sources that are uncorrelated with the input do not corrupt the system characterization.

The experiments were performed on bundles that separate and innervate specific areas of the crista of the guitarfish, *Rhinobatos productus*. Isolated labyrinths were prepared for afferent response recording by pithing the brain, removing the cranium and cartilage at the rear of the orbit to expose the horizontal ampullary nerve, and mounting the labyrinth on a rotating table. Single-unit spike trains were recorded by suspending severed nerve sub-bundles in air with a forceps electrode. The preparation was aligned on the rotational axis of a rotating table with the horizontal semicircular canal plane oriented parallel to that of the table (Fig. 10.14). The pseudorandom binary stimulus is generated by a circulating shift register that employs exclusive OR gates in feedback configuration such as shown in Fig. 10.15. The statistical properties of the generated signal have been discussed in Sec. 5.2. The binary signal in this experiment is directly proportional to the angular acceleration of the rotating table. Thus, in this system formulation, the input is acceleration and the output is the evoked spike train recorded with the forceps electrode.

The step length Δt of the binary stimulus was selected to correspond to the required high-frequency cutoff, and the binary sequence length N (number of bits in one period of the signal) was then selected to correspond to the required frequency band. Values of $\Delta t = 92$ msec and $N = 255$ were used, which resulted in a period of 23.5 sec and an input bandwidth approximately from 0.04 to 5 Hz, which are appropriate for this system.

To obtain the first-order (linear) kernel, crosscorrelation between the pseudorandom binary stimulus (6–16 periods of it) and the response was performed. A typical example is shown in Fig. 10.16. The linear kernel is shown plotted in Fig. 10.16B as computed by the crosscorrelation of the binary input with the experimental spike train output shown plotted in Fig. 10.16C. The latter is the average response trajectory obtained by averaging 18 periods of the output. Figure 10.16D is the response trajectory predicted by convolution of the linear kernel shown in Fig. 10.16B with the binary input. This differed from the experimental output shown in Fig. 10.16C by a percentage mean-square error of 7.3%. This implies that the linear kernel was a relatively good model for this afferent. A similar analysis of 62 afferents from this receptor resulted in an averaged mean-square error for this population of 10.2%. As a further test of the accuracy of the linear kernel for the afferent shown in Fig. 10.16, an impulse response of a low-order linear system was fitted to the experimental impulse response shown in Fig. 10.16B. The result, shown in Fig. 10.16A, was then used to predict by linear convolution the response to the binary input. The resulting prediction, shown in 10.16E, differed from the experimental output trajectory shown in 10.16C by 8.1% mean-square error, which again suggests excellent accuracy for the linear model (cf. O'Leary and Honrubia, 1975).

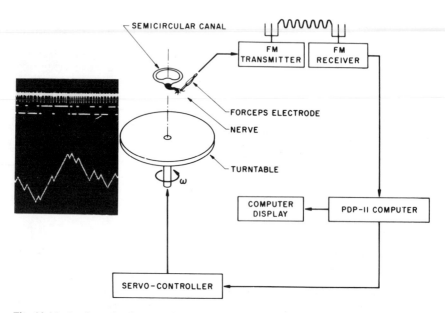

Fig. 10.14. A schematic diagram of the experimental apparatus used for on-line analysis of first-order afferent responses from the semicircular canal to controlled rotational ac-celeration inputs. Isolated guitarfish labyrinths were mounted at the center of rotation of a servo-controlled turntable shown at the left. A pseudorandom binary stimulus, generated by a PDP-11 computer program, controlled the direction of rotational acceleration of the table. A stainless-steel forceps was the active electrode for extracellular recording from dendrites innervating the horizontal semicircular canal. Single-unit spike trains were preamplified and broadcast using frequency modulation telemetry. A single PDP-11 assembly language pro-gram generated the white-noise stimulus, digitized the spike trains, crosscorrelated the input with the output, and displayed the resulting first-order kernel estimates on an oscilloscope display (on-line).

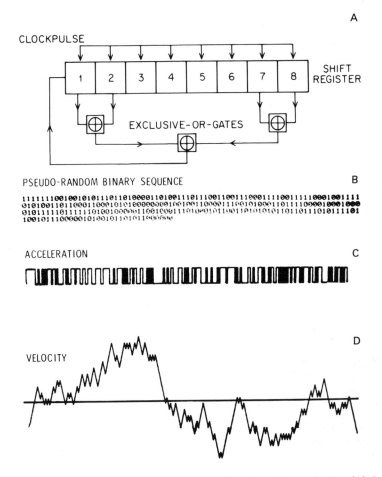

Fig. 10.15. The generation and interfacing of a pseudorandom binary stimulus. (A) A shift register formed from 8 flip-flops is shown with the output of selected pairs of bits fed back through exclusive OR gates to the first stage. A maximum length sequence of $2^8 - 1 = 255$ binary states (bits) is generated and repeats periodically as the register is shifted serially by a regularly timed clockpulse. (B) One stimulus period of 255 bits is shown as generated. (C) The output of a relay controller is shown as driven by the binary sequence. (D) The rotational velocity profile of the stimulus is shown as obtained by an integration of the acceleration pattern in (C). [From O'Leary, D. P., and V. Honrubia (1975). *Biophys. J.*, **15**, 505–532, by permission.]

10.5. Identification of One-Input Neural System Using CSRS Stimulus

In this section, we will illustrate the application of CSRS in identification of a physiological system, which is part of the visual neuron

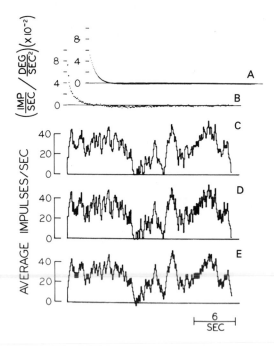

Fig. 10.16. Parametric and nonparametric impulse response models and their respective linear convolution output predictions to the binary input. (A) The parametric model is shown plotted from the equation $h(\tau) = 0.057 \exp(-1.11\tau) = 0.003 \exp(-0.047\tau)$, in which the numerical parameters were determined by a nonlinear least-squares regression technique. The parametric model was fitted on the experimental unit impulse response shown in (B). (C) The experimental afferent response of this unit is shown as averaged over 10 periods of the binary stimulus. (D) The response as predicted by linear convolution from the estimated impulse response shown in (B). This is in agreement with the experimental response shown in (C) with a mean-square error of 7.3%. (E) The response as predicted from the parametric linear system model shown in (A). It is in agreement with the experimental response shown in (C) within a mean-square error of 8.1%. [From O'Leary, D. P., and V. Honrubia (1975). *Biophys. J.*, **15**, 505–532, by permission.]

chain of the fly *Calliphora erythrocephala* (cf. V. Z. Marmarelis and McCann, 1977).

The physiological system under study is the very initial portion of a visual neuron chain, which operates as light-potential transducer in the photoreceptor cell 1–6. The input of the system is temporally varying light intensity applied to the eye of the fly and the output is a slow (continuous) potential recorded in the photoreceptor cell body. This system transforms photon energy to a slow potential through the isomerization of rhodopsin. This physicochemical process takes place within the membranes of micro-villi, which constitute the rhabdomere of the photoreceptor. The rhabdomere constitutes the site of the physiological processes that occur within the system.

In order to be able to employ the crosscorrelation technique in the identification of this system, we must show that the system satisfies the three basic requirements of stationarity, finite memory, and analyticity of the Volterra series expansion (cf. Sec. 4.1).

As far as the stationarity of the system is concerned, we test the stationarity hypothesis using the "run test" for the system response to a stationary Gaussian process, as outlined in Sec. 5.5. The outcome of the test is that we do not reject the stationarity hypothesis. The finite memory of the system is checked through the computation of the autocorrelation of the system response to a quasiwhite stimulus; and in a final check through the inspection of the system kernels themselves. The analyticity of the system is assumed on the basis of the expectable differential smoothness of a physical system, and it can only be checked indirectly through the identification and synthesis results obtained.

The CSRS stimuli used in this illustration are three members of the equirandom CSRS group (the members of this group are multilevel CSRS with a uniform probability distribution profile). These stimuli have various numbers of levels (namely, 2, 3, and 8 levels), the same operational range, the same step length, and the same record length.

The test parameters that we have used for all the stimuli are given in Table 10.4.

The first- and second-order CSRS kernel estimates for the CSRS stimuli with 2, 3, and 8 levels are shown in Figs. 10.17, 10.18, and 10.19 respectively. Portions of the CSRS stimuli with 2, 3, and 8 levels, the corresponding system responses and the second-order CSRS model-predicted responses are shown in Figs. 10.20, 10.21, and 10.22, respectively.

An interesting observation is that the size of the CSRS kernel estimate does not change significantly as the number of levels (and consequently the generalized power levels) change. This indicates the minor role of nonlinearities higher than the second order in the system.

Table 10.4. Test Parameters for CSRS Experiment

Step length	$\Delta t = 0.005$ sec
Record length	$T = 100$ sec
Sampling interval	$Dt = 0.001$ sec
Half operational range	$A = 1.85$ V (measured through a photocell)
First-order kernel memory	$\mu_1 = 0.05$ sec
Second-order kernel memory	$\mu_2 = 0.05$ sec

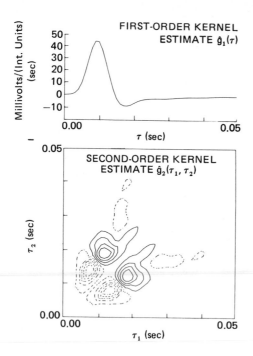

Fig. 10.17. First- and second-order kernel estimates of the photoreceptor of *Calliphora erythrocephala* (with white eyes) as obtained through the use of a two-level CSRS stimulus.

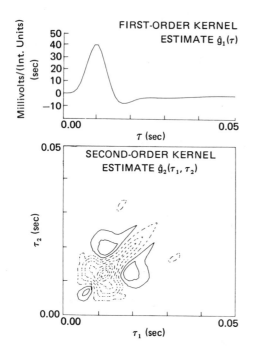

Fig. 10.18. First- and second-order kernel estimates of the photoreceptor of *Calliphora erythrocephala* (with white eyes) as obtained through the use of a three-level CSRS stimulus.

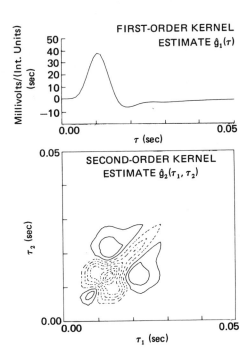

Fig. 10.19. First- and second-order kernel estimates of the photoreceptor of *Calliphora erythrocephala* (with white eyes) as obtained through the use of an eight-level CSRS stimulus. [From Marmarelis, V. Z., and G. D. McCann (1977). *Biol. Cyb.*, **27**, 57–62, by permission.]

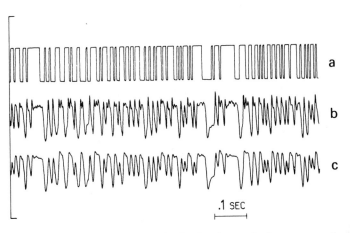

Fig. 10.20. Portion of the two-level CSRS stimulus (trace a), the corresponding system response (trace b), and the second-order model-predicted response (trace c). [From Marmarelis, V. Z., and G. D. McCann (1977). *Biol. Cyb.*, **27**, 57–62, by permission.]

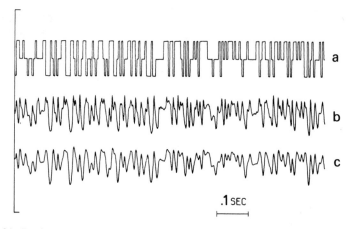

Fig. 10.21. Portion of the three-level CSRS stimulus (trace a), the corresponding system response (trace b), and the second-order model-predicted response (trace c). [From Marmarelis, V. Z., and G. D. McCann (1977). *Biol. Cyb.*, **27**, 57–62, by permission.]

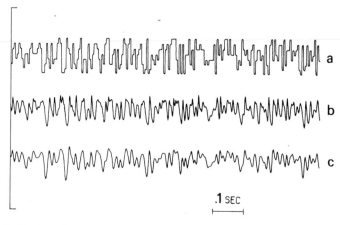

Fig. 10.22. Portion of the eight-level CSRS stimulus (trace a), the corresponding system response (trace b), and the second-order model-predicted response (trace c). [From Marmarelis, V. Z., and G. D. McCann (1977). *Biol. Cyb.*, **27**, 57–62, by permission.]

    The percentage MSE of the model-predicted response is found to be 12.28%, 11.43%, and 12.56% in the respective cases of equirandom CSRS stimuli with 2, 3, and 8 levels. This accuracy can be improved either by increasing the record length or by choosing the optimum step length Δt for the given record length (cf. Sec. 8.8). The optimization procedure outlined in Sec. 8.8 is actually followed and it yields an optimum step length of approximately 1.8 msec for a 100-sec-long record. This optimum step length is significantly smaller than the one used in the experiments above (5 msec).

10.6. Applications of Alternate Identification Techniques to Neural Systems with Discrete Input or Output

Variations of the white-noise method have been used in identification of discrete-output (impulse train) systems. Two of these variations as applied to neural systems are presented in this section.

10.6.1. System with Continuous Input and Discrete Output*

Bryant and Segundo (1976) applied the method described in Sec. 6.4 to the abdominal ganglion of *Aplysia californica* in an attempt to characterize the relation between neuron firing and transmembrane currents.

The basic experimental procedure was as follows: An identified cell was impaled intracellularly with two electrodes, one a single-barrel electrode for recording, the other a double-barrel electrode, one barrel for passing a continuously varying GWN current stimulus (Fig. 10.23).

*Initial material provided by H. L. Bryant and J. P. Segundo.

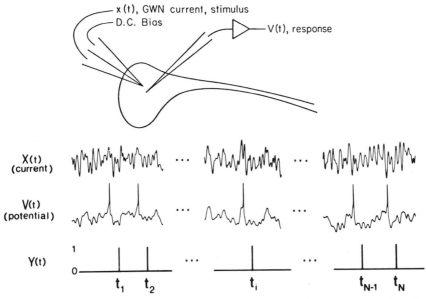

Fig. 10.23. Schematic of the experiment on the *Aplysia* cells. The response waveform is abstracted into an impulse train.

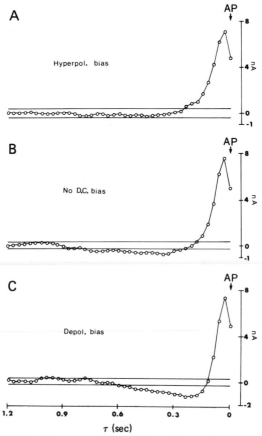

Fig. 10.24. First-order kernels corresponding to three different dc polarization levels of the *Aplysia* cell. [From Bryant, H. L., and J. P. Segundo (1976). *J. Physiol.*, **260**, 279–314, by permission.]

Figure 10.24 shows three first-order kernels corresponding to three different dc polarization levels. In A, the cell was subjected to GWN current stimulation during which a 10-nA hyperpolarizing dc current bias was imposed. In B, the GWN stimulation was repeated, but no dc bias was imposed. In C, the GWN stimulation was again repeated, but this time with a 10-nA depolarizing bias. The horizontal lines along the abscissa represent 98% confidence bands centered about the overall average of the noise, which was 0 nA. Any average value falling outside these limits does so by chance with a probability of only 2%.

As is clear from Fig. 10.24, the average of the effective stimulating epochs changes as a function of the presence and polarity of an imposed dc bias. This implies that the average stimulating epoch that the cell chooses from the ensemble of all possible epochs in producing an action potential is dependent on the dc current bias. (For a complete discussion of the results and their interpretation, cf. Bryant and Segundo, 1976.)

10.6.2. System with Discrete Input and Continuous Output*

The original white-noise method, as proposed for continuous-input–continuous-output systems, can be also used to identify discrete-input–continuous-output systems.

Krausz (1975) suggested a modification of the Wiener series to simplify this procedure if a Poisson impulse train is used as a stimulus. This modification amounts to the elimination of the lower-order integral terms of each Wiener functional, with simultaneous exclusion of the diagonal points from the integration range of the leading integral term. Krausz applied this technique experimentally to the characterization of the lobster cardiac ganglion (cf. Krausz, 1975).

The estimates of the first-, second-, and third-order kernels of the system are shown in Figs. 10.25, 10.26, and 10.27 respectively. Figure 10.28 shows a portion of the experimental system response (trace a), the response processed as to remove the high-frequency artifact (trace b), the response predicted by the second-order model (trace c), and the resposne predicted by the third-order model (trace d). The agreement between the actual and model responses is satisfactory and improves significantly with the inclusion of the third-order functional term.

*Initial material provided by H. Krausz.

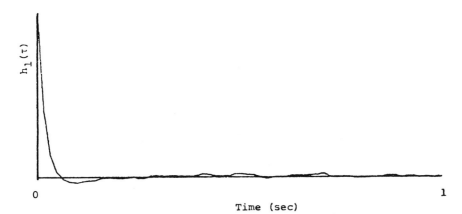

Fig. 10.25. First-order kernel of lobster cardiac ganglion.

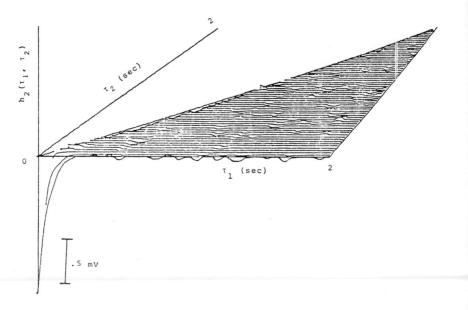

Fig. 10.26. Second-order kernel of lobster cardiac ganglion.

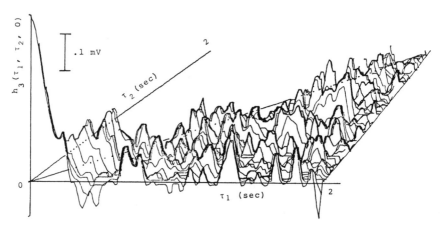

Fig. 10.27. Cross section of third-order kernel of lobster cardiac ganglion.

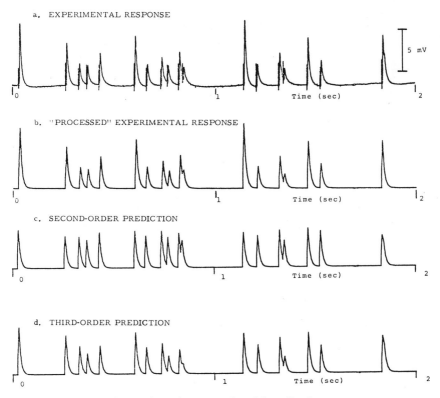

Fig. 10.28. Portions of system and model-predicted responses.

The fluctuation in the values of the third-order kernel estimate (cross section shown in Fig. 10.27) is largely of a statistical nature and appears so pronounced because of the limited length of the experimental record.

Physiological Systems Requiring Special Treatment

Introduction

In this chapter we discuss the identification procedures to be followed when the system does not fall into any of the categories covered in the previous chapters; for example, systems whose characteristics change with time (nonstationary systems), or whose inputs are functions of more than one independent variable (e.g., spatiotemporal stimuli). Several alternative methods of treating systems with point process (discrete) inputs and outputs (e.g., neural systems) are also presented.

11.1. Physiological Systems with Point Process Inputs and Outputs

In the study of neural systems the stimulus and response variables can be in the form of either continuous signals ("slow," analog potentials) or discrete signals (spike trains).

For example, consider the study of the *synapse* as shown in Fig. 11.1. In studying the synapse through stimulus–response experiments, we will be faced with the following types of situations (systems): (a) a system with input (presynaptic) a spike train and output (postsynaptic) a spike train; (b) input a spike train and output a continuous potential (PSP); (c) input a continuous signal (for example, current injected presynaptically) and output a spike train (presynaptic or postsynaptic); and (d) input a continuous signal and output a continuous signal. In these cases of discrete (spike train) input or output or both, several methods of treatment of the discrete data may be employed (cf. P. Z. Marmarelis and Naka, 1973; V. Z. Marmarelis and McCann, 1975). If the neural system has a high rate of firing (input, output or both), then a method such as the average histogram used by P. Z. Marmarelis and Naka (1973a) would be useful and, in fact, efficient. However, if the firing rate is low then a histogramming technique may tend to "obscure" a lot of the information contained in the *structure* of the spike train. Then the following techniques may be used.

Figure 11.2 shows a spike train and different ways of representing it. For each one way a somewhat different identification method and system representation would result. Since the waveform of the neural spike usually does not carry information, representation A is hardly ever used. Representation B, which just marks in time the occurrence of a spike (a "time of event") is used quite often. Representation C results by plotting as the waveform a constant value in the interval between spikes, this value being $1/\Delta t_s$, where Δt_s is the interspike interval. Representation D corresponds to counting the spikes within a fixed time interval and plotting the resulting number, i.e., forming a time histogram. Finally, in representation E the spike train is represented by a function $\varepsilon(t - t_i)$ in which, analogous to an impulse function, a spike is represented by a narrow pulse of width b and height $1/b$.

If the system input and output are represented as continuous functions, then the original white-noise method can be used directly. However, if the signals are represented as discrete functions (impulse trains), then variations of the original method can also be used. One such variation was presented in Sec. 6.4.

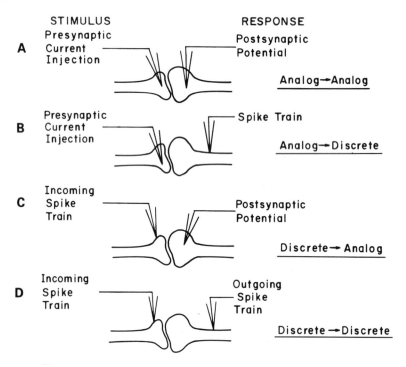

Fig. 11.1. The various types of system input/output encountered in the study of the synaptic mechanism.

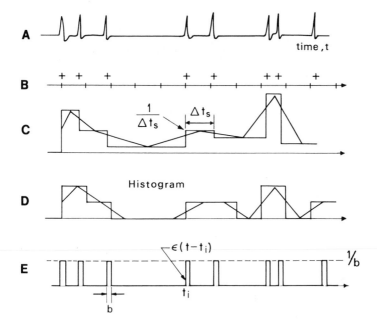

Fig. 11.2. Various modes of spike (impulse) train representation.

In the case of a system with impulse train input the question of interest is: What should the statistical properties (in terms of the autocorrelation functions of the process) of this point process be, so that we can estimate the system kernels in a computationally efficient way, given the limited lifetime of the experiment? Brillinger (1975b) and Krausz (1975) have answered this question by showing that a Poisson spike train possesses statistical properties equivalent to a white-noise stimulus.

Let us now consider the computation of the crosscorrelation functions in each of the cases (B, C, D) of Fig. 11.1, using representation E (of Fig. 11.2) for the discrete data. The operational role of each pulse $\varepsilon(t-t_i)$ is considered to coincide approximately with the one of an impulse.

11.1.1. Continuous-to-Discrete System

The stimulus and response records are as shown in Fig. 11.3. Assume the record length is R. Then the first-order crosscorrelation is

$$\phi_{yx}(\tau) = \frac{1}{R-\tau} \int_0^R y(t)x(t-\tau)\, dt$$

$$= \frac{1}{R-\tau} \int_0^R x(t-\tau) \sum_i \varepsilon(t-t_i)\, dt \approx \frac{1}{R-\tau} \sum_i x(t_i-\tau) \quad (11.1)$$

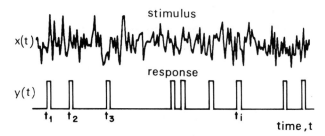

Fig. 11.3. Continuous white-noise stimulus and discrete response.

The extent to which τ is taken is equal to the system memory μ. Therefore, for any τ, the procedure for finding $\phi_{yx}(\tau)$ involves simply averaging the $x(t_i - \tau)$ waveforms of the stimulus for all t_i at which a response spike occurs. This is illustrated in Fig. 11.4. Notice that no multiplication is necessary in computing this correlation, only addition.

Similarly, we compute the second-order crosscorrelation

$$\phi_{yxx}(\tau_1, \tau_2) = \frac{1}{R - \max\{\tau_1, \tau_2\}} \int_0^R y(t)x(t - \tau_1)x(t - \tau_2)\, dt$$

$$= \frac{1}{R - \max\{\tau_1, \tau_2\}} \int_0^R x(t - \tau_1)x(t - \tau_2) \sum_i \varepsilon(t - t_i)\, dt$$

$$\simeq \frac{1}{R - \max\{\tau_1, \tau_2\}} \sum_i x(t_i - \tau_1)x(t_i - \tau_2) \tag{11.2}$$

where $\{t_i\}$ is the set of times at which a spike occurs. The procedure for computing this correlation is shown in Fig. 11.5. Again portions of the stimulus, chronologically preceding the response spikes for as long as the system memory, are averaged. What is measured is the crosstalk between

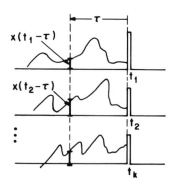

Fig. 11.4. First-order kernel estimation for continuous-to-discrete system.

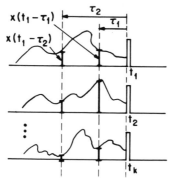

Fig. 11.5. Second-order kernel estimation for continuous-to-discrete system.

$x(t_i - \tau_1)$ and $x(t_i - \tau_2)$ in producing a spike at t_i. The extent to which τ_1, τ_2 are taken is equal to the system memory μ.

It should be noted that the computation is considerably shorter since for the second-order crosscorrelation $\phi_{yxx}(\tau_1, \tau_2)$ only one multiplication is required $[x(t_i - \tau_1)$ by $x(t_i - \tau_2)]$ instead of two $[y(t)$ by $x(t - \tau_1)$ by $(t - \tau_2)]$ (cf. also Sec. 6.4).

11.1.2. Discrete-to-Continuous System

In this case the response is continuous and the stimulus is discrete (e.g., presynaptic spikes, postsynaptic potential), as shown in Figs. 11.1C and 11.6. We have for the first-order crosscorrelation

$$\phi_{yx}(\tau) = \frac{1}{R - \tau} \int_0^R y(t)x(t - \tau)\, dt$$

$$= \frac{1}{R - \tau} \int_0^R y(t) \sum_i \varepsilon(t - t_i - \tau)\, dt$$

$$= \frac{1}{R - \tau} \sum_i y(t_i + \tau) \tag{11.3}$$

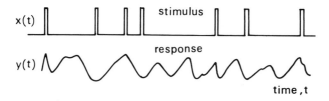

Fig. 11.6. Discrete stimulus and continuous response.

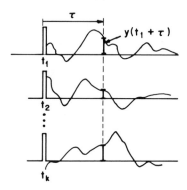

Fig. 11.7. First-order kernel estimation for discrete-to-continuous system.

Of course, as before, τ is taken to a maximum of μ sec, the system memory. Therefore, in this case, averaging of the response waveform shifted positively (into the future) is involved for all spikes at the stimulus (Fig. 11.7).

Similarly, we have for the second-order crosscorrelation

$$\phi_{yxx}(\tau_1, \tau_2) = \frac{1}{R - \max\{\tau_1, \tau_2\}} \int_0^R y(t)x(t - \tau_1)x(t - \tau_2)\, dt$$

$$= \frac{1}{R - \max\{\tau_1, \tau_2\}} \int_0^R y(t)\sum_i \varepsilon(t - t_i - \tau_1)\sum_j \varepsilon(t - t_j - \tau_2)\, dt$$

$$(11.4)$$

where $\{t_i\}$ is the set of times for which a spike occurs at the stimulus. We can visualize that the integral is computed as follows: The stimulus spike train is copied twice, one under the other (Fig. 11.8). One (the lower) is shifted to the left by $\Delta = \tau_1 - \tau_2$. Then we count coincidences. For each coincidence the integrand has a nonzero value. The response values are summed for all coincidences to give the crosscorrelation:

$$\phi_{yxx}(\tau_1, \tau_2) = \frac{1}{R - \max\{\tau_1, \tau_2\}} \sum_{\substack{k \\ \text{[over all} \\ \text{coincidences} \\ \text{for } (\tau_1 - \tau_2) \\ \text{shift]}}} y(t_k) \qquad (11.5)$$

The summation is carried, as before, up to $\tau_1 = \tau_2 = \mu$, the system memory.

This approach achieves remarkable economy in computation: Only additions are required. The detection of coincidence of spikes in $x(t - \tau_1)x(t - \tau_2)$, etc., can be carried out simply by digitally fast logical (conjunction) operations.

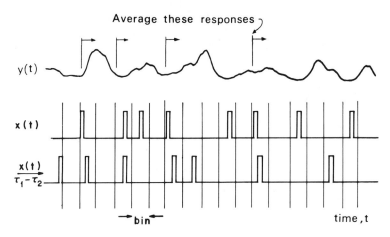

Fig. 11.8. Second-order kernel estimation for discrete-to-continuous system.

11.1.3. Discrete-to-Discrete System

This is the case in which both stimulus and response are spike trains, e.g., presynaptic spikes and postsynaptic spikes as shown in Figs. 11.1D and 11.9.

The first-order crosscorrelation is

$$\phi_{yx}(\tau) = \frac{1}{R - \tau} \int_0^R y(t)x(t - \tau)\, dt$$

$$= \frac{1}{R - \tau} \int_0^R \sum_i \varepsilon(t - t_i') \sum_j \varepsilon(t - t_j - \tau)\, dt \qquad (11.6)$$

The computation of this correlation is shown schematically in Fig. 11.10. For each spike at the stimulus, $\varepsilon(t - t_k)$, the spikes at the responses following t_k are considered up to time $t_k + \tau$ (maximum τ is μ, the system memory). All of the coincidences are summed up, as indicated by the above equation, and schematically shown in the figure.

The computation of the second-order correlation follows similar lines, as shown in Fig. 11.11. The same procedure is applicable in the case of two-input systems (Fig. 11.12).

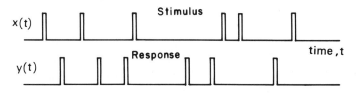

Fig. 11.9. Discrete stimulus and discrete response.

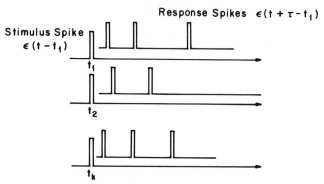

Fig. 11.10. First-order kernel estimation for discrete-to-discrete system.

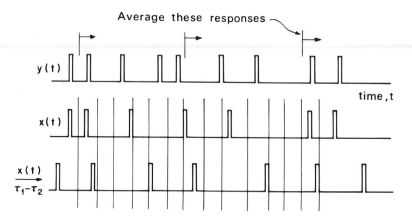

Fig. 11.11. Second-order kernel estimation for discrete-to-discrete system.

It should be noted again that the digital computation of these quantities is very fast since it does not involve multiplication. Thus high-order kernels can be easily computed.

11.2. Systems with Spatiotemporal Inputs

In studying certain types of sensory systems we are faced with stimuli that are functions of both *time* and *space*. Up to now we have considered systems with input stimuli that are functions of time only. We now turn our attention to systems whose inputs are functions of both space *and* time.

A natural instance of a physiological system with spatiotemporal inputs occurs in the study of visual systems. The retina is the part of the central nervous system whose basic function is to transform spatiotemporal light patterns falling on it into a complex array of ganglion spike train signals, which become the visual input to the brain. The basic unit of this transformation is the "concentric receptive field." This is a geometric area determined by the response elicited from the retinal neurons by photic stimulation. These receptive field responses may be thought of as the building blocks by which the brain reconstructs images of the outside world.

Therefore, in studying the system (receptive field stimulus) $\rightarrow$ (neuron response) we need to consider photic stimuli that cover the whole area (receptive field) and whose intensity is a function of time and position, i.e., the stimulus is $x^*(t, r, \theta)$, where r and θ are the polar coordinates of the plane. It has been found, for many retinas, that the stimulus position, in its effect on the neuron response, does not depend on the angle θ but only on the distance, r, from the center of the receptive field (cf. Levick, 1972; Naka, 1971; Stell, 1971; Chan, 1975; Rodieck and Stone, 1965; and Creutzfeldt *et al.*, 1970). This is, we can consider the stimulus as a function

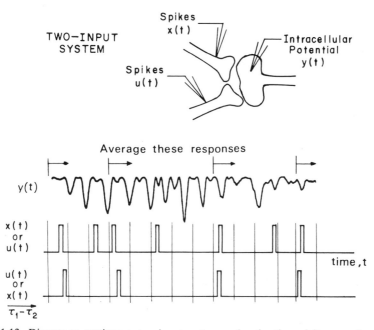

Fig. 11.12. Discrete-to-continuous two-input system and estimation of its second-order cross-kernel.

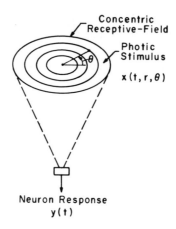

Fig. 11.13. Circular symmetry of the receptive field.

of time and only one space variable, the radial distance r, from the center, i.e., $x^*(t, r, \theta) = x(t, r)$ (Fig. 11.13).

Thus, a white-noise experiment in this case involves white-noise variations in light intensity that depend both on the radius r and time, i.e., both in the space and time dimensions. We can always consider this *multi-dimensional* white-noise stimulus as an extension of a *multi-input* white-noise experiment. Consider, in this example, that the receptive field is sliced into n concentric annular pieces as shown in Fig. 11.14. Then, since the photic stimulus effect on the neuron response is independent of the angle θ, we can visualize an n-input white-noise experiment in which each of the n rings is stimulated by *independent GWN photic signals*. Each of

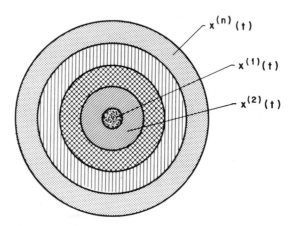

Fig. 11.14. Spatiotemporal stimulus with circular symmetry.

these stimuli has uniform intensity over the entire ring area. It is easily seen then that, in the limit, as the number n of rings in increased, we reach the case of white-noise stimulation both in time t and space r. The width of the ring (all of them have the same width) determines the bandwidth of the spatial stimulus, i.e., the highest spatial frequency present in the stimulus.

According to the multi-input formulation of the white-noise method (cf. Sec. 4.4) we can obtain Wiener kernels for the n-input system. The first-order Wiener kernels are

$$h_1^{(1)}(\tau), h_1^{(2)}(\tau), \ldots, h_1^{(n)}(\tau)$$

giving rise to the first-order response

$$y_1(t) = \sum_{k=1}^{n} \int_0^\infty h_1^{(k)}(\tau) x^{(k)}(t-\tau) \, d\tau \tag{11.7}$$

and as the number of rings is increased—while their width decreases—we obtain in the limit

$$y_1(t) = \int_0^R \int_0^\infty h_1(\tau, r) x(t-\tau, r) \, d\tau \, dr \tag{11.8}$$

where R is the maximum value of the radius, r. The integral above is the first-order functional of the extended spatiotemporal Wiener series.

The second-order terms can be found similarly. We recall that for a two-input system with inputs $x^{(1)}(t)$, $x^{(2)}(t)$—we have second-order kernels

self-kernels: $h_2^{(11)}(\tau_1, \tau_2), h_2^{(22)}(\tau_1, \tau_2)$, cross-kernel: $h_2^{(12)}(\tau_1, \tau_2)$

To simplify the following discussion let us adopt a slightly modified form of the second-order cross-term,

$$\int_0^\infty \int h_2^{*12}(\tau_1, \tau_2) x^{(1)}(t-\tau_1) x^{(2)}(t-\tau_2) \, d\tau_1 \, d\tau_2$$

$$= \int_0^\infty \int h_2^{12}(\tau_1, \tau_2) x^{(1)}(t-\tau_1) x^{(2)}(t-\tau_2) \, d\tau_1 \, d\tau_2$$

$$+ \int_0^\infty \int h_2^{21}(\tau_1, \tau_2) x^{(2)}(t-\tau_1) x^{(1)}(t-\tau_2) \, d\tau_1 \, d\tau_2 \tag{11.9}$$

where $h_2^{12}(\tau_1, \tau_2)$ and $h_2^{21}(\tau_1, \tau_2)$ are, in general, asymmetric functions of (τ_1, τ_2) but such that

$$h_2^{12}(\tau_1, \tau_2) = h_2^{21}(\tau_2, \tau_1) \tag{11.10}$$

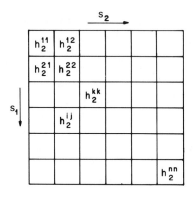

Fig. 11.15. Second-order kernels of *n*-input system.

and obviously their magnitude is one-half of that of the cross-kernel $h_2^{*12}(\tau_1, \tau_2)$.

With these minor adjustments made, we now consider the second-order kernels of the multi-input system (*n* inputs). Figure 11.15 shows the various second-order kernels obtained from the multi-input representation, arranged in a symmetric matrix form whose dimensions span the range of *r*. Notice that along the diagonal we have the self-kernels $h_2^{kk}(\tau_1, \tau_2)$, while off the diagonal are cross-kernels of the form $h_2^{ij}(\tau_1, \tau_2) = h_2^{ji}(\tau_2, \tau_1)$. We have for the response contributions of these kernels

$$y_2(t) = \sum_{j=1}^{n} \sum_{i=1}^{n} \int\int_0^\infty h_2^{ij}(\tau_1, \tau_2) x^{(i)}(t - \tau_1) x^{(i)}(t - \tau_2)\, d\tau_1\, d\tau_2$$

$$- \sum_{i=1}^{n} P_i \int_0^\infty h_2^{ii}(\tau_1, \tau_1)\, d\tau_1 \tag{11.11}$$

where P_i is the power level of the *i*th white-noise stimulus. And passing to the continuous case—as *n* increases while the width of each ring decreases—we obtain

$$y_2(t) = \int_0^R \int_0^R \int_0^\mu \int_0^\mu h_2(\tau_1, \tau_2, r_1, r_2) x(t - \tau_1, r_1) x(t - \tau_2, r_2)\, d\tau_1\, d\tau_2\, dr_1\, dr_2$$

$$- P \int_0^R \int_0^\mu h_2(\tau_1, \tau_1, r_1, r_1)\, d\tau_1\, dr_1 \tag{11.12}$$

assuming that the stimulus power level *P* is the same over all the receptive field. The integral above is the second-order functional term of the extended spatiotemporal Wiener series, where *R* is the spatial, and μ is the temporal, memory of the system. Thus the set of kernels $\{h_2^{ij}(\tau_1, \tau_2)\}$ is a quantized version of a single continuous kernel $h_2(\tau_1, \tau_2, r_1, r_2)$ that describes the second-order spatiotemporal dynamics of the system.

Proceeding similarly we can define the higher-order functional terms of the extended spatiotemporal Wiener series.

Let us now study rigorously the more general spatiotemporal case of a system with input a function of three independent variables (two spatial and one temporal) and output a function of one independent variable. This can be the case of a visual system (retina), the receptive field of which does not exhibit circular symmetry.

Suppose the stimulus is a square pattern consisting of elementary square spots of infinitesimal dimensions with the illumination of each one of them changing temporally. The response is temporally varying potential recorded intracellularly or extracellularly from the appropriate stage of the retinal neural structure.

The mathematical expression that we use to describe the stimulus–response functional relation has the form (cf. Yasui and Fender, 1975; Sutter, 1975)

$$r(t) = \sum_{n=0}^{\infty} \int_{-\infty}^{\infty} \cdots \int k_n(x_1, y_1, \tau_1; x_2, y_2, \tau_2; \ldots; x_n, y_n, \tau_n) s(x_1, y_1, \tau_1)$$

$$\times s(x_2, y_2, \tau_2) \cdots s(x_n, y_n, \tau_n)\, dx_1\, dy_1\, d\tau_1 \cdots dx_n\, dy_n\, d\tau_n \qquad (11.13)$$

where $r(t)$ is the response, $s(x, y, t)$ is the stimulus, and $\{k_n\}$ are the spatiotemporal Volterra kernels of the system. This is an extension of the original Volterra series to cover the case of a stimulus function of three independent variables. The validity of this expansion is based upon the same arguments as in the case of the original Volterra series, i.e., it is merely a generalization of a power series expansion as extended from the function space into the functional space. The differential smoothness of the system (analyticity) is assumed. Thus, the meaning of this functional series is that it represents the aggregate impact on the system response of all possible interactions of portions of the stimulus signal (considered in space and time). The pattern according to which these interactions take place is described by the spatiotemporal system kernels. Mathematically, these kernels correspond to partial functional derivatives with respect to space and time. The spatiotemporal kernels constitute a universal mathematical characterization of the spatial and temporal dynamics of the system, and they allow the prediction of the system response to any arbitrarily chosen spatiotemporal stimulus. Thus, the generality and the potency of this approach in studying the spatiotemporal dynamic properties of retinal organization becomes evident.

The direct estimation of the system spatiotemporal Volterra kernels, appearing in Eq. (11.13), is not presently possible. In order to estimate the system spatiotemporal kernels, we have to rewrite the functional series (11.13) so that it is orthogonal with respect to a spatiotemporal white-noise stimulus. This can be done routinely on the basis of a Gram–Schmidt orthogonalization procedure, in a way similar to the one followed by Wiener in the case of a stimulus with a single independent variable (cf. Sec. 4.2). Spatiotemporal white noise is defined as a stationary and ergodic random signal for which any two samples (in space and time) are statistically independent. In addition, the white-noise signal has a zero average value. Thus, for a spatiotemporal Gaussian white-noise signal $s(x, y, t)$, the three-dimensional autocorrelation functions are

$$E[\![s(x, y, t)]\!] = 0 \tag{11.14}$$

$$E[\![s(x_1, y_1, t_1)s(x_2, y_2, t_2)]\!] = P\delta(x_1 - x_2)\delta(y_1 - y_2)\delta(t_1 - t_2) \tag{11.15}$$

$$E[\![s(x_1, y_1, t_1)s(x_2, y_2, t_2)s(x_3, y_3, t_3)]\!] = 0 \tag{11.16}$$

$$E[\![s(x_1, y_1, t_1)s(x_2, y_2, t_2)s(x_3, y_3, t_3)s(x_4, y_4, t_4)]\!]$$

$$= P^2\delta(x_1 - x_2)\delta(y_1 - y_2)\delta(t_1 - t_2)\delta(x_3 - x_4)\delta(y_3 - y_4)\delta(t_3 - t_4)$$

$$+ P^2\delta(x_1 - x_3)\delta(y_1 - y_3)\delta(t_1 - t_3)\delta(x_2 - x_4)\delta(y_2 - y_4)\delta(t_2 - t_4)$$

$$+ P^2\delta(x_1 - x_4)\delta(y_1 - y_4)\delta(t_1 - t_4)\delta(x_2 - x_3)\delta(y_2 - y_3)\delta(t_2 - t_3)$$

$$\tag{11.17}$$

The odd-order autocorrelation functions are zero, while the even-order ones are expressible in terms of delta functions. These autocorrelation properties allow the easy orthogonalization of the functional series. The resulting orthogonal functionals are

$$G_0 = h_0 \tag{11.18}$$

$$G_1(t) = \int\limits_{-\infty}^{\infty}\!\!\!\int\!\!\!\int h_1(x, y, \tau)s(x, y, t - \tau)\, dx\, dy\, d\tau \tag{11.19}$$

$$G_2(t) = \int\limits_{-\infty}^{\infty}\!\!\!\int\!\!\!\int\!\!\!\int\!\!\!\int\!\!\!\int h_2(x_1, y_1, \tau_1; x_2, y_2, \tau_2)s(x_1, y_1, t - \tau_1)s(x_2, y_2, t - \tau_2)$$

$$\times dx_1\, dy_1\, d\tau_1\, dx_2\, dy_2\, d\tau_2$$

$$- P\int\limits_{-\infty}^{\infty}\!\!\!\int\!\!\!\int h_2(x, y, \tau; x, y, \tau)\, dx\, dy\, d\tau \tag{11.20}$$

etc., where

$$r(t) = \sum_{n=0}^{\infty} G_n(t) \tag{11.21}$$

The upper limit of integration is effectively the memory extent of the respective kernel. Effectively, then, the first-order functional becomes

$$G_1(t) = \int_0^{\mu} d\tau \int_0^{\lambda_x} dx \int_0^{\lambda_y} dy\, h_1(x, y, \tau) s(x, y, t-\tau) \tag{11.22}$$

where μ is the temporal, λ_x is the x-spatial, and λ_y is the y-spatial memory extent of h_1. Note that the spatial memory extent determines the area of the receptive field that appreciably affects the recorded response.

Estimation of the kernels of the orthogonal series is done through crosscorrelation, in a way similar to the technique that Lee and Schetzen (1965) proposed for the strictly temporal case (cf. Sec. 4.3). Thus the nth-order kernel can be estimated from the crosscorrelation of the nth-order response residual with n time-shifted versions of the stimulus:

$$h_n(x_1, y_1, \tau_1; \ldots; x_n, y_n, \tau_n)$$

$$= \frac{1}{n! P^n} E[\![r^{(n)}(t)\, s(x_1, y_1, t-\tau_1) \cdots s(x_n, y_n, t-\tau_n)]\!] \tag{11.23}$$

where

$$r^{(n)}(t) = r(t) - \sum_{k=0}^{n-1} G_k(t) \tag{11.24}$$

and P is the power level of the Gaussian white-noise stimulus.

Of course, the operator $E[\![\ ]\!]$ is implemented in practice through time averaging based on the ergodicity of the white-noise signal. The exact evaluation of the crosscorrelation would require an infinite integration interval. Therefore, in practice we obtain simply an estimate of this crosscorrelation by averaging over a finite time interval $[0, T]$. Thus, a kernel estimate is obtained as

$$\hat{h}_n(x_1, y_1, \tau_1; \ldots; x_n, y_n, \tau_n)$$

$$= \frac{1}{n! P^n} \frac{1}{T} \int_0^T r^{(n)}(t) s(x_1, y_1, t-\tau_1) \cdots s(x_n, y_n, t-\tau_n)\, dt \tag{11.25}$$

The variance of this estimate along with several other types of error that occur in the kernel estimation (like errors due to the finite stimulus bandwidth, etc.) have been studied thoroughly, and optimal procedures are now available for the accurate and efficient estimation of the system kernels (cf. V. Z. Marmarelis, 1976, 1977*a*).

The first-order spatiotemporal kernel $h_1(x, y, \tau)$ gives us a description of the first-order temporal dynamics of the neural activity channels that originate at the several points (x, y) of the receptive field and terminate at the recording location in the retinal structure. Thus, $h_1(x, y, \tau)$ constitutes a powerful tool to study the spatial properties of the receptive field (like excitatory and inhibitory regions). Also, being the simplest of the system kernels (in terms of number of arguments) it can be easily computed and inspected.

The second-order spatiotemporal kernel $h_2(x_1, y_1, \tau_1; x_2, y_2, \tau_2)$ provides the simplest mathematical description of the nonlinear spatiotemporal system dynamics. It gives us an idea of how two channels of neural activity interact in time within the retinal organization. By studying this kernel we can obtain valuable knowledge about the spatiotemporal interactions within the retina.

Since the dimensionality of the higher-order spatiotemporal kernels increases rapidly, we are limited by practical computational considerations to the first three kernels (h_0, h_1, h_2). If the study of these three kernels suggests an importance of higher-order interactions, then specialized tests can be performed using temporally varying spot stimuli applied to the appropriate locations of the receptive field.

The computation of spatiotemporal kernels through crosscorrelation is a burdensome task. However, our increasing computational capabilities due to the rapidly progressing computer technology, along with the development of more sophisticated and efficient procedures, make the spatiotemporal analysis of visual systems feasible. The optimal design of the experimental stimulus to minimize the kernel estimation error and the computational burden is the principal concern for a successful application of the method. The thorough study of the several types of estimation error and the complete understanding of the "mechanics" of the crosscorrelation technique allow the design of the optimum test.

To demonstrate the importance of optimizing our test parameters, let us consider the dependence of the computational load upon the stimulus bandwidths. The stimulus bandwidths (in spatial and temporal frequencies—the spatial bandwidth is otherwise called "resolution") determine the sampling rate of the data sets that are processed by the digital computer (on the basis of the Nyquist sampling theorem). Therefore the number of data points that have to be processed for a certain experimental duration and kernel memory extent depends directly on the stimulus bandwidths. More specifically, if ΔT is the temporal sampling interval, T is the experimental record length, μ is the temporal kernel memory, $\Delta \lambda$ is the spatial sampling interval, and λ is the spatial kernel memory (both in x and

y dimensions), then the computational burden is roughly proportional to

$$\left(\frac{T}{\Delta T}\right)\left(\frac{\mu}{\Delta T}\right)\left(\frac{\lambda^2}{\Delta\lambda^2}\right) \quad \text{for the first-order kernel}$$

$$\left(\frac{T}{\Delta T}\right)\left(\frac{\mu^2}{\Delta T^2}\right)\left(\frac{\lambda^4}{\Delta\lambda^4}\right) \quad \text{for the second-order kernel}$$

The expressions above demonstrate clearly the importance of using the optimal stimulus bandwidths, as well as of determining accurately the extent of spatiotemporal kernel memory. Analytical techniques for determining these test parameters in an optimum way have been developed (cf. V. Z. Marmarelis, 1976, 1977a).

11.3. Nonstationary Systems

The general problem of identifying nonstationary nonlinear systems is formally beyond the scope of this book, since the white-noise method requires that the system under study be stationary (cf. Sec. 4.1). However, we would like to discuss here certain cases of nonstationary systems that can be effectively handled with the white-noise method. These cases cover many situations of practical interest.

Case I. The notion of nonstationarity, as opposed to the notion of nonlinearity, implies that a portion of the system response is not causally linked to any stimulus but is a result of an independent course of the system in time. In that sense, we may be able in some cases to consider the system response consisting of two superimposed components:

$$y(t) = v(t) + y^*(t) \tag{11.26}$$

where $v(t)$ represents the stimulus-independent portion of the response (due to nonstationarities) and $y^*(t)$ represents the stimulus-dependent portion of the response, which reflects the stationary behavior of the system.

In this case the white-noise method can be employed (as in the stationary case) to identify the system kernels that characterize the stationary functional behavior of the system. The presence of the component $v(t)$ does not affect the kernel estimates except possibly at the full-diagonal points. This latter deficiency can be avoided if $v(t)$ is initially subtracted from $y(t)$. This is possible when in some practical cases $v(t)$ has a low-frequency content compared to the high-frequency content of $y^*(t)$ which is the stationary response to white-noise stimulus. Thus $v(t)$ can usually be extracted from $y(t)$ by high-pass filtering or by polynomial least-squares fitting, as discussed in Sec. 8.3. Note the analogy between the form of system response as given by Eq. (11.26), and the homogeneous (transient) and particular (steady-state) solutions of a differential equation.

Case II. The nonstationary character of the system response cannot be expressed as in Eq. (11.26), but it may be plausible to hypothesize that the system kernels are separable explicit functions of time, i.e.,

$$h_1(t, \tau) = A_1(t)g_1(\tau) \tag{11.27}$$

$$h_2(t, \tau_1, \tau_2) = A_2(t)g_2(\tau_1, \tau_2) \tag{11.28}$$

$$\vdots$$

where $A_1(t)$, $A_2(t)$ etc., are deterministic functions of time. Then, the the stationary part of the system kernels, i.e., $g_1(\tau)$, $g_2(\tau_1, \tau_2)$, etc., since the "expected value" operator is indifferent to deterministic functions [such as $A_1(t)$, $A_2(t)$, etc.] and consequently the autocorrelation functions of the stimulus (as they appear in the functionals of the Wiener series) are unaffected by the nonstationarities. For example, consider a linear system:

$$y(t) = \int_0^\infty A(t)h(\tau)x(t-\tau)\,d\tau \tag{11.29}$$

then the crosscorrelation yields

$$\phi_{yx}(t, \sigma) = E[y(t)x(t-\sigma)] = A(t)\int_0^\infty h(\tau)E[x(t-\tau)x(t-\sigma)]\,d\tau$$

$$= PA(t)h(\sigma) \tag{11.30}$$

where P is the power level of the white-noise stimulus. The practical drawback of this method is that it requires ensemble averaging instead of time averaging as in the stationary case. Of course $\phi_{yx}(t, \sigma)$ needs to be evaluated only for a single $t = t_0$, since the quantity

$$z(t) = \frac{1}{P}\int_0^\infty \phi_{yx}(t_0, \sigma)x(t-\sigma)\,d\sigma \tag{11.31}$$

can then be computed, and $A(t)$ can be found directly (except for a scaling factor) as

$$A(t) = A(t_0)y(t)/z(t) \tag{11.32}$$

The scaling factor $A(t_0)$ can be specified arbitrarily, since it will reflect only on the scaling of $h(\sigma)$, which is not differentiable from the scaling of $A(t)$.

Case III. The kernels of the system are deterministic functions of time. The ensemble averaging method still gives desirable results. The only complication here is that an ensemble averaging is required for every time instant t of interest. For example in the linear case

$$y(t) = \int_0^\infty h(t, \tau)x(t - \tau)\, d\tau \qquad (11.33)$$

and the crosscorrelation gives

$$\phi_{yx}(t, \sigma) = E[y(t)x(t - \sigma)]$$

$$= \int_0^\infty h(t, \tau)E[x(t - \tau)x(t - \sigma)]\, d\tau$$

$$= Ph(t, \sigma) \qquad (11.34)$$

Therefore, nonstationary systems can be identified in some cases with the white-noise method, if the required experimental and computational capacity is available to obtain the ensemble averages indicated above.

11.4. Systems with Nonwhite Random Inputs

Often, in practical applications of the method, it is not possible to provide white-noise input stimuli. In such cases the analysis can be performed on the basis of the nonwhite spectral characteristics of the inputs, as shown below (cf. Schetzen, 1974).

Let us consider a second-order nonlinear system with input $x(t)$ and output $y(t)$, such that

$$y(t) = \int_0^\infty g_1(\tau)x(t - \tau)\, d\tau + \int\int_0^\infty g_2(\tau_1, \tau_2)x(t - \tau_1)x(t - \tau_2)\, d\tau_1\, d\tau_2 \qquad (11.35)$$

Let us also evaluate the following crosscorrelations:

$$\phi_{yx}(\sigma) = E[y(t)x(t - \sigma)]$$

$$= \int_0^\infty g_1(\tau)\phi_{xx}(\sigma - \tau)\, d\tau$$

$$+ \int\int_0^\infty g_2(\tau_1, \tau_2)\phi_{xxx}(\sigma - \tau_1, \sigma - \tau_2)\, d\tau_1\, d\tau_2 \qquad (11.36)$$

$$\phi_{yxx}(\sigma_1, \sigma_2) = E[[y(t) - E[y(t)]]x(t - \sigma_1)x(t - \sigma_2)]$$

$$= \int_0^\infty g_1(\tau)\phi_{xxx}(\sigma_1 - \tau, \sigma_2 - \tau)\, d\tau$$

$$+ \int\int_0^\infty g_2(\tau_1, \tau_2)\phi_{xxxx}(\tau_1 - \tau_2, \tau_1 - \sigma_1, \tau_1 - \sigma_2)\, d\tau_1\, d\tau_2$$

$$- \phi_{xx}(\sigma_1 - \sigma_2)E[y(t)] \tag{11.37}$$

If the stimulus $x(t)$ is a stationary Gaussian nonwhite signal with zero mean, then

$$\phi_{xxx}(\sigma_1 - \tau, \sigma_2 - \tau) = 0 \tag{11.38}$$

and

$$\phi_{xxxx}(\tau_1 - \tau_2, \tau_1 - \sigma_1, \tau_1 - \sigma_2) = \phi_{xx}(\sigma_1 - \sigma_2)\phi_{xx}(\tau_1 - \tau_2)$$

$$+ \phi_{xx}(\sigma_1 - \tau_1)\phi_{xx}(\sigma_2 - \tau_2)$$

$$+ \phi_{xx}(\sigma_1 - \tau_2)\phi_{xx}(\sigma_2 - \tau_1) \tag{11.39}$$

Keeping in mind that $g_2(\tau_1, \tau_2) = g_2(\tau_2, \tau_1)$ and

$$E[y(t)] = \int\int_0^\infty g_2(\tau_1, \tau_2)\phi_{xx}(\tau_1 - \tau_2)\, d\tau_1\, d\tau_2 \tag{11.40}$$

Eqs. (11.36) and (11.37) become

$$\phi_{yx}(\sigma) = \int_0^\infty g_1(\tau)\phi_{xx}(\sigma - \tau)\, d\tau \tag{11.41}$$

$$\phi_{yxx}(\sigma_1, \sigma_2) = 2\int\int_0^\infty g_2(\tau_1, \tau_2)\phi_{xx}(\sigma_1 - \tau_1)\phi_{xx}(\sigma_2 - \tau_2)\, d\tau_1\, d\tau_2 \tag{11.42}$$

Taking the Fourier transforms of Eqs. (11.41) and (11.42), we obtain

$$\Phi_{yx}(\omega) = G_1(\omega)\Phi_{xx}(\omega) \tag{11.43}$$

$$\Phi_{yxx}(\omega_1, \omega_2) = 2G_2(\omega_1, \omega_2)\Phi_{xx}(\omega_1)\Phi_{xx}(\omega_2) \tag{11.44}$$

from which the system kernels $G_1(\omega)$ and $G_2(\omega_1, \omega_2)$ can be found since $\Phi_{xx}(\omega)$, $\Phi_{yx}(\omega)$ and $\Phi_{yxx}(\omega_1, \omega_2)$ are all directly computable from the stimulus–response data. Specifically,

$$G_1(\omega) = \frac{\Phi_{yx}(\omega)}{\Phi_{xx}(\omega)} \tag{11.45}$$

$$G_2(\omega_1, \omega_2) = \frac{1}{2}\frac{\Phi_{yxx}(\omega_1, \omega_2)}{\Phi_{xx}(\omega_1)\Phi_{xx}(\omega_2)} \tag{11.46}$$

If the stimulus amplitude distribution is not Gaussian, then a considerable savings in the complexity of the solution is achieved if it is at least symmetric with zero mean. In such a case, again $\phi_{xxx}(\ )=0$ but $\phi_{xxxx}(\ )$ cannot be decomposed, in general, in terms of $\phi_{xx}(\ )$. However, the two integral equations can always be solved (in principle) despite computational and numerical complications.

Similar expressions hold in the case of multi-input systems. For example, consider a second-order nonlinear system with two inputs $x(t)$ and $u(t)$; then

$$y(t)=\int_0^\infty g_{1x}(\tau)x(t-\tau)\,d\tau+\int_0^\infty g_{1u}(\tau)u(t-\tau)\,d\tau$$

$$+\int\int_0^\infty g_{2xx}(\tau_1,\tau_2)x(t-\tau_1)x(t-\tau_2)\,d\tau_1\,d\tau_2$$

$$+\int\int_0^\infty g_{2uu}(\tau_1,\tau_2)u(t-\tau_1)u(t-\tau_2)\,d\tau_1\,d\tau_2$$

$$+\int\int_0^\infty g_{2xu}(\tau_1,\tau_2)x(t-\tau_1)u(t-\tau_2)\,d\tau_1\,d\tau_2 \qquad (11.47)$$

If $x(t)$ and $u(t)$ are zero-mean Gaussian and independent then we obtain for the various crosscorrelations

$$\phi_{yx}(\sigma)=\int_0^\infty g_{1x}(\tau)\phi_{xx}(\sigma-\tau)\,d\tau \qquad (11.48)$$

$$\phi_{yu}(\sigma)=\int_0^\infty g_{1u}(\tau)\phi_{uu}(\sigma-\tau)\,d\tau \qquad (11.49)$$

$$\phi_{yxx}(\sigma_1,\sigma_2)=\int\int_0^\infty g_{2xx}(\tau_1,\tau_2)[\phi_{xx}(\sigma_1-\tau_1)\phi_{xx}(\sigma_2-\tau_2)$$

$$+\phi_{xx}(\sigma_1-\tau_2)\phi_{xx}(\sigma_2-\tau_1)]\,d\tau_1\,d\tau_2 \qquad (11.50)$$

$$\phi_{yuu}(\sigma_1,\sigma_2)=\int\int_0^\infty g_{2uu}(\tau_1,\tau_2)[\phi_{uu}(\sigma_1-\tau_1)\phi_{uu}(\sigma_2-\tau_2)$$

$$+\phi_{uu}(\sigma_1-\tau_2)\phi_{uu}(\sigma_2-\tau_1)]\,d\tau_1\,d\tau_2 \qquad (11.51)$$

$$\phi_{yxu}(\sigma_1, \sigma_2) = \int\limits_0^\infty\!\!\int g_{2xu}(\tau_1, \tau_2)\phi_{xx}(\sigma_1 - \tau_1)\phi_{uu}(\sigma_2 - \tau_2)\,d\tau_1\,d\tau_2 \qquad (11.52)$$

Note that the average value of the response has been subtracted before ϕ_{yxx} and ϕ_{yuu} are evaluated (as before). Taking the Fourier transforms of these quantities and solving for the system kernels we have

$$G_{1x}(\omega) = \frac{\Phi_{yx}(\omega)}{\Phi_{xx}(\omega)} \qquad (11.53)$$

$$G_{1u}(\omega) = \frac{\Phi_{yu}(\omega)}{\Phi_{uu}(\omega)} \qquad (11.54)$$

$$G_{2xx}(\omega_1, \omega_2) = \frac{1}{2}\frac{\Phi_{yxx}(\omega_1, \omega_2)}{\Phi_{xx}(\omega_1)\Phi_{xx}(\omega_2)} \qquad (11.55)$$

$$G_{2uu}(\omega_1, \omega_2) = \frac{1}{2}\frac{\Phi_{yuu}(\omega_1, \omega_2)}{\Phi_{uu}(\omega_1)\Phi_{uu}(\omega_2)} \qquad (11.56)$$

$$G_{2xu}(\omega_1, \omega_2) = \frac{\Phi_{yxu}(\omega_1, \omega_2)}{\Phi_{xx}(\omega_1)\Phi_{uu}(\omega_2)} \qquad (11.57)$$

Thus, even in the multi-input case the kernels can be found if the stimuli are nonwhite but Gaussian and independent. If, in addition, the stimuli are non-Gaussian or dependent, the kernels can still be found, in principle, by solving simultaneous integral equations.

Dialogue for Epilogue

Question. What is our principal objective in system functional identification?

Answer. To be able to describe quantitatively the response of the system to an arbitrary stimulus.

Question. How can this be achieved?

Answer. By examining the system's responses to several stimuli and trying to derive a quantitative relation between stimulus and response. Of course, the way the bioscientist often interprets his experience is more or less intuitive and sometimes arbitrary. For this activity to become a scientific discipline, we must assure ourselves that a systematic and rigorous method of interpretation is established; to this end, we resort to mathematical methods.

Question. Fine, we have to use some kind of mathematical representation of the concepts involved in our problem; but what are the ways that such a mathematical formulation may follow that will be proper and convenient in the study of physiological systems?

Answer. First, it should aim to describe in "dynamic terms" the transformation of stimuli into responses. By saying, in "dynamic terms," we mean that the description would involve the past and present values of the stimulus related to past and present values of the response in such a way that prediction of the present value of the response is possible.

There are two main ways in which such a description can be achieved, and the applicability of each depends on the information available on the "internal structure" of the system or the accessibility of the system's internal structure (i.e., observability, experimentability, etc.).

(1) If sufficient information on the system's internal structure is available, and experimentation (stimulus–response data acquisition) is possible for the component elements of the system, an analysis procedure can be established by following the driving signal from the input to the output site—thus obtaining a description of each successive step (subsystem). It is evident that each component element is itself a system and therefore can be, in principle, analyzed into its component elements, and so on. Thus we perform our analysis on a certain level of system-elements

conceptualization (one out of an infinite number of such levels) that appears to be suitable for the application at hand.

This exhaustive type of analysis is the one most rarely encountered in present research on physiological systems. The reason for this is that the requirements for its applicability can only rarely be met in practice. For example, studying the vertebrate retina as a system by this approach would require the ability to stimulate and record from all neurons in the retinal network.

(2) The other way to go about our problem is by facing the system as a "black box" with several input and output paths of interaction with the environment and trying to derive some overall description of the relation between the stimulus and response signals. Clearly, the black-box approach appears to be conceptually and experimentally simpler. It should be noted that the "black-box" and the "open-box" approach are *not* mutually exclusive and, in fact, can complement each other.

Question. O.K., let's get down to some specific problems. I am faced with a nonlinear system with one input and one output; is there always a mathematical relation of known form relating the input and output signals?

Answer. Under the assumptions of stationarity, finite-memory, and analyticity of the system, there is always the Volterra-series representation of the output in terms of a sum of multiple integrals involving the input.

Question. Does stationarity mean time invariance of the functional characteristics of the system?

Answer. Yes. I noted that "functional characteristics" refers to the *"pattern"* according to which the response is constructed from the past and present values of the stimulus. This "pattern" is described in the Volterra series by various kernels. So stationarity implies that this "pattern" remains invariant in time. However it can be shown (cf. Sec. 11.3) that several nonstationary cases can be accommodated by a similar type of formulation.

Question. What does finite memory mean?

Answer. It refers to this pattern according to which the present value of the response is constructed from the past and present values of the stimulus. In this process, the system "remembers" the recent history of the input and responds according to it. *Finite memory* means that the system does not "remember" very remote past values of the input when it constructs its present response. Mathematically, finite memory is expressed as a condition of absolute integrability of all the kernels in the Volterra series.

Question. And what about analyticity?

Answer. Analyticity of the system implies that the differential behavior of the system is smooth. It also means that the output doesn't contain subharmonics of the input. It must be noted, however, that some nonanalytic systems can be satisfactorily approximated by the Volterra-series representation.

Question. Are these assumptions very strict for physical systems?

Answer. Finite memory is a property that the overwhelming majority of systems exhibit. In principle, finite memory seems an inescapable property of physical systems, connected originally with the second thermodynamic law and entropy considerations. Analyticity is also a very common characteristic of physical systems, but not universal.

Stationarity is the less common characteristic of the three. In some cases it is in principle valid, and in most cases can be approximately assumed within specified periods of time with good practical results.

Question. How can we represent a nonlinear system with a Volterra series?

Answer. According to the Stone–Weierstrass theorem, if the system is analytic—i.e., its output does not change abruptly for a small change in the stimulus—then, using a Volterra series of finite degree n, we can represent the system functional to an arbitrary degree of accuracy.

Question. Besides the mathematical anxieties concerning convergence of the series, the important consideration is: How *fast* does the series converge so that a truncation after a few terms will give a respectable representation of the system response?

Answer. In Sec. 8.5, we presented an approximate method of answering this question (in terms of harmonic analysis of the system response to sine waves). Fortunately, a lot of physiological systems seem to be adequately described by the first two or three kernels within their normal range of operation. This is indicative of the operational smoothness of a lot of physiological systems. One additional reason for this is the linearizing effect of noise (abundantly present in the operation of physiological systems) as described in Sec. 3.6. It should be noted that such linearizing noise is manifested not only as measurement noise, but also as intrinsic noise of the system.

Question. Can you give an intuitive mathematical justification of the Volterra-series representation?

Answer. Yes. I think the best way to think of it is as a generalization of the Taylor series expansion of a function with multiple arguments. In the limiting case, the function becomes a functional and the infinite number of arguments becomes a continuous function, while the coefficients of the Taylor series become accordingly the kernels of the Volterra series.

Question. Well, do you think that would make me feel better about the Volterra series? But now that it seems we are inescapably involved, what is the Wiener series?

Answer. The Wiener series is a series of functionals constructed as linear combinations of Volterra-type functionals. The terms of this series are made mutually orthogonal with respect to a Gaussian white-noise input. The species of this construction (which is basically a Gram–Schmidt orthogonalization procedure) can be found in Sec. 4.2.

Question. Are the Wiener kernels the same as the Volterra kernels?
Answer. In general, no. Only in the case of a second-order system, the first- and second-order Wiener and Volterra kernels are, respectively, identical. The relation between Wiener and Volterra kernels is discussed in Sec. 4.2.

Question. Are both representations valid?
Answer. Of course, yes.

Question. What is their basic difference?
Answer. Wiener's functionals are orthogonal with respect to Gaussian white-noise input, while this is not true for the Volterra series. However, it cannot be excluded that the Volterra series may give better approximates—in the mean-square-error sense—than the Wiener for *some* kinds of input signals. Note of course, that Gaussian white noise is a very rich stimulus (in waveforms) and thus the Wiener model should be expected to do better for most stimuli.

Question. Why is the Wiener series so widely used instead of the Volterra series?
Answer. There are two main reasons:

(1) The orthogonality of the Wiener functionals allows use of the crosscorrelation technique for the practical and efficient computation of the kernels.

(2) The Wiener series, being orthogonal, gives a system model of some order (if truncated) that is a better approximation than the Volterra model of the same order. It must be emphasized, however, that the region of orthogonality of the Wiener functionals is determined by the power level of the Gaussian white-noise stimulus and thus optimality of the Wiener model is referred to this specific orthogonality region. In other words, if a stimulus is used that does not conform to the orthogonality region of the available Wiener model, then the Wiener-model-predicted response may not be the best (in the mean-square-error sense). Thus, it is evident that the Wiener kernels and functionals depend on the power level of the Gaussian white-noise stimulus with respect to which the Wiener series has been

orthogonalized. This is not the case for the Volterra kernels and functionals, which are independent of any stimulus characteristics.

Question. Since white noise satisfies in general the requirement of a rich stimulus (many different waveforms) why do we use *Gaussian* white noise?

Answer. Because Gaussian white noise possesses the convenient decomposition property of its even-order autocorrelation functions, which simplifies the expressions for the orthogonal functional series and facilitates the estimation of the system kernels. However, the Gaussian amplitude distribution is not vital for the application of the white-noise method, as discussed in Sec. 5.3.

Question. Of course, white noise is not a physically realizable signal. What do we do in practice?

Answer. In practical applications band-limited white noise (quasiwhite) is used which, under some conditions, approximates satisfactorily the ideal white noise. Experience has shown that for most physical systems this approximation gives very satisfactory results. History has also shown that the successful applied scientist must achieve a balance between mathematical rigor and practical feasibility.

Question. I think your last statement summarizes the chronicle of applied scientific research. But tell me, why is the white-noise approach suitable for the identification and analysis of physiological systems?

Answer. I am glad you asked this because the answer is the *raison d'être* of this book. Let me take an example. When we go into the lab and are faced with a neural system, the function of which we wish to identify, we are confronted with a host of unpleasant considerations; namely, that the system is probably nonlinear, that we cannot hold the unit (from which we record) for a long time, and that our recorded signals will be corrupted by noise (electrode noise, preparation noise, etc.). The white-noise approach provides us with a *systematic* way of treating and alleviating all these difficulties. We have discussed this point throughout the book, so I will not go into details about it. I will only state in conclusion that for the purpose of functional identification of such systems, the white-noise approach is the best we can do in the present state of the art!

References

Balcomb, D. J., H. B. Demuth, and E. P. Gyftopoulos (1961). "A crosscorrelation method for measuring the impulse response of reactor systems," *Nucl. Sci. Eng.*, 11, 159–166.

Barker, H. A., and T. Pradisthayon (1970). "High-order autocorrelation functions of pseudorandom signals based on M-sequences," *Proc. IEE*, 117, 1857–1863.

Barker, H. A., S. N. Obidegwu, and T. Pradisthayon (1972). "Performance of antisymmetric pseudorandom signals in the measurement of second-order Volterra kernels by crosscorrelation," *Proc. IEE*, 119, 353–362.

Barrett, J. R. (1963). "The use of functionals in the analysis of nonlinear physical systems," *J. Electron Control*, 15, 567–615.

Bendat, J. S., and A. G. Piersol (1971). *Random Data: Analysis and Measurement Procedures*, Wiley Interscience, New York.

Blackman, R. B., and J. W. Tukey (1958). *The Measurement of Power Spectra*, Dover, New York.

Boer, E. de, and P. Kuyper (1968). "Triggered correlation," *IEEE Biomed. Eng.*, 15, 169–179.

Bogdanoff, J. L., and F. Kozin (eds.) (1963). *Symposium on Engineering Applications of Random Function Theory and Probability*, Wiley, New York.

Bose, A. G. (1956). "A theory of nonlinear systems," Technical Report No. 309, Research Laboratory of Electronics, M.I.T., Cambridge, Massachusetts.

Brandstetter, A., and J. Amorocho (1970). "Generalized analysis of small watershed responses," *Water Science and Engineering*, No. 1035, University of California, Davis.

Briggs, P. A., K. R. Godfrey, and P. H. Hammond (1967). "Estimation of process dynamic characteristics by correlation methods using pseudorandom signals," *IFAC Symposium on Identification in Automatic Control Systems*, Prague, pp. 1–12.

Brilliant, M. B. (1958). "Theory of the analysis of nonlinear systems," Technical Report No. 345, Research Laboratory of Electronics, M.I.T., Cambridge, Massachusetts.

Brillinger, D. R. (1975a). *Time Series: Data Analysis and Theory*, Holt, Rinehart and Winston, New York.

Brillinger, D. R. (1975b). "The identification of point process systems," *Ann. Probability*, 3, 909–929.

Brillinger, D. R., H. Bryant, and J. P. Segundo (1976). "Identification of synaptic interactions," *Biol. Cyb.*, 22, 213–228.

Brownlee, K. A. (1965). *Statistical Theory and Methodology in Science and Engineering* (2nd edition), Wiley, New York.

Bryant, H. L., and J. P. Segundo (1976). "Spike initiation by transmembrane current: a white-noise analysis," *J. Physiol.*, 260, 279–314.

Chan, R. Y. (1975). "Spatial dynamics of vertebrate retinal neurons," Ph.D. Thesis, California Institute of Technology.

Church, R. (1935). "Tables of irreducible polynomials for the first four prime moduli," *Ann. Math.*, 36, 198.

Clynes, M., and J. H. Milsum (1970). *Biomedical Engineering Systems*, McGraw-Hill, New York.

Cooley, J. W., and J. W. Tukey (1965). "An algorithm for the machine calculation of complex Fourier series," *Math. Comp.*, **19**, 297–301.

Creutzfeldt, O., B. Sakmann, H. Scheich, and A. Korn (1970). "Sensitivity distribution and spatial summation within receptive-field center of retinal on-center ganglion cells and transfer function of the retina," *J. Neurophysiol.*, **33**, 654–671.

Davenport, W. D., and W. L. Root (1958). *Random Signals and Noise*, McGraw-Hill, New York.

Davies, G. L. (1961). *Magnetic Tape Instrumentation*, McGraw-Hill, New York.

Davies, W. D. T. (1970). *System Identification for Self-Adaptive Control*, Wiley, New York.

Elgerd, O. I. (1967). *Control Systems Theory*, McGraw-Hill, New York.

Fender, D. H. (1964a). "Techniques of systems-analysis applied to feedback pathways in the control of eye movements," *Symp. Soc. Exp. Biol.*, **18**, 401–419.

Fender, D. H. (1964b). "The eye-movement control system; evolution of a model," *Neural Theory and Modeling*, R. F. Reiss (ed.), Stanford University Press, Stanford, California, pp. 306–324.

French, A. S. (1974). "Synthesis of low-frequency noise for use on biological experiments," *Trans. IEEE Biomed. Eng.*, **21**, 251–252.

French, A. S., and E. G. Butz (1973). "Measuring the Wiener kernels of a nonlinear system using the fast Fourier transform algorithm," *Int. J. Control*, **17**, 529–539.

French, A. A., and E. G. Butz (1974). "The use of Walsh functions in the Wiener analysis of nonlinear systems," *IEEE Trans. Computers*, **C-23**, 225–232.

George, D. A. (1959). "Continuous nonlinear systems," Technical Report No. 355, Research Laboratory of Electronics, M.I.T.

Godfrey, K. R., and W. Murgatroyd (1965). "Input-transducer errors in binary cross-correlation experiments," *Proc. IEE*, **112**, 565–573.

Godfrey, K. R., D. Everett, and P. R. Bryant (1966). "Input-transducer errors in binary crosscorrelation experiments—2," *Proc. IEE*, **113**, 185–189.

Gyftopoulos, E. P., and R. J. Hooper (1964). "Signals for transfer function measurement in nonlinear systems," *Noise Analysis in Nuclear Systems*, USAEC Symposium series 4, TID-7679.

Hooper, R. J., and E. P. Gyftopoulos (1967). "On the measurement of characteristic kernels of a class of nonlinear systems," *Neutron Noise, Waves and Pulse Propagation*, USAEC Conference Report No. 660206.

Jenkins, G. M., and D. G. Watts (1968). *Spectral Analysis*, Holden-Day, San Francisco.

Katzenelson, J., and L. A. Gould (1962). "The design of nonlinear filters and control systems, Part I," *Inform. Control*, **5**, 108–143.

Katzenelson, J., and L. A. Gould (1964). "The design of nonlinear filters and control systems, Part II," *Inform. Control*, **7**, 117–145.

Korenberg, M. J. (1973a). "Identification of biological cascades of linear and static nonlinear systems," *Proc. 16th Midwest Symp. Circuit Theory*, 18.2, pp. 1–9.

Korenberg, M. J. (1973b). "Crosscorrelation analysis of neural cascades," *Proc. 10th Ann. Rocky Mountain Bioeng. Symp.*, pp. 47–52.

Korn, G. A. (1966). *Random-Process Simulation and Measurements*, McGraw-Hill, New York.

Krausz, H. I. (1975). "Identification of nonlinear systems using random impulse train inputs," *Biol. Cyb.*, **19**, 217–230.

Lanczos, C. (1956). *Applied Analysis*, Prentice-Hall, New Jersey.

Laning, J. H., and R. H. Battin (1956). *Random Processes in Automatic Control*, McGraw-Hill, New York.

Lee, Y. W., and M. Schetzen: "Measurement of the Wiener kernels of a nonlinear system by cross-correlation," *Int. J. Control*, **2**, 237–254.

Levick, W. R. (1972). "Receptive fields of retinal ganglion cells," *Handbook of Sensory Physiology: Physiology of Photoreceptor Organs*, 7/2, M. G. F. Fuortes (ed.), Berlin, pp. 531–566.

Lipson, E. D. (1975a). "White noise analysis of Phycomyces light growth response system I. Normal intensity range," *Biophys. J.*, **15**, 989–1012.

Lipson, E. D. (1975b). "White noise analysis of Phycomyces light growth response system II. Extended intensity ranges," *Biophys. J.*, **15**, 1013–1031.

Lipson, E. D. (1975c). "White noise analysis of Phycomyces light growth response system III. Photomutants," *Biophys. J.*, **15**, 1033–1045.

Marmarelis, P. Z. (1972). "Nonlinear Identification of bioneuronal systems through white-noise stimulation," *Thirteenth Joint Automatic Control Conference*, pp. 117–126, Stanford University, Stanford, California.

Marmarelis, P. Z. (1975). "The noise about white-noise: Pros and cons," *Proc. 1st Symp. on Testing and Identification on Nonlinear Systems*, pp. 56–75, California Institute of Technology, Pasadena, California.

Marmarelis, P. Z., and G. D. McCann (1973). "Development and application of white-noise modeling techniques for studies of insect visual nervous systems," *Kybernetik*, **12**, 74–89.

Marmarelis, P. Z., and G. D. McCann (1975). "Errors involved in the practical estimation of nonlinear system kernels," *Proc. 1st Symp. on Testing and Identification of Nonlinear Systems*, California Institute of Technology, Pasadena, California.

Marmarelis, P. Z., and K.-I. Naka (1972). "White noise analysis of a neuron chain: An application of the Wiener theory," *Science*, **175**, 1276–1278.

Marmarelis, P. Z., and K.-I. Naka: (1973a) "Nonlinear analysis and synthesis of receptive-field responses in the catfish retina, Part I: Horizontal cell → ganglion cell chain," *J. Neurophysiol.* **36**, 605–618.

Marmarelis, P. Z., and K.-I. Naka (1973b). "Nonlinear analysis and synthesis of receptive-field responses in the catfish retina, Part II: One-input white-noise analysis," *J. Neurophysiol.* **36**, 619–633.

Marmarelis, P. Z., and K.-I. Naka (1973c). "Nonlinear analysis and synthesis of receptive-field responses in the catfish retina, Part III: Two-input white-noise analysis," *J. Neurophysiol.*, **36**, 634–648.

Marmarelis, P. Z., and K.-I. Naka (1973d). "Mimetic model of retinal network in catfish," *Proc. Conf. on Regulation and Control in Physiological Systems*, A. S. Iberall and A. C. Guyton (eds.), Rochester, New York, pp. 159–162.

Marmarelis, P. Z., and K.-I. Naka (1974a). "Identification of multi-input biological systems," *IEEE Trans. Biomed. Eng.*, **BME-21**, 88–101.

Marmarelis, P. Z., and K.-I. Naka (1974b). "Experimental analysis of a neural system: Two modeling approaches," *Kybernetik*, **15**, 11–26.

Marmarelis, P. Z., and K.-I. Naka (1974c). "Visual signal control and processing in a vertebrate retina," *Proc. 27th Ann. Conf. Engineering in Medicine and Biology*, p. 106, Philadelphia, Pennsylvania.

Marmarelis, P. Z., and K.-I. Naka (1974d). "Multi-input statistical testing on physiological systems," *Proc. 27th Ann. Conf. Engineering in Medicine and Biology*, p. 306, Philadelphia, Pennsylvania.

Marmarelis, V. Z. (1975). "Identification of nonlinear systems through multi-level random signals," *Proc. 1st Symp. on Testing and Identification of Nonlinear Systems*, California Institute of Technology, Pasadena, California, pp. 106–124.

Marmarelis, V. Z. (1976). "Identification of nonlinear systems through quasi-white test signals," Ph.D. Thesis, California Institute of Technology, Pasadena, California.

Marmarelis, V. Z. (1977). "A family of quasi-white random signals and its optimal use in biological system identification. Part I: Theory," *Biol. Cyb.*, **27**, 49–56.

Marmarelis, V. Z., and G. D. McCann (1975). "Optimization of test parameters for identification of spike train responses of biological systems through random test signals," *Proc. 1st Symp. on Testing and Identification of Nonlinear Systems*, California Institute of Technology, Pasadena, California, pp. 325–338.

Marmarelis, V. Z., and G. D. McCann (1977). "A family of quasi-white random signals and its optimal use in biological system identification. Part II: Application to the photoreceptor of Calliphora Erythrocephala," *Biol. Cyb.*, **27**, 57–62.

McCann, G. D., and J. C. Dill (1969). "Fundamental properties of intensity, form and motion perception in the visual nervous systems of *Calliphora phaenicia* and *Musca domestica*," *J. Gen. Physiol.*, **53**, 385–413.

McCann, G. D. (1974). "Nonlinear identification theory models for successive stages of visual nervous systems in flies," *J. Neurophysiol.*, **37**, 869–895.

McCann, G. D., Y. Sasaki, and M. C. Biedebach (1966). "Correlated studies of insect visual nervous systems," *Proc. Int. Symp. on Functional Organization of Compound Eye*, Stockholm, Sweden, Pergamon Press, Oxford, pp. 559–583.

Møller, A. R. (1975a). "Latency of unit responses in cochlear nucleus determined in two different ways," *J. Neurophysiol.*, **38**, 812–821.

Møller, A. R. (1976a). "Dynamic properties of excitation and two-tone inhibition in the cochlear nucleus studied using amplitude-modulated tones," *Exp. Brain Res.*, **25**, 307–321.

Møller, A. R. (1976b). "Dynamic properties of the responses of single neurones in the cochlear nucleus of the rat," *J. Physiol.*, **259**, 63–82.

Moore, G. P., D. H. Perkel, and J. P. Segundo (1966). "Statistical analysis and functional interpretation of neuronal spike data," *Ann. Rev. Physiol.*, **28**, 493–522.

Moore, G. P., D. G. Stuart, E. K. Stauffer, and R. Reinking (1975). "White-noise analysis of mammalian muscle receptors," *Proc. 1st Symp. on Testing and Identification of Nonlinear Systems*, G. D. McCann and P. Z. Marmarelis (eds.), California Institute of Technology, Pasadena, California, pp. 316–324.

Naka, K.-I. (1971). "Receptive field mechanism in the vertebrate retina," *Science*, **171**, 691–693.

Naka, K.-I., and P. W. Nye (1970). "Receptive-field organization of the catfish retina: Are at least two lateral mechanisms involved?," *J. Neurophysiol.*, **33**, 625–642.

Naka, K.-I., and P. W. Nye (1971). "Function of horizontal cells," *J. Neurophysiol.*, **34**, 785–801.

Naka, K.-I., P. Z. Marmarelis, and R. Y. Chan (1975). "Morphological and functional identifications of catfish retinal neurons. III. Functional identifications," *J. Neurophysiol.*, **38**, 92–131.

O'Leary, D. P., and V. Honrubia (1975). "On-line identification of sensory systems using pseudorandom binary noise perturbations," *Biophys. J.*, **15**, 505–532.

O'Leary, D. P., R. Dunn, and V. Honrubia (1974): "Functional and anatomical correlation of afferent responses from the isolated semicircular canal," *Nature*, **251**, 225–227.

Otnes, R. K., and L. Enochson (1972). *Digital Time Series Analysis*, Wiley-Interscience, New York.

Parzen, E. (1962). *Stochastic Processes*, Holden-Day, San Francisco.

Poggio, T. (1973). *Processing of Visual Information in Insects: A Theoretical Characterization*, H. Drischel (ed.), Fischer-Verlag, Leipzig.

Poggio, T., and W. Reichardt (1973a). "A theory of the pattern induced flight orientation of the fly *Musca domestica*," *Kybernetik*, **12**, 185–203.

Poggio, T. and W. Reichardt (1973b). "Considerations on models of movement detection," *Kybernetik*, **13**, 223–227.

Poggio, T., and W. Reichardt (1976). "Visual control of orientation behaviour in the fly. Part II: Towards the underlying neural interactions," *Quart. Rev. Biophys.*, **9**, 377–448. [For Part I see Reichardt and Poggio (1976).]

Rabiner, L. R., and C. M. Rader (eds.) (1972). *Digital Signal Processing*, IEEE Press.

Ream, N. (1967). "Testing a two-input linear system with periodic binary sequences," *Proc. IEE*, **114**, 305–307.

Ream, N. (1970). "Nonlinear identification using inverse-repeat m-sequences," *Proc. IEE*, **117**, 213–218.

Reichardt, W. (1961). *Sensory Communication*, Wiley, New York.

Reichardt, W. (1970). "The insect eye as a model for analysis of uptake, transduction and processing of optical data in the nervous system," *Neurosciences; Second Study Program*, F. O. Schmitt (ed.).

Reichardt, W., and T. Poggio (1975). "A theory of the pattern induced flight orientation of the fly *Musca domestica*: II," *Biol. Cyb.*, **18**, 69–80.

Reichardt, W., and T. Poggio (1976). "Visual control of orientation behaviour in the fly. Part I: A quantitative analysis," *Quart. Rev. Biophys.*, **9**, 311–375. [For Part II see Poggio and Reichardt (1976).]

Rice, S. O. (1945). "Mathematical analysis of random noise," *Bell Syst. Tech. J.*, **24**, 46–156.

Rodieck, R. W., and J. Stone (1965). "Analysis of receptive fields of cat retina ganglion cells," *J. Neurophysiol.*, **28**, 832–849.

Sandberg, A., and L. Stark (1968). "Wiener G-function analysis as an approach to nonlinear characteristics of human pupil reflex," *Brain Res.*, **11**, 194–211.

Schetzen, M. (1965a). "Measurements of the kernels of a nonlinear system of finite order," *Int. J. Control*, **1**, 251–263.

Schetzen, M. (1965b). "Synthesis of a class of nonlinear systems," *Int. J. Control*, **1**, 401–414.

Schetzen, M. (1974). "A theory of nonlinear system identification," *Int. J. Control*, **20**, 557–592.

Simpson, H. R. (1966). "Statistical properties of a class of pseudorandom sequences," *Proc. IEE*, **113**, 2075–2080.

Spekreijse, H. (1969). "Rectification in the goldfish retina: Analysis by sinusoidal and auxilliary stimulation," *Vision Res.*, **9**, 1461–1472.

Spekreijse, H., and H. Oosting (1970). "Linearizing: A method for analyzing and synthesizing nonlinear systems," *Kybernetik*, **7**, 22–31.

Stark, L. (1968). *Neurological Control Systems, Studies in Bioengineering*, Plenum Press, New York.

Stark, L. (1969). "The pupillary control system: Its nonlinear adaptive and stochastic engineering design characteristics," *Automatica*, **5**, 655–676.

Stark, L., F. W. Campbell, and J. Atwood (1958). "Pupil unrest: An example of noise in a biological servomechanism," *Nature*, **182**, 857–858.

Stein, R. B., A. S. French, and A. V. Holden (1972). "The frequency response coherence, and information capacity of two neuronal models," *Biophys. J.*, **12**, 295–322.

Stell, W. K. (1971). "The morphological organization of the vertebrate retina," *Handbook of Sensory Physiology*, *7/1b*, M. G. F. Fuortes (ed.), Berlin.

Sutter, E. (1975). "A revised conception of visual receptive fields based upon pseudorandom spatio-temporal pattern stimuli," *Proc. 1st Symp. on Testing and Identification of Nonlinear Systems*, California Institute of Technology, Pasadena, California, pp. 353–365.

Udwadia, F. E., and P. Z. Marmarelis (1976). "The identification of building structural systems, I. The linear case; II. The nonlinear case," *Bull. Seismol. Soc. Am.*, **66**, 125–171.

Valdiosera, R., C. Clausen, and R. S. Eisenberg (1974). "Measurement of the impedance of frog skeletal muscle fibers," *Biohpys. J.*, **14**, 295–314.

Volterra, V. (1959). *Theory of Functionals and of Integral and Integro-Differential Equations,* Dover Publications, New York.

Wiener, N. (1942). "Response of a nonlinear device to noise," Report No. 129, Radiation Laboratory, M.I.T., Cambridge, Massachusetts.

Wiener, N. (1958). *Nonlinear Problems in Random Theory*, Wiley, New York.

Yasui, S., and D. H. Fender (1975). "Methodology for measurement of spatiotemporal Volterra and Wiener kernels for visual systems," *Proc. 1st Symp. on Testing and Identification of Nonlinear Systems*, California Institute of Technology, Pasadena, California, pp. 366–383.

Young, L. R., D. M. Green, J. I. Elkind, and J. A. Kelly (1964). "Adaptive dynamic response characteristics of the human operator in simple manual control," *IEEE Trans. Human Factors Electron.*, **5**, 6–13.

Zierler, N. (1959). "Linear recurring sequences," *J. Soc. Indust. Applied Math.*, **7**, 31–49.

Related Literature

Amorocho, J., and A. Brandstetter (1971): "Determination of nonlinear functional response functions in rainfall-runoff processes," *Water Resour. Res.*, **7**, 1087–1101.

Aracil, J. (1970). "Measurement of Wiener kernels with binary random signals," *IEEE Trans. Autom. Control*, **AC-15**, 123–125.

Balakrishnan, A. V. (1963). "Prediction and filtering," *IRE Trans. Inform. Theory*, **9**, 237–240.

Balakrishnan, A. V. (1963). "Determination of nonlinear systems from input-output data," *Proceedings of the Princeton Conference on Identification Problems in Communication and Control*, Academic Press, New York.

Barker, H. A. (1967). "Choice of pseudorandom binary signals for system identification," *Electron. Lett.*, **3**, 524–526.

Barker, H. A. (1968). "Elimination of quadratic drift errors in system identification by pseudorandom binary signals," *Electron. Lett.* **4**, 255–256.

Barker, H. A. (1969). "Reference phase of pseudorandom signals," *Proc. IEE*, **116**, 429–435.

Barker, H. A., and R. W. Davy (1975). "System identification using pseudorandom signals and the discrete Fourier transform," *Proc. IEE*, **122**, 305–311.

Barker, H. A., and S. N. Obidegwu (1973). "Combined crosscorrelation method for the measurement of 2nd-order Volterra kernels," *Proc. IEE*, **120**, 114–118.

Barker, H. A. and S. N. Obidegwu (1973). "Effects of nonlinearities on the measurement of weighting functions by crosscorrelation using pseudorandom signals," *Proc. IEE* **120**, 1293–1300.

Barlow, H. B., R. Narasimhan, and A. Rosenfield (1972). "Visual pattern analysis in machines and animals," *Science*, **177**, 567–575.

Barrett, T. W. (1973). "Information processing in the inferior colliculus of cat using high frequency acoustical stimulation and direct electrical stimulation of the osseous spiral laminae," *Behav. Biol.*, **9**, 189–219.

Barrett, T. W. (1975). "On linearizing nonlinear systems," *J. Sound Vib.*, **39**, 265–268.

Baylor, D., M. Fuortes, and P. O'Bryan (1971). "Receptive fields of cones in the retina of the turtle," *J. Physiol.*, **215**, 265–294.

Bedrosian, E., and S. O. Rice: "The output properties of Volterra systems (nonlinear systems with memory) driven by harmonic and Gaussian inputs," *Proc. IEEE*, **59**, 1688–1707.

Bekey, G. A. (1973). "Parameter estimation in biological systems: A survey," *Proceedings of the Third IFAC Symposium—Identification and System Parameter Estimation*, North-Holland Publication Company, Amsterdam, pp. 1123–1130.

Bekey, G. A., and C. B. Neal (1968). "Identification of sampling intervals in sampled-data models of human operators," *IEEE Trans. Man-Machine Syst.*, **MMS-9**, 138–142.

Bellman, R., and K. J. Astrom (1969). "On structural identifiability," *Math. Biosci.*, **1**, 329–339.

Bendat, J. S. (1958). *Principles and Applications of Random Noise Theory*, Wiley, New York.

Bendat, J. S. (1976). "Solutions for the multiple input/output problem," *J. Sound Vib.*, **44**, 311–325.

Bendat, J. S. (1976). "System identification from multiple input/output data," *J. Sound Vib.*, **49**, 293–308.

Briggs, P. A., and K. R. Godfrey (1966). "Pseudorandom signals for the dynamic analysis of multivariable systems," *Proc. IEE*, **113**, 1259–1267.

Brillinger, D. R. (1970). "The identification of polynomial systems by means of higher order spectra," *J. Sound Vib.*, **12**, 301–313.

Brillinger, D. R. (1976). "Measuring the association of point processes: A case history," *Am. Math. Mon.*, **83**, 16–22.

Brindley, G. S., and G. Westheimer (1968). "How deeply nonlinear is the electroretinogram?", *J. Physiol.*, **196**, 78–79.

Brown, J. H. V., and D. S. Gann (eds.) (1973). *Engineering Principles in Physiology*, Academic Press, New York.

Brown, R. F. (1968). "Drift correction in periodic crosscorrelation schemes," *Electron Lett.*, **4**, 478–479.

Bryant, H. L., A. R. Marcos, and J. P. Segundo (1973). "Correlations of neural spike discharges produced by monosynaptic connections and by common inputs," *J. Neurophysiol.* **36**, 205–225.

Bussgang, J. J. (1952). "Crosscorrelation functions of amplitude distorted Gaussian signals," *M.I.T. Research Laboratory of Electronics*, Technical Report No. 216.

Bussgang, J. J., L. Ehrman and J. W. Graham (1974), "Analysis of nonlinear systems with multiple inputs," *Proc. IEEE*, **62**, 1088–1119.

Cameron, R. H., and W. T. Martin (1947). "The orthogonal development of nonlinear functionals in series of Fourier–Hermite functionals," *Ann. Math.*, **48**, 385–392.

Chen, W. J., and R. E. Poppele (1973). "Static fusimator effect on the sensitivity of mammalian muscle spindles," *Brain Res.*, **57**, 244–247.

Coggshall, J. C. (1973). "Linear models for biological transducers and impulse train spectra: General formulation and review," *Kybernetik*, **13**, 30–37.

Cosgriff, R. L. (1958). *Nonlinear Control Systems*, McGraw-Hill, New York.

Cox, D. R., and P. A. W. Lewis (1966). *The Statistical Analysis of Series of Events*, Methuen Monographs, London.

Cox, D. R., and P. A. W. Lewis (1970). "Multivariate Point Process," Yorktown Heights, New York. IBM Report No. RC 3029, 1970.

Crum, L. A., and J. A. Heinen (1974). "Simultaneous reduction and expansion of multidimensional Laplace transform kernels," *SIAM J. Appl. Math.*, **26**, 753–771.

Davies, W. D. T., and J. L. Douce (1967). "On-line system identification in the presence of drift," *IFAC Symposium on Identification in Automatic Control Systems*, paper 3.10, Prague.

DeFelice, L. J., and J. P. L. M. Michalides (1972). "Electrical noise from synthetic membranes," *J. Membrane Biol.*, **9**, 261–290.

DeFelice, L. J., E. Wanke, and F. Conti (1975). "Potassium and sodium current noise from squid axon membranes," *Federation Proc.*, **34**, 1338–1342.

Deutsch, R. (1955). "On a method of Wiener for noise through nonlinear devices," *IRE Convention Record*, Part 4, pp. 186–192.

Deutsch, R. (1962). *Nonlinear Transformation of Random Processes*, Prentice-Hall, New Jersey.

DeVoe, R. D. (1963). "Linear relations between stimulus amplitudes and amplitudes of retinal action potentials from the eye of the wolf spider," *J. Gen. Physiol.*, **47**, 13–32.

Dixon, W. J., and F. J. Massey (1969). *Introduction to Statistical Analysis*, 3rd edition, McGraw-Hill, New York.

Dodge, F. A., B. W. Knight, and J. Toyoda (1968). "Voltage noise in *Limulus* visual cells," *Science*, **160**, 88–90.

Dodge, F. A., R. M. Shapley, and B. W. Knight (1970). "Linear systems analysis of the *Limulus* retina," *Behav. Sci.*, **15**, 24–36.

Doeblin, E. O. (1966). *Measurement Systems: Application and Design*, McGraw-Hill, New York.

Eckert, H., and L. G. Bishop (1975). "Nonlinear dynamic transfer characteristics of cells in the peripheral visual pathway of flies, Part I: The retinula cells," *Biol. Cyb.*, **17**, 1–6.

Eisenberg, R. S. (1967). "Equivalent circuit of crab muscle fibers as determined by impedance measurements with intracellular electrodes," *J. Gen. Physiol.*, **50**, 1785–1812.

Evanich, M. J., A. O. Newberry, and L. D. Partridge (1972). "Some limitations on the removal of periodic noise by averaging," *J. Appl. Phys.*, **33**, 536–541.

Eykhoff, P. (1963). "Some fundamental aspects of process-parameter estimation," *IEEE Trans. Autom. Control*, **AC-8**, 347–357.

Eykhoff, P. (1974). *System Identification: Parameter and State Estimation*, John Wiley & Sons, New York.

Fishman, H. M. (1973). "Relaxation spectra of potassium channel noise from squid axon membranes," *Proc. Natl. Acad. Sci. USA*, **70**, 876–879.

French, A. S. (1976). "Practical nonlinear system analysis by Wiener kernel estimation in the frequency domain," *Biol. Cyb.*, **24**, 111–119.

French, A. S., and Holden, A. V. (1971). "Frequency domain analysis of neurophysiological data," *Comp. Prog. Biomed.*, **1**, 219–234.

Fricker, S. J., and J. J. Sanders (1974). "ERGS and noise: Detection probability, time and amplitude errors," *Proc. 11th I.S.C.E.R.G. Symp. Documenta Ophthalmologica*.

Fukurotani, K., and K.-I. Hara (1976). "A dynamic model of the receptive field of horizontal cells for monochromatic light," *Biol. Cyb.*, **21**, 221–226.

Gemperlein, R., and G. D. McCann (1975). "A study of the response properties of retinula cells of flies using nonlinear identification theory," *Biol. Cyb.*, **19**, 147–158.

Gentleman, W. M., and G. Sande (1966). "Fast Fourier transforms—for fun and profit," *Proc. Fall Joint Computer Conf.*, pp. 563–578.

Gerstein, G. L. (1970). "Functional Association of neurons: Detection and interpretation," in: *The Neurosciences: Second Study Program*, G. C. Quarton, T. Melnechuk, and G. A. Adelman (eds.), Rockefeller University Press, New York, pp. 648–660.

Godfrey, K. R. (1966). "Input-transducer errors in binary crosscorrelation experiments. Part 3," *Proc. IEE*, **113**, 1095–1102.

Godfrey, K. R., and P. A. N. Briggs (1972). "Identification of processes with direction-dependent dynamic responses," *Proc. IEE*, **119**, 1733–1739.

Graham, D., and D. McRuer (1961). *Analysis of Nonlinear Control Systems*, John Wiley, New York.

Guttman, R., and L. Feldman (1975). "White noise measurement of squid axon membrane impedance," *Biochem. Biophys. Res. Commun.*, **67**, 427–432.

Guttman, R., L. Feldman, and H. Lecar (1974). "Squid axon membrane response to white noise stimulation," *Biophys. J.*, **14**, 941–955.

Halpern, W., and N. R. Alpert (1971). "A stochastic signal method for measuring dynamic mechanical properties of muscle," *J. Appl. Physiol.*, **31**, 913–925.

Hannan, E. J. (1960). *Time Series Analysis*, J. Wiley and Sons, New York.

Hara, K.-I., and M. Kurose (1976). "A model for the mechanisms of sensitivity control in the submammalian vertebrate retina," *Biol. Cyb.*, **22**, 121–128.

Harmon, L. D., and E. R. Lewis (1966). "Neural modeling," *Physiol. Rev.*, **46**, 513–591.

Harris, G. H. (1965). "The identification of nonlinear systems with two-level inputs," Ph.D. Thesis, Princeton University, Princeton, New Jersey.

Hinich, M. (1967). "Estimation of spectra after hard clipping of Gaussian processes," *Technometrics*, **9**, 391–400.

Ho, Y. C., and R. C. K. Lee (1965). "Identification of linear dynamic systems," *Inf. Control*, **8**, 93–110.

Iberall, A. S. (1972). *Toward a General Science of Viable Systems*, McGraw-Hill, New York.

Izawa, K., and K. Kuruta (1965). "Simultaneous identification of multi-input and output systems," *Proc. of IFAC Tokyo Symposium*, pp. 229–236.

Kalman, R. E., and R. S. Bucy (1961). "New results in linear filtering and prediction theory," *J. Basic Eng. (ASME Trans.)*, **83**, 95–108.

Knight, B. (1973). "The horseshoe crab eye: A little nervous system that is solvable," In: *Some Mathematical Questions in Biology, IV. Lectures on Mathematics in the Life Sciences*, Vol. 5, The American Mathematical Society, Providence, Rhode Island, pp. 113–144.

Knox, C. K. (1974). "Crosscorrelation functions for a neuronal model," *Biophys. J.*, **14**, 567–582.

Knox, C. K., and R. E. Poppele (1973). "A neuronal circuit modeling program," *Comp. Biomed. Res.*, **6**, 487–497.

Koenderink, J. J., and A. J. Doorn (1974). "Event train decoders with many inputs, pulse density versus momentaneous frequency," *Kybernetik*, **13**, 215–222.

Korenberg, M. J. (1972). "Aspects of time-varying and nonlinear systems theory with biological applications," Ph.D. Thesis, McGill University, Montreal, Canada.

Korenberg, M. J. (1973). "Identification of nonlinear differential systems," *Proc. Joint Automatic Control Conf.*, pp. 597–603.

Korenberg, M. J. (1973). "New methods in the frequency analysis of linear time-varying differential equations," *Proc. of IEEE International Symp. on Circuit Theory*, pp. 185–188.

Korenberg, M. J. (1973). "A statistical method for directly identifying Volterra kernels of finite or infinite order systems," *Proc. 7th Ann. Princeton Conf. Inform. Sci. Syst.*

Korenberg, M. J. (1973). "Obtaining differential equation functional expansion, or cascade representations for nonlinear biological systems," *New England Bioengineering Conference*.

Korenberg, M. J. (1973). "Identification of neural pulse modulators," *Proc. International Symp. Dynamics and Controls in Physiological Systems*.

Krause, D. J., J. W. Steadman, and T. W. Williams (1972). "Effect of record length on noise-induced error in the crosscorrelation estimate," *IEEE Trans. Syst., Man Cyb.*, **SMC-2**, 255–261.

Krausz, H. I. (1976). "Nonlinear analysis of synaptic transmission using random stimulation of a presynaptic axon," Ph.D. Thesis, University of California at San Diego, La Jolla, California.

Kuffler, S. W. (1952). "Neurons in the retina: Organization, inhibition and excitation problems," *Cold Spring Harbor Symp. Quant. Biol.*, **17**, 281–292.

Lecar, H., and R. Nossal (1971). "Theory of threshold fluctuations in nerves. I. Relationships between electrical noise and fluctuations in axon firing," *Biophys. J.*, **11**, 1048–1065.

Lecar, H., and R. Nossal (1971). "Theory of threshold fluctuations in nerves. II. Analysis of various sources of membrane noise," *Biophys. J.*, **11**, 1068–1084.

Lee, Y. W. (1960). *Statistical Theory of Communication*, J. Wiley and Sons, New York.

Lee, Y. W. (1964). "Contributions of Norbert Wiener to linear theory and nonlinear theory in engineering," In: *Selected Papers of Norbert Wiener*, SIAM, MIT Press, pp. 17–33.

Levett, J. (1970). "Nonlinear-linear transition in the frog intraretinal electroretinogram," *Vision Res.*, **10**, 1347–1353.

Lewis, P. A. W. (1970). "Remarks on the theory, computation and application of the spectral analysis of series of events," *J. Sound Vib.*, **12**, 353–375.

Lichtenberger, W. W. (1961). "A technique of linear system identification using correlating filters," *IRE Trans. Autom. Control*, **AC-6**, 183–199.

Maffei, L., and R. E. Poppele (1967). "Frequency analysis of the late receptor potential," *J. Neurophysiol.*, **30**, 993–999.

Maffei, L., and R. E. Poppele (1968). "Transient and steady state electroretinal responses," *Vision Res.*, **8**, 229–246.

Maffei, L., A. Fiorentini, and L. Cervetto (1971). "Homeostasis in retinal receptive fields," *J. Neurophysiol.*, **34**, 579–587.

McCann, G. D., and P. Z. Marmarelis, (eds.) (1975). *Proceedings of the First Symposium on Testing and Identification of Nonlinear Systems*, California Institute of Technology, Pasadena, California.

McFee, R. (1961). "Determining the response of nonlinear systems to arbitrary inputs," *Trans. AIEE, Part II*, **80**, 189.

Mesarovic, M. D. (ed.) (1968). *Systems Theory and Biology*, Springer, Berlin.

Mihram, G. A. (1972). "The modeling process," *IEEE Trans. Syst. Man Cyb.*, **SMC-2**, 621–629.

Milsum, J. H. (1966). *Biological Control Systems Analysis*, McGraw-Hill, New York.

Møller, A. R. (1973). "Statistical evaluation of the dynamic properties of cochlear nucleus units using stimuli modulated with pseudorandom noise," *Brain Res.*, **57**, 443–456.

Møller, A. R. (1975b). "Dynamic properties of excitation and inhibition in the cochlear nucleus," *Acta Physiol. Scand.*, **93**, 442–454.

Moore, G. P., J. P. Segundo, and D. H. Perkel (1963). "Stability patterns in interneuronal pacemaker regulation," *Proc. San Diego Symp. for Biomed. Eng.*, pp. 184–193.

Moore, G. P., J. P. Segundo, D. H. Perkel, and H. Levitan (1970). "Statistical signs of synaptic interaction in neurons," *Biophys. J.*, **10**, 876–900.

Naka, K.-I., and N. R. G. Caraway (1975). "Morphological and functional identifications of catfish retinal neurons. I. Classical morphology," *J. Neurophysiol.*, **38**, 53–71.

Naka, K.-I., and T. Ohtsuka (1975). "Morphological and functional identifications of catfish retinal neurons. II. Morphological identification," *J. Neurophysiol.*, **38**, 72–91.

Naka, K.-I., and W. A. H. Rushton (1967). "The generation and spread of S-potentials in fish (Cyprinidae)," *J. Physiol.*, **192**, 437–461.

Ogura, H. (1972). "Orthogonal functions of the Poisson process," *IEEE Trans. Inform. Theory*, **IT-18**, 473–481.

O'Leary, D. P., R. F. Dunn, and V. Honrubia (1976). "Analysis of afferent responses from isolated semicircular canal of the guitarfish using rotational acceleration white-noise inputs. Part I: Correlation of response dynamics with receptor innervation. Part II: Estimation of linear system parameters and gain and phase spectra," *J. Neurophysiol.*, **39**, 631–659.

Papoulis, A. (1965). *Probability, Random Variables, and Stochastic Processes*, McGraw-Hill Book Co., New York.

Partridge, L. D. (1965). "Modifications of neural output signals by muscles: A frequency response study," *J. Appl. Physiol.*, **20**, 150–156.

Partridge, L. D. (1966). "Signal-handling characteristics of load-moving skeletal muscles," *Am. J. Physiol.*, **210**, 1178–1191.

Partridge, L. D. (1973). "Integration in the central nervous system," In: *Engineering Principles in Physiology*, J. H. V. Brown and D. S. Gann (eds.), Academic Press, New York.

Partridge, L. D., and J. H. Kim (1969). "Dynamic characteristics of response in a vestibulomotor reflex," *J. Neurophysiol.*, **32**, 485–495.

Pavlidis, T. (1966). "Design of neural nets with intermittent response and certain other relevant studies," *Bull. Math. Biophys.*, **28**, 51–74.

Perkel, D. H., G. L. Gerstein, and G. P. Moore (1967). "Neuronal spike trains and stochastic point processes. I. The single spike train," *Biophys. J.*, **7**, 391–418.

Perkel, D. H., G. L. Gerstein, and G. P. Moore (1967). "Neuronal spike trains and stochastic point processes. II. Simultaneous spike trains," *Biophys. J.*, **7**, 419–440.

Poppele, R. E., and W. J. Chen (1972). "Repetitive firing behavior of mammalian muscle spindle," *J. Neurophysiol.*, **35**, 357–364.

Poussart, D. (1971). "Membrane current noise in lobster axon under voltage damp," *Biophys. J.*, **11**, 211–234.

Pradisthayon, T. (1971). "Identification of nonlinear systems using pseudorandom signals," Ph.D. Thesis, University of Glasgow.

Price, R. A. (1958). "A useful theorem for nonlinear devices having Gaussian inputs," *IRE Trans. Inform. Theory*, **IT-4**, 69–72.

Ream, N. (1968). "Proof of the drift-resistant property of binary *m*-sequences," *Electron. Lett.*, **4**, 380–381.

Reichardt, W. (1961). "Autocorrelation, a principle for the evaluation of sensory information by the central nervous system," In: *Sensory Communication*, W. A. Rosenblith (ed.), MIT Press, Cambridge, Massachusetts, pp. 303–317.

Rescigno, A., R. B. Skin, R. L. Purple, and R. E. Poppele (1970). "A neuronal model for the discharge patterns produced by cyclic inputs," *Bull. Math. Biophys.*, **32**, 338–353.

Robinson, D. (1973). "Models of saccadic eye movement control system," *Kybernetik*, **14**, 71.

Rodieck, R. W., N. Y.-S. Kiang, and G. L. Gerstein (1962). "Some quantitative methods for the study of spontaneous activity of single neurons," *Biophys. J.*, **2**, 351–368.

Rosenblueth, A., and N. Wiener (1945). "The role of models in science," *Philos. Sci.*, **12**, 316–321.

Schellart, N. A. M. and H. Spekreijse (1973). "Origin of the stochastic nature of ganglion cell activity in isolated goldfish retina," *Vision Res.*, **13**, 337–345.

Schetzen, M. (1962). "Some problems in nonlinear theory," Technical Report No. 390, Research Laboratory of Electronics, M.I.T., Cambridge, Massachusetts.

Seelen, W. von, and K.-P. Hoffmann (1976). "Analysis of neuronal networks in the visual system of the cat using statistical signals; Part I," *Biol. Cyb.*, **22**, 7–20.

Segundo, J. P., and D. H. Perkel (1969). "The nerve cell as an analyzer of spike trains," In: *The Interneuron*, M. A. B. Brazier (ed.), UCLA Forum in the Medical Sciences, No. 11, University of California Press, Los Angeles, California, pp. 349–389.

Segundo, J. P., D. H. Perkel, H. Wyman, H. Hegstad, and G. P. Moore (1968). "Input-output relations in computer-simulated nerve cells. Influence of the statistical properties, strength, number and interdependence of excitatory presynaptic terminals," *Kybernetik*, **4**, 157–171.

Simpson, R. J., and H. M. Power (1972). "Correlation techniques for the identification of nonlinear systems," *Meas. Control*, **5**, 316–321.

St.-Cyr, G. J., and D. H. Fender (1969). "Nonlinearities of the human oculomotor system: Time delays," *Vision Res.*, **9**, 1491–1503.

Stein, R. B. (1965). "A theoretical analysis of neuronal variability," *Biophys. J.*, **5**, 173–194.

Stevens, C. F. (1972). "Inferences about membrane properties from electrical noise measurements," *Biophys. J.*, **12**, 1028–1047.

Stockham, T. G., Jr. (1966). "High-speed convolution and correlation," *Proc. Spring Joint Computer Conf.*, pp. 229–233.

Stromeyer, C. F., and S. Klein (1974). "Spatial frequency channels in human vision as asymmetric (edge) mechanisms," *Vision Res.*, **14**, 1409–1420.

Taylor, L. W., and A. V. Balakrishnan (1967). "Identification of human response models in manual control systems," *IFAC Symp. on Identification in Automatic Control Systems*, Prague, paper 1.7.

Taylor, M. G. (1966). "Use of random excitation and spectral analysis in the study of frequency-dependent parameters of the cardiovascular system," Circ. Res., **18**, 585–595.

Terzuolo, C. (ed.) (1969). *Systems Analysis in Neurophysiology*, University of Minnesota Press, Minneapolis, Minnesota.

Thaler, G. J., and M. P. Pastel (1962). *Analysis and Design of Nonlinear Feedback Control Systems*, McGraw-Hill, New York.

Toyoda, J. I. (1974). "Frequency characteristics of retinal neurons in the carp," *J. Gen. Physiol.*, **63**, 214–234.

Verveen, A. A., and L. J. DeFelice (1974). "Membrane noise," *Progr. Biophys. Molec. Biol.*, **28**, 189–265.

Watanabe, A. (1972). "Characterization of nonlinear systems by discrete Volterra series and its application to a biological system," Ph.D. Thesis, University of California at Berkeley.

Watanabe, A., and L. Stark (1975). "Kernel method for nonlinear analysis: Identification of a biological control system," *Math. Biosci.*, **27**, 99–108.

Wax, N. (ed.) (1954). *Selected Papers on Noise and Stochastic Processes*, Dover Publications, New York.

Werblin, F. S. (1974). "Control of retinal sensitivity. II. Lateral interactions at the outer plexiform layer," *J. Gen. Physiol.*, **63**, 62–87.

Werblin, F. S., and J. E. Dowling (1969). "Organization of the retina of the mudpuppy, Nocturus Maculosus. II. Intracellular recording," *J. Neurophysiol.*, **32**, 339–355.

Widnall, W. S. (1962). "Measurement of a second order Wiener kernel in a nonlinear system by crosscorrelation," *Quarterly Progress Report No. 65*, Research Laboratory of Electronics, M.I.T., Cambridge, Massachusetts.

Wiener, N. (1949). *Extrapolation, Interpolation and Smoothing of Stationary Time Series*, J. Wiley and Sons, New York.

Wyman, R. (1965). "Probabilistic characterization of simultaneous nerve impulse sequences controlling dipteran flight," *Biophys. J.*, **5**, 447–471.

Yates, F. E. (1973). "Systems biology as a concept," In: *Engineering Principles in Physiology*, Vol. 1, J. H. V. Brown and D. S. Gann (eds.), Academic Press, New York.

Zadeh, L. A. (1956). "On the identification problem," *IRE Trans. Circuit Theory*, **3**, 277–281.

Zadeh, L. A. (1957). "On the representation of nonlinear operators," *IRE Wescon Conv. Rec., Part 2*, pp. 105–113.

Index